Methods in Biomedical Informatics

A Pragmatic Approach

Methods in Biomedical Informatics
A Pragmatic Approach

Edited by

Indra Neil Sarkar

University of Vermont, Burlington, USA

AMSTERDAM • BOSTON • HEIDELBERG • LONDON
NEW YORK • OXFORD • PARIS • SAN DIEGO
SAN FRANCISCO • SINGAPORE • SYDNEY • TOKYO

Academic Press is an Imprint of Elsevier

Academic Press is an imprint of Elsevier
32 Jamestown Road, London NW1 7BY, UK
225 Wyman Street, Waltham, MA 02451, USA
525 B Street, Suite 1800, San Diego, CA 92101-4495, USA

Notice
No responsibility is assumed by the publisher for any injury and/or damage to persons or property as a matter of products
liability, negligence or otherwise, or from any use or operation of any methods, products, instructions or ideas contained in the
material herein. Because of rapid advances in the medical sciences, in particular, independent verification of diagnoses and drug
dosages should be made.

British Library Cataloguing-in-Publication Data
A catalogue record for this book is available from the British Library

Library of Congress Cataloging-in-Publication Data
A catalog record for this book is available from the Library of Congress

ISBN: 978-0-12-401678-1

For information on all Academic Press publications
visit our website at elsevierdirect.com

Typeset by Scientific Publishing Services (P) Ltd., Chennai
www.sps.co.in

Printed and bound in United States of America
13 14 15 16 17   10 9 8 7 6 5 4 3 2 1

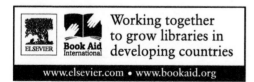

Working together
to grow libraries in
developing countries

www.elsevier.com • www.bookaid.org

Contents

CHAPTER 13 Putting Theory into Practice **425**
Indra Neil Sarkar

APPENDIX A Unix Primer **433**
Elizabeth S. Chen

APPENDIX B Ruby Primer **451**
Elizabeth S. Chen

Contributors

Gil Alterovitz
Children's Hospital Informatics Program at Harvard-MIT Division of Health Science, Boston, MA, USA.
Center for Biomedical Informatics, Harvard Medical School, Boston, MA, USA.
Computer Science and Artificial Intelligence Laboratory, Department of Electrical Engineering and Computer Science, MIT, Cambridge, MA, USA.

Riccardo Bellazzi
Dipartimento di Ingegneria Industriale e dell'Informazione, Università di Pavia, Pavia, Italy.

Elizabeth S. Chen
Center for Clinical and Translational Science, University of Vermont, Burlington, VT, USA
Department of Medicine, Division of General Internal Medicine, University of Vermont, Burlington, VT, USA
Department of Computer Science, University of Vermont, Burlington, VT, USA

Hsun-Hsien Chang
Children's Hospital Informatics Program at Harvard-MIT Division of Health Science, Boston, MA, USA.

Kevin Bretonnel Cohen
Computational Bioscience Program, University of Colorado School of Medicine, Department of Linguistics, University of Colorado at Boulder, USA.

Trevor Cohen
University of Texas School of Biomedical Informatics at Houston, Houston, TX, USA.

Joshua C. Denny
Department of Biomedical Informatics and Medicine, Vanderbilt University, Nashville, TN, USA.

Matteo Gabetta
Dipartimento di Ingegneria Industriale e dell'Informazione, Università di Pavia, Pavia, Italy.

Kathleen Gray
Health and Biomedical Informatics Centre, Melbourne Medical School, Faculty of Medicine, Dentistry & Health Sciences and Department of Computing and Information Systems, The University of Melbourne, Melbourne, VIC, Australia.

John H. Holmes
University of Pennsylvania, Philadelphia, PA, USA.

Giorgio Leonardi

Dipartimento di Ingegneria Industriale e dell'Informazione, Università di Pavia, Pavia, Italy.

Haiquan Li

Department of Medicine, University of Illinois at Chicago, Chicago, IL, USA.

Guillermo Lopez-Campos

Health and Biomedical Informatics Centre, Melbourne Medical School, Faculty of Medicine, Dentistry & Health Sciences, The University of Melbourne, Melbourne, VIC, Australia.

Yves A. Lussier

Department of Medicine, University of Illinois at Chicago, Chicago, IL, USA. Department of Bioengineering, University of Illinois at Chicago, Chicago, IL, USA.
Cancer Center, University of Illinois, Chicago, IL, USA.

Luis N. Marenco

Yale University School of Medicine, New Haven, CT, USA.

Fernando Martin-Sanchez

Health and Biomedical Informatics Centre, Melbourne Medical School, Faculty of Medicine, Dentistry & Health Sciences, The University of Melbourne, Melbourne, VIC, Australia.

Jason H. Moore

Dartmouth College Department of Genetics, Hanover, NH, USA.

Mark A. Musen

Stanford Center for Biomedical Informatics Research, Stanford University, Stanford, CA, USA.

Prakash M. Nadkarni

Yale University School of Medicine, New Haven, CT, USA.

Indra Neil Sarkar

Center for Clinical and Translational Science, University of Vermont, Burlington, VT, USA.

Ryan J. Urbanowicz

Dartmouth College Department of Genetics, Hanover, NH, USA.

Dominic Widdows

Microsoft Bing, Serendipity, Palo Alto, CA, USA.

Hua Xu

School of Biomedical Informatics, University of Texas Health Science Center at Houston, Houston, TX, USA.

Introduction

Indra Neil Sarkar

Center for Clinical and Translational Science, University of Vermont, Burlington, VT, USA

1.1 BIOMEDICAL INFORMATICS AND ITS APPLICATIONS

Biomedicine is a complex ecosystem of foundational and applied disciplines. Generally, researchers and practitioners in biomedicine are specialized in a particular area of emphasis that can be described as either: (1) "bench"—aiming to understand the underpinning principles of dysfunction leading to compromised health status; (2) "bedside"—aiming to develop preventative approaches for the maintenance of normal health status or addressing abnormal health status through clinical intervention and quantifying the effect on individuals; or (3) "community"—aiming to quantify the effect of preventative measures or treatment regimens across defined population groups and developing systematic approaches to promote effective practices. There has been increased discussion in recent years about these areas of emphasis and the need for strategies to promote synergies between them [1–3].

This book is focused on describing methodologies that underpin the discipline of *Biomedical Informatics*, which is defined as a field "that studies and pursues the effective uses of biomedical data, information, and knowledge for scientific inquiry, problem solving and decision making, motivated by efforts to improve human health [4]." Biomedical informatics has evolved into a discipline that encompasses the bench, bedside, and community areas of biomedicine and represents a synergy between foundational and applied aspects of biomedical science [4]. The foundational aspects of biomedical informatics are derived from a wide array of fundamental disciplines, including those from formal science (e.g., logic, mathematics, and statistics) and basic science (e.g., physics, chemistry, biology, psychology, and economics). Additional applied disciplines also contribute key foundational elements to biomedical informatics (e.g., medical science, computer science, engineering, and epidemiology).

From the foundational sciences that contribute to biomedical informatics, methodologies are developed and applied to specific biomedical areas. For example, biomedical informatics methods may be applied to specific domain areas, like: biology (termed "bioinformatics"), medicine and nursing (termed "clinical informatics"), and public health (termed "public health informatics"). In contemporary biomedical informatics parlance, "health informatics" is often used as an umbrella term for clinical informatics and public health informatics. There are many other areas of informatics that traverse domain boundaries (e.g., "imaging informatics" involves the application of biomedical informatics approaches to areas that span biological and clinical domains) or are aligned with particular specialties (e.g., "pathology informatics"). A comprehensive survey of biomedical informatics and its application areas can be found in *Biomedical Informatics: Computer Applications in Health Care* (edited by Shortliffe and Cimino) [5].

Biomedical informatics methods may also be applied to areas that focus on the translation of innovations from one part of the biomedicine spectrum to another [6]. In recent years, this area of emphasis has collectively been referred to as "translational sciences." Working alongside translational medicine, the translational sciences aim to enable greater synergy between basic and applied sciences [7,8]. Within the context of biomedical informatics, "translational informatics" is the use of informatics approaches to support translational science and medicine [9]. Translational informatics is divided into two major sub-specialties: (1) "translational bioinformatics"—which is focused on the development of informatics approaches that facilitate the translation of basic science findings into ones that may be utilized in clinical contexts [10,11]; and (2) "clinical research informatics"—which is focused on the development of informatics approaches for evaluating and generalizing clinical innovations [12]. Translational bioinformatics and clinical research informatics work in tandem to increase the likelihood of basic science innovations being put into clinical practice and improving the health of communities—thus directly addressing the translational bottlenecks, such as those that are often seen at the transition of knowledge from bench to bedside or bedside to community. Figure 1.1 provides a graphical overview biomedical informatics and its sub-disciplines that span the full breath of biomedicine.

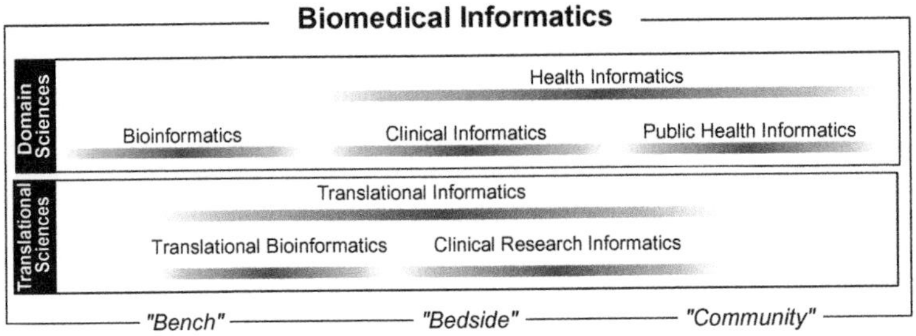

Biomedical Informatics

Domain Sciences			
	Health Informatics		
	Bioinformatics	Clinical Informatics	Public Health Informatics

Translational Sciences		
	Translational Informatics	
	Translational Bioinformatics	Clinical Research Informatics

———— *"Bench"* ———————— *"Bedside"* ———————— *"Community"* ————

■ **FIGURE 1.1** Overview of Biomedical Informatics. Major application areas of biomedical informatics are shown, aligned according to their general emphasis to develop solutions for bench, bedside, or community stakeholders. The major application areas are also segregated according to their domain or translational science centricity. Note that not all application areas are shown.

The expansiveness of biomedical informatics in many ways requires a polymathic approach to developing approaches for the betterment of health. Formal training in biomedical informatics thus requires a unique combination of formal, basic, and applied science [4]. It therefore is not uncommon for one to first attain formal, graduate-level scholarly or professional training in at least one area of science before embarking on additional training in biomedical informatics. In addition to these cross-trained individuals, there are also a growing number of formally trained biomedical informaticians whose entire graduate-level education is done in biomedical informatics. In most cases, biomedical informaticians choose at least one application area of specialization (e.g., bioinformatics, clinical informatics, or public health informatics). Regardless of the path to becoming a biomedical informatician, the approaches used to address biomedical problems are built on a common set of methodologies [4]. It must be noted that the highly specialized training required for success in biomedical informatics has resulted in a significant shortage of biomedical informaticians across the entire spectrum of biomedicine. To address this challenge, there are an increasingly growing number of formal training opportunities that strive to help provide the biomedical enterprise with biomedical informaticians [13].

In contrast to multi- or inter-disciplinary disciplines, where foundational elements are respectively combined in additive or interactive ways, biomedical informatics is a trans-disciplinary discipline, where foundational elements are holistically combined in ways that result in the emergence of entirely new concepts [14–16]. To this end, biomedical informatics is a unique discipline in that it brings together an array of diverse expertise and experience, but remains with the singular purpose to develop methods to improve the process of health maintenance and treatment of deviations from normal health. The development and use of these methodologies can be organized according to the *Scientific Method* (described in Section 1.2), with the goal of transforming biomedical data into information that leads to actionable knowledge and therefore leading to wisdom (collectively referred to as the *DIKW framework*, described in Section 1.3). This book provides an introduction to a number of key methodologies used in biomedical informatics that hone the Scientific Method in the context of the DIKW framework (an overview of the chapters is provided in Section 1.4, along with expectations in Section 1.5).

1.2 THE SCIENTIFIC METHOD

Like all scientific disciplines, biomedical informatics is strongly grounded in the Scientific Method. The Scientific Method can be traced back to Artistotle, who introduced the principles of logic coming in two forms [17]: (1) inductive—which makes postulations based on observation of universal concepts; and (2) deductive—which makes postulations based on relationships between already accepted universal concepts (called "syllogisms"). It was not, however, until the Arab polymath al-Hasan ibn al-Haytham (often referred to in the Western world as "Alhazen" or "Alhacen") described the principles of optics in a systematic manner that the contemporary Scientific Method became a formally described process [18]. Ibn al-Haytham's *Book of Optics* was one of the main sources used by the Englishman Roger Bacon (not to be confused with Francis Bacon, who described an alternative inductive methodology referred to as the "Baconian Method," which in many ways rejected the hypothesis-driven Scientific Method [19]) to formally describe the Scientific Method to the Western world [20].

The Scientific Method consists of five major activities: (1) Question formulation; (2) Hypothesis Generation; (3) Prediction; (4) Testing; and (5) Analysis. The first activity of *question formulation* aims to identify a query of interest relative to a specific observation (e.g., "will this treatment regimen cure the patient of this illness?"). Question formulation can involve the consultation of existing knowledge sources or other experts for determining the validity of the question. Question formulation, in many ways, is the most difficult step of the Scientific Method; however, it is also the most crucial step because all the consequent steps are dependent on a well-formed question. Once a question is developed, the next stage of the Scientific Method strives to add focus by postulating a specific *hypothesis* (e.g., "this treatment will treat the patient of their illness.").

The generation of a hypothesis is often done in two parts, which together make the hypothesis *testable*: (1) defining the *null hypothesis* (H_0)—a contemplation of the hypothesis in a statistical framework that presents the default conclusion (e.g., "this treatment regimen does not cure the patient of their illness compared to a placebo."); and (2) defining the *alternative hypothesis* (H_1)—a contemplation of the hypothesis in a statistical framework that presents the desired outcome (e.g., "this treatment, when compared to a placebo, cures the patient of their illness"). An important feature of a well-formed hypothesis is that it is *falsifiable*. Falsifiability is defined as the ability to identify potential solutions that could disprove a stated hypothesis (e.g., "the patient is cured by a placebo."). Thus, the testability of a hypothesis is inherently a feature of its falsifiability [21].

After it is deemed that a hypothesis is testable, the next stage in the Scientific Method is to propose some *predictions* that help determine the plausibility of the hypothesis relative to alternatives, including coincidence (e.g., "this treatment cures the patient of their illness compared to doing nothing"). The predictions are then *tested* through the gathering of evidence, which support or refute the hypothesis of interest (e.g., "for a sample of chosen patients who have the same illness, measure the effect of the treatment versus a placebo versus nothing"). As noted earlier, an important feature of developed tests is that they aim to address the falsifiability of the hypothesis.

The results of the tests are then *analyzed* to determine if the hypothesis was indeed proved true (rejection of the null hypothesis and thus acceptance of the alternative hypothesis). This is commonly done using a statistical comparison test such as one that can be derived from a confusion matrix [which delineates verifiable ("true positive" and "true negative") and unexpected ("false positive" and "false negative") results based on previous knowledge]. Common comparison tests include the Pearson's chi-square [22] and Fisher's exact test [23]. The final outcome of the analysis is a statement relative to the original question (e.g., "yes, this treatment regimen will cure patients of this illness.").

The Scientific Method does not necessarily conclude at the completion of the analysis step; the analysis of one hypothesis may lead to additional questions that can consequently be examined through an additional iteration of the Scientific Method. Indeed, the Scientific Method as classically implemented can be perceived as an infinite process. Within the context of biomedicine, a modern interpretation of the Scientific Method is often used, termed the "hypothetico-deductive approach." The hypothetico-deductive approach is a cornerstone in clinical education and practice [24–26]: (1) gather data about a patient; (2) develop questions that lead to hypotheses for the patient's state; (3) propose predictions based on the suggested hypotheses that explain the patient's state; and (4) test the hypotheses through attempts at falsifying them to explain the patient's state. It is important to once again underscore that clinical inquiry into patient status is not a verification of a particular condition; evidence to support a proposed set of hypotheses is done through a series of falsification tests (in clinical parlance, these are often termed "rule-in" or "rule-out" tests). As in many clinical scenarios, it must be acknowledged that the absolute true diagnosis for a given patient may not be known or even knowable (e.g., to determine whether a patient actually has Alzheimer disease, the most definitive method of detection is a neuropathological analysis done post-mortem [27]); however, the development of hypotheses and tests to prove or refute them enables a clinician to get closer to the true diagnosis.

1.3 DATA, INFORMATION, KNOWLEDGE, AND WISDOM

Data are composed of individual datum points that may originate from a plethora of sources (it is for this reason that in scientific writing the term "data" should be treated as a plural noun; the singular form is "datum"). Simply put, data are the raw substrate that can be transformed through formal science methods to acquire meaning. Data may come in many forms, from any part of the biomedical spectrum. Data are the essential building blocks wherefrom the Scientific Method begins and may lead to the gathering of additional data in the testing of hypotheses. In biomedicine, data are generated from a wide range of sources—as artifacts of digital systems (e.g., as might be generated from automated laboratory systems) or as recorded events from human-human interactions (e.g., as might be generated from a clinician-patient interview). Data are an essential component of modern science, and can acquire different meanings depending on their interpretation. These interpretations are dependent on the use of appropriate formal science techniques—most often a combination of logic and statistics.

It is important for one to be aware of the assumptions made in both the logic (e.g., the definition of *true* versus *false*) and statistics (e.g., the data distributed in a Gaussian manner). An additional layer of complexity is that data can, and often do, suffer from unavoidable inconsistencies, which may be an artifact of either the generation, collection, or interpretation of data. Even with all these issues, data form the basis for all derived interpretations and thus form the foundation for the biomedical sciences. It is the study and improvement of formal science techniques that also form the basis of biomedical informatics methods.

As data are transformed into *information*, which is the result of the application of formal science techniques, hypotheses may be generated about the meaning of the observed data that form the basis for basic science. The basic sciences, which have a strong basis in the Scientific Method (built around the generation, testing, and validation of hypotheses), impart interpretations of data based on a specific domain focus. For example, physics is focused on the interpretation of data to understand the physical world in terms of matter and its motion; chemistry is focused on analyzing data to understand the composition of matter; biology is focused on understanding extinct and extant organisms; and economics is focused on the understanding of data associated with goods or services that form the basis for inter-personal relationships. The basic sciences form the foundation for biomedicine, and provide the insights about the underlying cause of dysfunction and its detection as well as provide the tools for tracking treatment outcomes from both clinical and economical perspectives.

As information about health is collected and analyzed, it can be coalesced into reusable constructs (e.g., a particular treatment regimen that has been shown to improve health). These constructs form the basis of *knowledge*, which require a systematic understanding and use of data that have been transformed into interpretable information. Knowledge can be used to guide decisions or subsequent analyses—this type of knowledge is referred to as "actionable knowledge [28]." Actionable knowledge is of the most utility in biomedicine when data can be used in a way to guide clinical decisions in a manner to positively affect patient health outcomes. The study and evaluation of knowledge leads to *wisdom*, which promotes the development of best practices and guidance for how to interpret future encounters with biomedical data.

The applied sciences provide the scaffolding to systematically transform information from biomedical data into knowledge and retain it as wisdom that can be used to guide disease diagnoses, treatment regimens, or outcomes analyses. For example, medical science approaches can be used to consistently interpret a laboratory result in combination with a collection of signs and symptoms to determine the health status of a patient; engineering approaches can be used to develop a process to provide consistent levels of care to patients as they interact with the health care system; and epidemiology approaches can be used to analyze the effect of vaccinations across susceptible populations.

Data, information, knowledge, and wisdom and their relationships to each other are collectively referred to as the Data-Information-Knowledge-Wisdom (DIKW) framework, and the most common interpretations are credited to Ackoff [29, 30]. The DIKW framework (where data are transformed into wisdom) can certainly be applied to each individual scientific discipline; however, as noted earlier, what sets biomedical informatics apart from other disciplines is that its scope is trans-disciplinary. The DIKW framework can be applied in specific formal, basic, or applied science contexts; however, in the context of biomedical informatics, the DIKW framework is used to bridge formal, basic, and applied sciences toward a single purpose—to improve the diagnosis, care, and treatment of illness. Furthermore, the DIKW framework in biomedical informatics formalizes the implementation of the Scientific Method towards the discovery and implementation of biomedical innovations. Like the Scientific Method, the DIKW framework does not necessarily conclude at the establishment of wisdom; the wisdom gained from one set of data can be used as data for a subsequent study. The relationships between the sciences, the Scientific Method, and the DIKW framework are graphically depicted in Figure 1.2.

The DIKW framework can be used to formally organize, study, and innovate at different levels of inquiry. Put into the context of biomedicine, the DIKW framework is an essential process that transverses the aforementioned major areas of bench, bedside, and community. The results of transforming data into wisdom in one area may very well lead to data for another area. Of course, the boundaries between the suggested areas of biomedicine are not always apparent. Recently, there has been a concerted effort in the biomedical research enterprise to acknowledge that much of biomedicine innovation does suffer from a "siloed" approach that force the bench, bedside, and community researchers into disjointed endeavors [1–3].

From the earliest days of biomedical informatics, it was proposed that concepts and approaches, such as those that could be implemented in computers, could be used to better integrate the bench, bedside, and community areas of research and practice [31–33]. Biomedical informaticians thus necessarily

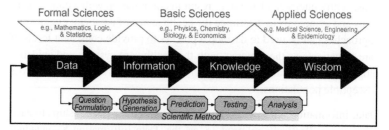

■ **FIGURE 1.2** DIKW Framework. The Data-Information-Knowledge-Wisdom (DIKW) framework is depicted as a process that unifies the formal, basic, and applied sciences. The graphic also shows how the major steps of the Scientific Method can be aligned with the transformation of data into wisdom.

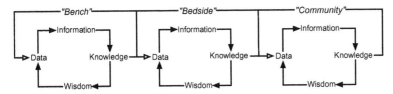

■ **FIGURE 1.3** Iterative DIKW Process to Translation. The DIKW framework is shown as an iterative process where wisdom that is derived from bench, bedside, or community-based data can be used as source data for generation of additional testable hypotheses.

work together as teams of formal, basic, and applied scientists to develop solutions that aim to address specific bench, bedside, or community challenges. Whilst a given approach may be originally designed for one particular area, biomedical informatics espouses that it may be generalized to another area. The realization of the DIKW framework in the practice of biomedical informatics is thus intertwined in a manner that suggests a holistic approach that uniquely unifies the many facets of biomedicine (as depicted in Figure 1.3).

1.4 OVERVIEW OF CHAPTERS

The main goal of this book is to present biomedical informatics methods that are used to focus the Scientific Method to transform data into wisdom, along the aforementioned DIKW framework. Where possible, practical examples are provided that aim to help the reader appreciate the methodological concepts within "real world" bench, bedside, or community scenarios. It is impossible to provide complete coverage of the entire range of biomedical informatics methods. Therefore, this book aims to provide a foundation for many of the commonly used and discussed approaches. Similarly, it is impossible to fully describe all the nuances of a given methodology across all possible biomedical scenarios in a single book chapter. The chapters of this book thus focus on presenting key features of a given area of biomedical informatics methodology with emphasis on a chosen set of biomedical contexts. All of the authors are established leaders in the development and application of biomedical informatics methods, and present examples from their own work and experience. The overall order of chapters in this book aims to present methodologies according to the DIKW framework, and a given chapter may span multiple facets of the framework.

As described earlier, the substrate wherefrom biomedical informatics innovations emerge to address challenges in biomedicine is composed of data. It is not uncommon for one to bring together multiple streams of data to develop transformative approaches further along the DIKW framework. Chapter 2 (by Prakash M. Nadkarni and Luis N. Marenco) thus focuses on the methodologies associated with data integration. Particular attention is given to comparing competing approaches for integrating data from disparate sources, while accounting for political and resource realities. Chapter 3 (by Mark A. Musen) then shifts the attention to how one might represent knowledge that can be attributed to gathered data. Within the context of the DIKW framework, this chapter highlights important methodological considerations and challenges with representing the meaning and preserving the knowledge associated with data. As continual improvements are seen in data generation technologies, such as next generation molecular sequencing, there is an increased need to harness biomedical informatics methodologies to identify potential testable hypotheses. To this end, Chapter 4 (by Yves A. Lussier and Haiquan Li) explores the challenges with generating hypotheses from heterogeneous data sets that span the spectrum of biomedicine.

It is essential to acknowledge that a significant volume of biomedical knowledge is not readily searchable or available for computational analyses. The next two chapters thus aim to introduce the reader to key methods associated with retrieval of knowledge from traditionally text based sources. The first of these, Chapter 5 (by Trevor Cohen and Dominic Widdows), presents contemporary biomedical informatics approaches that utilize geometric techniques to explore or analyze multi-faceted biomedical knowledge. Chapter 6 (by Kevin B. Cohen) provides an overview of natural language processing, which continues to mature within the realm of biomedical informatics for extracting potentially usable information from a range of sources across biomedicine.

As data are gathered from a plethora of sources and potentially represented as knowledge that can be of utility for future use, one must consider how one performs the transformation from data into information and knowledge such that it might enter into the stage of wisdom. Chapter 7 (by John H. Holmes) provides a foundational overview of data mining techniques, which are used to realize the DIKW framework. The next two chapters then present specific techniques that are used in biomedical informatics to impute information and knowledge from biomedical data. Chapter 8 (by Hsun-Hsien Chang and Gil Alterovitz) presents Bayesian methods that represent a major foundational category of techniques used in biomedical informatics to impute knowledge from biomedical data. Chapter 9 (by Ryan J. Urbanowicz and Jason H. Moore) then introduces learning classifier systems, which are increasingly becoming essential to decipher complex phenomena from potentially undecipherable data that can be perceived as knowledge.

As biomedical informatics solutions are developed, largely through the harnessing of formal and basic science techniques, their biomedical utility can only be realized through the implementation and contextualization through applied science. The next set of chapters aim to provide examples of methodologies that harness the applied aspects of biomedical informatics. The first of these chapters, Chapter 10 (by Riccardo Bellazzi, Matteo Gabetta, and Giorgio Leonardi), describes fundamental engineering principles that are germane to the design, development, and ultimate implementation of biomedical informatics innovations. Chapter 11 (by Fernando Martin-Sanchez, Guillermo Lopez-Campos, and Kathleen Gray) follows by exploring the biomedical informatics landscape associated with personalized medicine and participatory health, which reflects a holistic biomedical revolution that seamlessly integrates classical biomedical data with patient centered data to result in a new cadre of biomedical knowledge. Chapter 12 (by Joshua C. Denny and Hua Xu) then focuses on the development of personalized care regimens that harness increasingly digitally available genomic and health data that can be used to develop informed clinical decisions.

Chapter 13 provides a concluding perspective of biomedical informatics and its continued relevance in the emerging "Big Data" era. The chapters of the main book are followed by four mini-primers (Appendices A–D by Elizabeth S. Chen) that aim to provide hands-on experience with basic technical skills that are often used in the implementation of biomedical informatics methods: Unix (Appendix A); Ruby (Appendix B); Databases (Appendix C); and Web Services (Appendix D).

1.5 **EXPECTATIONS AND CHALLENGE TO THE READER**

As with any multi-authored book, there will be varying styles in presenting content. Each of the authors was charged with taking what are traditionally complex and difficult concepts in biomedical informatics and presenting them in a manner that is accessible but still of utility in the context of contemporary biomedicine. To this end, each chapter should be approached with the aim to understand the principles of the concepts described within the context of the examples from within a given chapter. The reader should then aim to address three questions:

1. What are the key aspects of the methodological concepts described?
2. How can the methodological concepts be applied to my area of interest (e.g., bioinformatics, clinical informatics, or public health informatics)?
3. What are potential advantages/disadvantages of the methods presented?

The reader should then aim to identify additional peer-reviewed literature (starting with other articles written by the chapter authors) that further describes the methodological aspects of the techniques presented within a given chapter.

For this book to be used as an effective educational instrument or as an introduction to the broad range of methodologies that are used in biomedical informatics, it must be used as a starting point and not as a comprehensive reference for a given methodology. Many of the chapter authors have included references that may be consulted for additional details. Whilst a book of this nature will never be comprehensive (or even complete in topics covered), it is expected that it will provide a foundation for the methodological principles of biomedical informatics that can be applied across the spectrum of biomedicine.

REFERENCES

[1] Keramaris NC, Kanakaris NK, Tzioupis C, Kontakis G, Giannoudis PV. Translational research: from benchside to bedside. Injury 2008;39(6):643–50.

[2] Woolf SH. The meaning of translational research and why it matters. J Am Med Assoc 2008;299(2):211–3.

[3] Westfall JM, Mold J, Fagnan L. Practice-based research–"Blue Highways" on the NIH roadmap. J Am Med Assoc 2007;297(4):403–6.

[4] Kulikowski CA, Shortliffe EH, Currie LM, Elkin PL, Hunter LE, Johnson TR, et al. AMIA board white paper: definition of biomedical informatics and specification of core competencies for graduate education in the discipline. J Am Med Inform Assoc 2012;19(6):931–8.

[5] Shortliffe EH, Cimino JJ, editors. Biomedical informatics: computer applications in health care and biomedicine. 4th ed. New York: Springer; 2013.

[6] Sarkar IN. Biomedical informatics and translational medicine. J Transl Med 2010;8:22. PubMed PMID: 20187952.

[7] Lean ME, Mann JI, Hoek JA, Elliot RM, Schofield G. Translational research. BMJ 2008;337:a863.

[8] Wehling M. Principles of translational science in medicine: from bench to bedside. Cambridge, New York: Cambridge University Press; 2010. xxii, 382 p., 24 p. of plates p.

[9] Payne PR, Embi PJ, Sen CK. Translational informatics: enabling high-throughput research paradigms. Physiol Genomics 2009;39(3):131–40.

[10] Altman RB. Translational bioinformatics: linking the molecular world to the clinical world. Clin Pharmacol Ther 2012;91(6):994–1000.

[11] Sarkar IN, Butte AJ, Lussier YA, Tarczy-Hornoch P, Ohno-Machado L. Translational bioinformatics: linking knowledge across biological and clinical realms. J Am Med Inform Assoc 2011;18(4):354–7.

[12] Embi PJ, Payne PR. Clinical research informatics: challenges, opportunities and definition for an emerging domain. J Am Med Inform Assoc 2009;16(3):316–27.

[13] Shortliffe EH. The future of biomedical informatics: a perspective from academia. Stud Health Technol Inform 2012;180:19–24.

[14] Choi BC, Pak AW. Multidisciplinarity, interdisciplinarity and transdisciplinarity in health research, services, education and policy: 1. Definitions, objectives, and evidence of effectiveness. Clin Invest Med. Medecine clinique et experimentale 2006;29(6):351–64.

[15] Choi BC, Pak AW. Multidisciplinarity, interdisciplinarity, and transdisciplinarity in health research, services, education and policy: 2. Promotors, barriers, and

strategies of enhancement. Clin Invest Med. Medecine clinique et experimentale 2007;30(6):E224–32.

[16] Choi BC, Pak AW. Multidisciplinarity, interdisciplinarity, and transdisciplinarity in health research, services, education and policy: 3. Discipline, inter-discipline distance, and selection of discipline. Clin Invest Med. Medecine clinique et experimentale 2008;31(1):E41–8.

[17] Barnes J. The Cambridge companion to Aristotle. Cambridge, New York: Cambridge University Press; 1995. xxv, p. 404.

[18] Omar SB. Ibn al-Haytham's optics: a study of the origins of experimental science. Minneapolis: Bibliotheca Islamica; 1977. p. 168.

[19] Bacon F, Jardine L, Silverthorne M. The new organon. Cambridge U.K., New York: Cambridge University Press; 2000. xxxv, p. 252.

[20] Hackett J. Roger Bacon and the sciences: commemorative essays. Leiden, New York: Brill; 1997. x, p. 439.

[21] Popper KR. The logic of scientific discovery. London, New York: Routledge; 1992. p. 479.

[22] Pearson K. On the criterion that a given system of deviations from the probable in the case of a correlated system of variables is such that it can be reasonably supposed to have arisen from random sampling. Philos Mag Ser 5 1900;50(302):157–75.

[23] Fisher RA. On the interpretation of χ^2 from contingency tables, and the calculation of P. J Roy Stat Soc 1922;85(1):87–94.

[24] Barrows HS, Tamblyn RM. Problem-based learning: an approach to medical education. New York: Springer Pub. Co.; 1980. xvii, p. 206.

[25] Mandin H, Jones A, Woloschuk W, Harasym P. Helping students learn to think like experts when solving clinical problems. Acad Med: J Assoc Am Med Coll 1997;72(3):173–9.

[26] Connelly DP, Johnson PE. The medical problem solving process. Hum Pathol 1980;11(5):412–9.

[27] Beach TG, Monsell SE, Phillips LE, Kukull W. Accuracy of the clinical diagnosis of Alzheimer disease at National Institute on Aging Alzheimer Disease Centers, 2005–2010. J Neuropathol Exp Neurol 2012;71(4):266–73.

[28] Cao L. Domain driven data mining. New York, London: Springer; 2010. xvi, p. 248

[29] Ackoff RL. From data to wisdom. J Appl Syst Anal 1989;16:3–9.

[30] Rowley J. The wisdom hierarchy: representations of the DIKW hierarchy. J Inf Sci 2007;33(2):163–80.

[31] Ledley RS, Lusted LB. Reasoning foundations of medical diagnosis; symbolic logic, probability, and value theory aid our understanding of how physicians reason. Science 1959;130(3366):9–21.

[32] Lusted LB, Ledley RS. Mathematical models in medical diagnosis. J Med Educ 1960;35:214–22.

[33] Blois MS. Information holds medicine together. MD Comput: Comput Med Practice 1987;4(5):42–6.

Data Integration: An Overview

Prakash M. Nadkarni and Luis N. Marenco

Yale University School of Medicine, New Haven, CT, USA

2.1 OBJECTIVES OF INTEGRATION

The broad objective of integration is to be able to answer questions of combined data that would be otherwise very difficult and/or tedious to address if each individual data source had to be accessed separately or in sequence. We can look at these goals in the context of *Health information exchanges* (HIE) [1], which are data repositories created geographically related to a consortium of stakeholders (e.g., hospitals, insurance companies, and group practices). HIEs, whose data can be accessed when needed by any authorized stakeholder, are intended to maintain an up-to-date pool of essential information on patients within the geographical region who are associated with any stakeholder-caregiver.

The specific goals of data integration are to:

1. *Be able to look at the "Big Picture":* Organizations that carry out identical or highly similar operations at different geographical locations need to be able to look at consolidated summaries of structurally identical, pooled data to know how they are performing. In other scenarios (e.g., research consortia), different sites that function autonomously may be generating different kinds of primary data that focus on a broad overall problem, or with the same sources (e.g., a common pool of patients and biospecimens): here, being able to inspect or analyze the pooled dataset can help answer research questions. With HIEs, pooled data facilitate epidemiological and outcomes research.

2. *Identify shared elements within different sources, which can then be used as the basis of interoperation between systems that make use of individual sources:* An example of such an operational national effort is the National Library of Medicine's Unified Medical Language System (UMLS) [2]. The UMLS is primarily a compendium ("meta-thesaurus") of individual controlled vocabularies that have achieved the status of standards for specific biomedical applications, or within certain biomedical areas. Different areas overlap, and therefore many elements (here, biomedical concepts) are shared across multiple vocabularies, often with different names. The UMLS maintains a list of biomedical concepts, a list of synonyms (terms) for each concept and their occurrence in individual vocabularies, along with vocabulary-specific information such as the alphanumeric codes assigned to individual concepts. In the context of HIEs, identification of functionally similar elements across different systems simplifies the task of updating the patient's medical history in that patient's primary medical record when the patient has been treated somewhere else within the HIE's geographical area.

3. *Eliminate duplicated effort and errors due to non-communicating systems:* Many businesses (including hospitals), which use software from multiple vendors, are still notorious for maintaining multiple, often non-synchronized or out-of-date copies of essential customer/patient data, e.g., demographics, insurance, and vital parameters such as blood group, allergies, current ailments, current medications. In emergency cases where a patient is seen by a caregiver/institution different from the usual caregiver (a problem that is particularly acute in the US, where the

healthcare system is fragmented), laboratory tests must sometimes be repeated because data are unobtainable expeditiously from the original source. The benefits in an HIE context are obvious: for patients in an emergency situation being treated at a site other than the usual provider, the new providers accessing HIE content can access the patient's medical history, and can focus on treating the present complaint rather than losing precious time in gathering old information.

2.2 **INTEGRATION APPROACHES: OVERVIEW**

Integration may be achieved using two broad strategies:

1. *Physical Data Integration:* Copies of the primary data are restructured and moved to one or more data repositories. Depending on the scope and volume of the data, this repository can either constitute a *data warehouse* [3] or a *data mart* [4]. The differences between the two lie primarily in scope, orientation, and purpose, and secondarily in the choice of design and technology. Data warehouses have organization-wide scope, are oriented toward business analysts or statisticians, and store every possible type of data of interest across the organization. Data marts have departmental-level scope, are typically end-user oriented, and are special-purpose (e.g., they may be concerned only with clinical data or only with administrative/financial data). The significantly greater challenges of devising warehouses relate to the difficulty of the implementation team's being able to thoroughly understand the greater diversity of the data that they must integrate.

   Extraction, Transformation, and Load (ETL) is the process of migrating data from their original source into a warehouse or mart. This process can be extremely involved, as we now discuss. Note that ETL is not a one-time task: because the original sources are regularly updated during production operations, ETL must be performed at a regular frequency to ensure that the physically integrated data in the warehouse or marts are current. Historically, the ideal was to ensure that the integrated data were not more than 24 h out of date: the ETL processes were run at night in batch mode, when the production systems were mostly idle. Currently, many high-end DBMSs support technologies that allow updates of the integrated data at frequencies greater than nightly, or even in continuous, real-time mode.

   In organizations that employ data integration, there is one warehouse and multiple data marts: the contents of the marts are derived from the warehouse through secondary transformation and load processes.

2. *Virtual (or Logical) Data Integration:* Data reside in a distributed manner at their original sites. However, software that resides at a central site communicates with the hardware that houses the distributed data, via the Internet and using a specific query protocol. Users interact with the sources only via the intermediary software, which is therefore referred to as a *mediator*. The central site stores information that describes the data at individual sites. Users of the system only interact directly with the central site, which *mediates* their requests for data. That is, the central site acts as an intermediary between users and the distributed sites. In logical data integration, the analog of the data warehouse/mart is *data federation*.

Theoretically, one could implement a federation of data warehouses. Warehousing technology, however, is expensive enough (and expertise in warehousing processes scarce enough) that it is best applied at a single centralized location. Data mart technology, by contrast, is cheap enough to be deployed at multiple sites. In fact, data marts at multiple locations—e.g., departments within an organization—often act as end-user front-ends to a central warehouse: this set up, however, still involves physical integration.

In either circumstance, integration focuses primarily on *data query* rather than *interactive data updates*. In the federation scenario, where individual sites are autonomous, updates by anyone other than the sites' own users would not even be permitted. In the physical-integration scenario, warehouse technology is optimized for query, and not intended to support interactive transaction processing. Updates to the sources only occur during fixing of errors discovered during the integration effort, an issue discussed shortly.

2.2.1 Scope of this Chapter

The field of integration is too vast to be covered in a single chapter. Entire books cover various aspects of physical data integration (which is more mature than logical integration): practically every single book where Ralph Kimball shares authorship is worth reading, and Larry Greenfield's Web site, the Data Warehousing Information Center [5], is an invaluable resource that this chapter's authors used to commence learning about this field, and continue to consult. (Bill Inmon is justifiably credited as the father of the data warehouse. However, we find his post-1999 work far less useful than those of Kimball, with whom he occasionally has very public disagreements.) Reference books on logical integration are far fewer: they deal with specific products (e.g., by IBM), or with scenarios (e.g., "semantic web") where implementation lags greatly behind theory.

This chapter will therefore limit itself to provide an overview, with the objective of enabling the reader to better utilize resources such as the above. Specifically, this chapter will:

- Summarize and contrast approaches with respect to benefits and drawbacks.
- Characterize the subtasks that underlie all integration efforts irrespective of the approach.
- Summarize some efforts in biomedicine.
- Provide practical advice on integration.

While some overlap is unavoidable, we will focus on areas that are relatively underemphasized (or not discussed at all) in book-length references, incorporating our own experience where appropriate.

In our exploration of integration approaches, we will make the reasonable assumption that each data source ("database") will utilize some form of Database Management System (DBMS) to manage its content. The following subsection (Database Basics), which provides a foundation required to appreciate the rest of the chapter, can be skipped by those already familiar with DBMS technology.

2.3 **DATABASE BASICS**

Relational databases (RDBs) [6], invented in 1970 by E.F. Codd, currently form the basis of the most widely used DBMS technology. Here, the database can be thought of as a set of interconnected tables: each table has *columns* corresponding to fields and *rows* corresponding to records. A column is defined in terms of its *data type* (the type of data it holds, e.g., text, integers, decimal numbers, dates) and *constraints*—conditions that dictate what values are permitted in individual columns (or combinations of columns). We will discuss constraints shortly in the next section.

An RDB is typically designed using a methodology called *normalization* [7], which involves segregating the data to be represented across multiple tables with minimal duplication of elements across tables. For example, patients may be assigned a unique Patient ID (typically an auto-incrementing integer). A "Patient Demographics" table associates, with the Patient ID, details such as the patient's name, birth date, gender, current address, contact information, etc. A separate "Visits" table records a patient's (possibly numerous) visits using only the Patient ID without duplicating the name, gender, etc.: the latter data are looked up from the Patient Demographics table. The Demographics and Visits tables are thus *linked* by the Patient ID column. The link serves another purpose: maintaining *referential integrity*.

That is, in any row of the Visits table, the value of the "Patient ID" column must match an actual patient in the Demographics table. Similarly, a user working with the Demographics table is not permitted to accidentally delete a patient who has at least one Visit record.

The term *schema* refers to the structure or blueprint of a database. For an RDB, the schema comprises the definition of each table (primarily in terms of its columns) and the links (also called *relationships*) between individual tables. An RDB schema is typically specified using Structured Query Language (SQL), the *lingua franca* of RDB technology, which is used both to define a database and to manipulate its contents (query and record addition, deletion, and change).

2.3.1 **SQL Dialects**

The term "*lingua franca*" is partially misleading: SQL actually refers to a set of vendor-specific dialects based on a standard, whose differences may be significant enough to impact an integration effort, especially a data federation where different sites are likely to use different vendor DBMSs. The International Standards Organization (ISO) SQL committee, which defines the standard, has a process that generally lags behind business needs and development of commercial software: to a large extent the process has played catch-up rather than having a direct influence on commercial SQL development. The various commercial RDBMSs vary in how they manage basic data types such as dates, and functions with identical purpose (e.g., for basic math or string manipulation) may be invoked differently. Further, Extensible Markup Language (XML) content, geographic data, formatted text of arbitrary size are handled in vendor-specific ways.

Numerous third-party software vendors market tools that facilitate creating software applications that translate a "vendor-neutral" SQL into vendor-specific SQL. This allows the creation of front-end tools (e.g., analytical software or query interfaces) that can connect to a variety of database engines without their power-users having to worry about which DBMS engine they are connecting to. Among the "vendor-neutral" standards is Open Database Connectivity (ODBC), originally promulgated by Microsoft but made freely available, so that it has formed the basis of other standards, such as Java Database Connectivity (JDBC). "Vendor-neutral" SQL does not support manipulation of XML/formatted text/geographic data, and similarly, different DBMSs vary widely with respect to the built-in analytical functions that they support: for example, the standard statistical function, *standard deviation*, is an intrinsic function in some SQL dialects but not others. In all these circumstances, one still resorts to vendor-specific SQL: fortunately, ODBC allows software developers to designate "vendor-specific" code when this capability is needed.

2.3.2 **Design for High Performance**

Modern relational database technology achieves high performance using a variety of technological approaches. Chief among these are:

- *Indexes:* These are data structures on disk that can dramatically improve search performance. With an index, search operations on the table associated with the index are proportional to the logarithm of the record count or even better, thus greatly increasing speed of querying for large volumes of data. Indexing normally involves a trade-off: when data are interactively updated, with every addition or deletion of a record, the indexes on those data must be updated, which takes time, and therefore indexes are restricted only to those necessary for interactive operations (e.g., index on last names or dates of birth of patients). Most DBMSs employ "B-tree" indexes [8], which give balanced performance with respect to query versus update.
- *Caching:* DBMSs will take advantage of RAM, which is used to store portions of tables and indexes, as well as data previously requested.
- *Query Optimization:* The interpretation and execution of SQL data-retrieval statements has been refined over three decades: DBMSs will utilize information such as the presence of indexes, the availability of RAM, and even pre-computed statistics on the distribution of data within tables. Software developers can also inspect execution plans (which are typically displayed graphically) and use this information to identify bottlenecks and improve performance—e.g., by adding an index.

2.3.3 **Data Integration vs. Interoperation**

Data integration focuses primarily on query of the integrated data. The related term *systems integration* involves getting separate software or hardware systems to *interoperate*: e.g., propagating updates to one or more systems based on changes to another system [9]. It is possible to achieve data integration without interoperation, and vice versa.

Interoperation involves two or more systems communicating using a message-passing protocol, which may be *ad hoc* or based on some kind of standard. It involves two aspects: data interchange and distributed computing.

- In *data interchange*, the protocol is used to transmit data for export/ import. For healthcare systems, the interchange standard is Health

Level 7 (HL7). Among the problems with the current official version of HL7 (v 2.x) [10] are that it is somewhat underspecified, so that each vendor's flavor of HL7 differs somewhat, and exchanging data between systems created by separate vendors is non-trivial. The latest (non-official) version of HL7 (version 3) is not backward-compatible with v 2.x, and complaints of excessive complexity [11] have delayed its widespread acceptance. Another caveat is that HL7 interchange has sufficient overhead that if simpler means of exchange are available, they should be used preferentially (the Epic Electronic Health Record, for example, uses the medium of delimited text files as a mechanism for exporting data [12]). In any case, such streams are unsuited for the purpose of complex, *ad hoc* querying: their contents are best parsed, restructured, and imported into RDBMSs for that purpose.

- In *distributed computing*, two or more hardware units (which may be geographically separated) are involved in the solving of a problem. This configuration enables individual sites to contribute computing resources that can be accessed remotely, though they may also support data access. Here, the communication approach involves mechanisms such as Web Services [13], which may be regarded as subroutines executed remotely using Web-based technologies: data are passed to the subroutine, and results returned. Web services may use one of two approaches: the simple Representational State Transfer (REST) [14] and the complex SOAP, which originally stood for Simple Object Access Protocol, but now stands for nothing after it was discovered through experience that SOAP is anything but simple [15]. REST is more lightweight. The pros and cons of each approach are beyond the scope of this chapter; a good, accessible overview is provided by Steve Francia [16].

2.4 PHYSICAL VS. LOGICAL INTEGRATION: PROS AND CONS

A general rule of thumb is that physical integration is always preferable to virtual integration/federation except when it is not feasible for non-technical reasons (e.g., business or political). The following issues must be considered:

- *Query Performance and Technological Considerations:* Integrated data are ultimately intended to be queried. Users expect queries that are run on a regularly scheduled basis to execute rapidly. Queries run much faster when all data are hosted on a single machine, as opposed to having to deal with network (or Internet) latency inherent in having a mediator query multiple, geographically separated sources and moving intermediate results back and forth between locales in order to combine, filter, and format the results for the end-user. While network latency may also be an issue in querying a single, remotely located, integrated data store, it is less so because the query results are much less voluminous than the data that must be processed to yield the results.

Warehouses and data marts (marketed for the most part by organizations that also sell RDBMSs) utilize performance-enhancing technologies that take advantage of the read-only nature of the data (end-users do not update data interactively). Such data can be more extensively indexed, and certain types of indexes (hash-table based indexes [17], join indexes, and bitmap indexes [18,19]) employed that give significantly faster query performance than "B-tree" indexes, but whose performance would be unacceptable for data that is interactively updated frequently [20]. In addition, physical integration allows data to be *restructured* to speed performance of common queries, a topic we consider in Section 2.6, "Data restructuring."

Another way to improve query performance is to *pre-compute data aggregates* that form the basis of common data requests. For example, one can compute several statistics related to hospital care (such as median length of stay, total number of admissions in different departments, etc.) just once, and store them for future use. Most warehouse/mart vendors include "multi-dimensional database" technology that computes such aggregates either automatically, based on the data model, or with minimal developer intervention.

- *The existence of "black-box" legacy systems or non-database sources:* One or more of the data sources to be integrated may be poorly understood, decades-old "legacy" systems, whose original programmers may have long since retired, and which were created long-before modern DBMSs or modern communications protocols (or the Internet) existed. Integrating such systems logically with the others is impossible or prohibitively expensive: it is better to try to extract data (from their outputs, if necessary: see screen-scraping, later) and move it to a modern DBMS.

In addition, much of the data may reside in formats such as spreadsheets or statistical packages: suitable for their intended purpose, but not really intended to support multi-user queries. In this case, too, logical integration is infeasible, and transformation of copies of such data into DBMS structures is desirable.

- *Query Translation vs. Data Translation:* Integration of diverse data sources requires creating a *global data model* that represents the information that the integrated resource will store or provide access to. As stated later, this is typically not the union of all the elements in all data sources, but a subset of the union. Once the global data model is defined, the correspondences (*mappings*) between elements in individual sources and elements in the data model must then be defined. Such correspondence may not be a one-to-one match for reasons discussed in Section 2.5.2.2, and conversions (such as mathematical transformation) may need to be performed.

We now contrast how logical integration and physical integration work. In logical integration, a user issues a query against the global data model. The mediator looks up mapping information to identify which local sources contain the desired elements, and then *translates* the global query into queries that are meaningful to each individual source. (Thus, if a user asks for elements A, B, and C, but a particular source contains only elements A and B, then the translated query for that source will only ask for those elements.) The translated query must also conform to the syntax of the local DBMS's query language or dialect of SQL. The translation process can be streamlined to some extent by using *database views* (predefined queries, typically across multiple tables). Such translation must, of course, be performed each time a user issues a new query.

Physical integration, by contrast, is based on *data* translation. All the integrated data are ultimately converted (mathematically transformed, if needed) to the structures required by the global model (and into a single DBMS). Restructuring is performed as a batch process—i.e., only once during data load. Therefore the expense of translation is incurred only once, and issues of worrying about various SQL dialects do not arise.

Further, once physical homogenization is achieved, queries against a physically integrated system can be significantly more complex/powerful, and implementation of query capability significantly simpler, than for a federated system that may use different DBMSs at each site. With logical integration, by contrast, while simple browsing interfaces that show details of a single item of interest are feasible, sophisticated analytic queries involving complex Boolean logic that return numerous rows of data are rarely possible.

- *Authority and Organizational Structure:* Physical integration generally mandates that the integration team should be able to access all of the data sources (both data definitions as well as samples) freely, so as to understand each source and determine what can be integrated. This is feasible when integration is being performed within a single organization (assuming that divisional turf battles can be overridden by senior management). Here, the information technology (IT) staff responsible for the data-source sites report to the same authority as the central team.

In the case of consortia of independent organizations that may be competitors—this is also true for scientific efforts—it is politically infeasible to expect an integration team, even one comprised of members of every organization, to have this level of authority and access: certain data, and even the existence of certain data elements, may be considered proprietary. Also, lines of command are crossed: the site IT staff is not answerable to the integration team, and without their cooperation, integration will not happen. In this situation, federation is the only option.

- *Political issues* arise in any integration effort (see the references of Greenfield [21] and Demarest [22]), but are much worse in the consortium context. Some sites may believe, rightly or wrongly, that giving a remotely based integration team copies of their data might somehow lower their "control" over their own data: they would rather have end-users query their systems via a mediator. When physical integration was mandated, the authors have witnessed, due to individual sites' fear of getting "scooped" by their competitors, the deploying of passive-aggressive tactics to delay transmission of data copies, including the use of obscure and hard-to-parse data formats that require significant programming effort by the integration team.

  Again, federation may be the only choice: political minefields exist here as well. Funding authorities may have to employ a combination of incentives and strong-arming to ensure progress. The paranoia of certain investigators in at least one National Institutes of Health research consortium, coupled with limited direct involvement of NIH program staff, has doomed data integration efforts even before they began: the least-common-denominator data that was agreed to be shared was so rudimentary that it had little value to the broader scientific community.

- *Expertise:* Expertise in integration is not widespread. Consequently, in a federation scenario, where there were many more cooks (not all of them fully qualified) involved in making the broth, it is easier for things to go wrong: much more time must be spent in education and training, and the site with the least skills can play a rate-determining role. Also, if such expertise is unavailable and must be hired, it is less expensive to hire a team that operates centrally than multiple teams for each geographic site.

The too-many-cooks constraint, in our opinion, also reflects in the final product: consortium-created logically integrated resources that aim to provide access to heterogeneous data may be awkward to use and less likely to reflect a unifying, consistent vision. The hurdles in trying to arrive at, and impose such a vision (which may require significant overhaul and cleanup of the individual sources to serve new purposes for which they were not originally intended) are often insuperable, and may result in "lipstick on a pig": cosmetic changes that fail to achieve the desired result.

Occasionally, one may implement a *hybrid* approach, involving aspects of both strategies. Here, too, there are two possibilities.

- Primarily federated, but data fetched by the central site in response to user requests may be stored for reuse ("cached"), so that a subsequent request for the same data sends back the cached copy rather than reaching out to the distributed sites. Caching is especially applicable for subsets of the data that have *low volatility*, i.e., change infrequently. In this case, one must record the time-stamps (date/times) of last change to the source-data elements, and the time-stamps of last caching for those elements on the server. Prior to execution of a query that asks for the cached data, the time-stamps are compared to see if the source-data time-stamps are more recent than the cached time-stamps. If so, it is time for the source data to be "pulled" and cached again.
- Primarily physically integrated. However, data in the physical store is refreshed ("pulled") from multiple (possibly geographically separated) primary sources in as unobtrusive a manner as possible (as far as the owners of the remote systems are concerned). As above, time-stamps are used at both ends (sources and repository) to determine when to pull new data, and what rows of data to pull. Intra-organization warehouses may also use pull strategies: the difference here is that in a federation, primary sources are controlled independently, the data owners' IT teams need to specify to the "pull" software what elements in their systems they are making "public"—only these will be accessed, while all other elements will be "invisible."

No matter which strategy is used, certain subtasks are essential. We discuss the circumstances that determine feasibility, and the prerequisite subtasks, shortly.

2.5 **PREREQUISITE SUBTASKS**

The shared subtasks comprise the following:

1. Determining the objectives of the integration effort, in terms of specific desirable end-results. This in turn determines the scope of the effort.
2. Identifying the data elements that, when integrated, will help meet the objectives, and using these to define the "global" data model of the integrated system. This requires acquiring an understanding of the data sources. Among the activities to perform here are:
   a. Characterizing the sources in terms of redundancy and inconsistency of data elements.
   b. Characterizing the heterogeneity and modeling conflicts among the data sources.
3. Estimating data quality, and reducing data errors.
4. Creating detailed human- and machine-interpretable descriptions/ documentation of the data sources. As the integration effort proceeds, documentation extends to the processes used to extract and transform the data (for physical integration) and later, to the integrated end-result.

After prerequisites are completed, the integration process diverges depending on whether physical or logical integration is intended. In physical integration, the ETL process now commences. (ETL is too vast to do justice in a single book chapter, so we will refer the reader to Kimball et al.'s excellent text [23].) In logical integration, one defines correspondences (*mappings*) between the global model and components of the local models are defined, as discussed later, and the software that performs global-to-local query translation is implemented, or purchased: with the commercial option, mappings must be defined using the vendor-provided framework. Describing the nuts-and-bolts of logical integration is also beyond the scope of this chapter, but see the freely available articles by Marenco et al. [24,25] for such detail.

We will explore subtask in turn.

2.5.1 **Determining Objectives**

Integration efforts are expensive. Even if infinite time and resources were available, it would not be desirable to attempt to integrate every single item of data that exists within an organization or consortium. Many data elements will be used only by a particular division/department/laboratory for a variety of internal purposes, and will have little utility beyond it: in a consortium, some data may be considered proprietary and non-shareable by individual sites. Determining specific (i.e., detailed) goals and deliverables will identify what kinds of data elements must be integrated: prioritizing these goals determines the order in which integration-related tasks will be performed.

2.5.2 **Identifying Elements: Understanding the Data Sources**

Understanding data sources can be challenging, especially for legacy systems where the only documentation may comprise source code written in an unfamiliar programming language. Further, for any given data source, only some of the data elements that it records (or no elements at all) may be relevant to integration objectives. Integrators must be prepared for the possibility of an unpleasant discovery: the data that would otherwise meet the integration objectives may not actually be identifiable/ available, or be present in a form that is unusable (e.g., it may lack the requisite level of detail). Many integration efforts have resulted in modifications of source systems to capture such information in future.

The steps in understanding data sources are the following:

- *Identifying the purpose* of every table in source systems. If the table appears to be of interest to the integration effort, one identifies the purpose of the columns in the table.
- *Constraints* or *checks* are rules that limit the permissible values in a column (or set of columns). They need to be determined by inspecting the documentation and/or source code, from knowledge of the area (which is often gleaned by interviewing users), and examination of the data.

  Examination of data requires that data be extracted. Even for well-understood source systems, this task may not be trivial. While modern systems that rely on RDBMSs readily generate delimited text output, we have encountered commercial "black-box" hospital-accounting software that only generates 80-characters-per-line format (VT-52 terminal output that is spooled to disk), which must be "screen-scraped" to extract the needed data from the copious admixed whitespace and label content. Several third-party vendors provide graphical tools (e.g., Monarch™) that greatly simplify extraction from such output.

- *Rules* are a generalization of constraints: they have the general structure: if (condition) then (perform actions) where both the condition and the actions may be arbitrarily complex. Rules may be of two kinds: *absolute* and *heuristic*. Absolute rules are like constraints: they should never be violated. Heuristic rules embody judgment calls or "rules of thumb": they are probabilistic, though the probability may be stated on a crude qualitative scale rather than as a precise number. The term "business rules" applies to rules, implicit or explicit, that determine how processes in business applications are conducted. The process by which they are discovered is similar to that of constraints. It is important to note that rules change over time, because of legislation, evolving goals, and so forth.

Examples of constraints are:

- *Data-type:* E.g., dates should be valid, numeric fields should not contain alphabetical characters and be in a standardized format like YYYY-MM-DD.
- *Range:* Maximum and minimum permissible values. One may also record maximum and minimum *reasonable* values, where out-of-range values are possible but must be verified (e.g., human weight more than 900 lbs).
- *Enumerations:* The values of a column must belong to a modest-sized set of values: these values are typically (alpha-) numeric codes, each of which corresponds to a textual description. Sometimes, these values may represent ordering, so that the enumeration represents an ordinal scale: for example, pain may be coded as 0 (Absent), 1 (Mild), 2 (Moderate), and 3 (Severe).
- *Mandatory:* A column's value cannot be blank.
- *Unique:* For a given row in a table, the column's value must be unique. Thus, social security number and Patient ID must be unique for every patient.
- *Regular-expression* [26]*:* The column contents must match a pattern. For example, social security number must match the pattern nnn-nn-nnnn ($n =$ any digit).
- *Multi-column:* The sum of the individual components together must be valid. For example, differential white blood cell count across multiple columns must be equal to 100 (since they are all percentages). A simpler example may be that the time-stamp of hospital admission must be less than time-stamp of discharge. Multi-column constraints can often be arbitrarily complex and must be specified using programming code.
- *Computed columns:* Certain columns may be derived from others. For example, for humans, Body-Mass Index is calculated by (weight in kg)/(height in meters)^2.

2.5.2.1 *Identifying Redundancy and Inconsistency*

Exploration of the sources may reveal that the same information is recorded redundantly in multiple sources: this is often seen in pre-relational systems, or in systems that have not been designed to interoperate with others. Further, like multiple clocks in a house where each indicates a different time, the sources may be inconsistent: when a patient's contact information changes, for example, only one source may be current: when insurance information changes, only another source may be accurate. In such cases, it is important to identify the workflow to determine which sources are "authoritative" for which elements. In many cases, it is impossible to know which source is the accurate one, because the work processes for data update are haphazard.

A *Master Patient Index* (MPI) is a database application that facilitates consistency-maintenance for essential patient information. It records every patient's most current information, assigning a unique Patient ID. Ideally, all other software systems within the organization use this Patient ID, querying the MPI to obtain current information, or posting updates to specific MPI fields (such as current diagnoses or most recent hospital admissions) as needed. One can also query the MPI using a combination of criteria (name, date of birth, gender, contact info) to see whether a newly encountered patient is already in the system, so that a duplicate record for the same patient is not accidentally created. (To allow for name-spelling errors and changed contact info, the MPI software must support inexact or "probabilistic" matching.) In practice, many commercial black-box systems such as described above may refuse to interoperate with MPIs, making some duplication unavoidable.

In scientific contexts, inconsistency has other aspects.

- While detectable by computer programs, inconsistency may be resolvable only by domain expertise, not by integrators with primarily software expertise. An example is the UMLS, where interconcept relationships contradict each other across source vocabularies. The National Library of Medicine has a hands-off policy on content curation, merely tagging each fact with its source, so that you may encounter something equivalent to: "according to vocabulary X, sound travels faster than light." Users who lack domain expertise may have to rely on heuristics such as the authoritativeness of individual vocabularies.
- In other cases, inconsistency is a consequence of experimental uncertainty: the correct answer is not yet known, and all the results must be preserved (and tagged with their original source), until such time that the discrepancies can be resolved with further experiment. Examples of this type of inconsistency were seen in genomic maps in the mid-1990s, when yeast artificial chromosomes (YACs) were used as experimental reagents to clone human DNA. YACs have a high incidence of "chimerism": the cloned DNA, which is supposed to correspond to a single genomic region, may actually be a composite of DNA from two or more genomic regions, leading to errors in interpretation if the DNA is characterized or sequenced. The chimerism incidence was high enough that the Human Genome Project ultimately abandoned them.

2.5.2.2 *Characterizing Heterogeneity: Modeling Conflicts*

Even in cases where different sources do not contradict each other, they may say the same thing about the same data differently, and they may state slightly different things. Modeling conflicts pose an important challenge in integration, and it must be identified rigorously. Won Kim's classic 1991 article [27] provides a useful classification for the integration practitioner.

1. *Storage-engine conflicts:* While RDBMSs are widely used, they are not universal, and a wide variety of non-relational data stores may be encountered, especially in scientific data sets where performance is less importance than convenience for analysis. Data may be stored in the formats used by statistical and other analytic packages. Consequently, the data structures encountered may not match the designs of relational data stores.

   Even when DBMS-type stores are used, the data organization may violate the principles of "normalization" stated earlier. This violation may be either *deliberate*, to fix significant performance problems—an issue more likely to be encountered in the past than today, but still seen with Electronic Health Record (EHR) systems that use non-relational engines—or *accidental*—where the system's developers did not fully comprehend the consequences of the short-cuts that they took.

2. *Naming conflicts across tables, columns, and relationships:* Synonymy occurs when the same concept is named differently in two sources— thus laboratory procedures may be called *LABS* in one system and *LAB_PROCS* in another. *Homonymy* occurs when the same phrase is used to label related, but non-identical, or different concepts. For example, one EHR may use *PERSON* to refer to end-users of the system, and another to refer to patients. For payroll tables, a *Salary* column in one table may be a *Wage* column in another.

   Many biomedical databases, notably UMLS and the Systematized Nomenclature of Medicine Clinical Terms (SNOMED CT) [28], record associations between objects or concepts using triples of the form object-1/relationship/object-2. For example, finger/is-part-of/hand. Here, it is possible to record the same fact in a different way: hand/has-component/finger. A common class of relationship is the *hierarchy*, where one concept is more general or specific than another. For example, atrial flutter is a kind of (i.e., more specific than) heart rhythm disorder. The more general concept may also be called the *parent* or *ancestor*, while the more specific concept may be called a *child* or *descendant*. Most databases would differentiate between parent and ancestor in that a parent is a specific type of ancestor: thus, heart disease is a more remote ancestor of atrial fibrillation (e.g., a parent of the parent or grandparent). However, we have seen databases where "ancestor" is used as a synonym of "parent."

Also note that in biomedicine, strict hierarchies rarely occur: that is, a concept can be a "child" of more than one concept, so that, if we visualized all concepts and their inter-connections in a diagram, we would have a directed graph rather than a hierarchical tree. Thus, atrial flutter is a child of both "disorders of the atrium of the heart" and "heart disorders causing accelerated heart rate."

The precise semantics of a table, column, or relationship must be determined by inspecting both the documentation and the data, with the help of domain experts. In any case, trying to find correspondences between separate source schemas by relying on exact-name matches (an approach actually advocated in some theoretical computer-science papers) is extremely naïve. In real life, column names may be quasi-gibberish, heavily abbreviated, and their names may follow arbitrary conventions that are idiosyncratic to the system designer or organization.

3. *Structural Conflicts* arise when the same concept or set of concepts is represented using different modeling constructs in different databases. For example, some EHRs may store all laboratory findings associated with a patient in a giant table, while others may segregate clinical chemistry, microbiology, immunology, etc., into separate tables.

4. *Different levels of detail:* Even when two sources are modeling the same concept (e.g., olfactory receptors), the degree to which they do so may vary markedly. In scientific databases, this is understandable because different researchers are interested in different aspects of a broad problem. Therefore, the number and nature of the columns within a pair of tables serving the same broad purpose will differ. The approaches used to unify such data—these are also used to deal with structural conflicts, above—fall on a spectrum of two extremes:

   a. Semantically identical, shared columns are moved to a common table while separate source-specific tables record the information that varies.

   b. Entity-Attribute-Value (EAV) modeling [29]: In principle, multiple tables that have numerous columns are converted to a single table with fewer columns and many more rows. (This data transformation is an example of *homogenization*, discussed later in Section 2.6.) To illustrate this, consider a clinical chemistry table that recorded a serum electrolyte panel, with the columns: Patient ID, date-time of sample collection, serum sodium, serum potassium, serum bicarbonate, serum chloride, etc. Another table records liver function tests, with the columns: Patient ID, date-time of sample collection, alanine transaminase, aspartate transaminase, conjugated bilirubin, etc. The unified table model would have the columns: Patient ID, date-time of sample collection, laboratory parameter name, value of parameter. The Patient ID plus sample-collection date-time represent the "Entity"—the thing being described. The laboratory parameter is the Attribute—an aspect of the Entity. The "Value" column would refer to the value of the particular parameter. For a given patient, there would be as many rows of data as there are tests performed for that patient. Note that for a given row of data, the value is not interpretable in isolation—one needs to inspect the corresponding Attribute.

The EAV design is seldom taught in undergraduate computer-science courses, even though it is invariably used to record clinical data within EHRs and clinical research information systems. It is a natural fit for such data because the universe of clinical parameters (history and clinical exam findings, laboratory tests, and investigations) is enormous and constantly expanding, but only a relatively modest proportion of these parameters will apply to a given patient. That is, the attributes are *sparse*. A guide to the appropriate use of EAV modeling is provided in Dinu and Nadkarni [30].

A modification of the EAV approach is used in the UMLS, which needs to amalgamate around 150 source vocabularies, many of which use schemas that reflect particular biomedical domains (e.g., adverse drug reactions, clinical measurements). The UMLS "Attributes" table records this information. The end-result has pros and cons. The homogenized content is extremely useful when one wants to perform queries across multiple vocabularies. The drawback is that, as with sausage, the original components become hard to identify: if you are intending to work with a single vocabulary component, you may find it much simpler to work with the original source, if you can access it.

An intermediate approach may also be used. For example, in unified demographics tables, common information, such as Name, Date of Birth, Gender, present Address, etc., are stored in a common table, while database-specific variations, such as the specific army tours served in (this needs to be recorded in the Veterans Administration databases), are recorded in EAV form.

5. *Different units and/or different precision for quantitative measurements:* Different units impact the recording of clinical and laboratory parameters. The USA is among a few countries that use the British system for basic measurements (weight and height): the same laboratory parameter may be measured in mg/100 ml or (milli-, nano-) mol/l. Distances on chromosomal genetic maps are typically measured physically in base pairs (kilo- or mega-bases), but if predisposition for inheritance is considered, linkage distance (measured in centiMorgans) is used.

Even when the same unit is being used, the "normal" range for a parameter may vary modestly with the laboratory where the assay is performed—thus, a blood glucose value of 108 mg/dl may be normal for one lab, but slightly above normal for another. This is why the normal range always needs to be reported.

6. *Measures defined differently on minimally compatible or incompatible scales:* This is also a function of scientific objectives. Thus, smoking may be recorded in cigarettes per day (current consumption) or in pack-years (cumulative consumption). When pooling such data, such measures are reduced to the least common denominator: all that one can say is that someone has never smoked, been an ex-smoker, or is a current smoker.

This issue may also be encountered for subjective symptoms: these may be recorded on an interval scale of 0–10, or on an ordinal scale.

2.5.3 Data Quality: Identifying and Fixing Errors

Like death and taxes, the presence of data errors is inevitable. However, in the typical transactional operations involved in the system's daily use, many errors may have little consequence: the people responsible for daily operations may notice an error, but, unless they can fix it expeditiously (e.g., when interacting with a customer/patient to whom the error applies), may simply ignore the erroneous value(s) in their decision making. It is only when one tries to use the data as the basis for system-wide reporting does the impact of errors become significant: errors in numerical values, for example, propagate to aggregates such as sums or averages.

Data Profiling refers to the ascertaining of data quality through a mixture of automated and manual processes. Extremely poor data quality may act as a show-stopper: integration cannot occur unless errors are reduced to a tolerable level.

One aspect of profiling is to check for constraint violation: the mere existence of constraints does not guarantee that existing data obeys them. Constraints may have been added to already operational systems, but not actually implemented, or implemented incorrectly. Especially with old data in legacy systems, a kind of Murphy's Law may prevail: any constraint that can be violated will be. Errors due to constraint violation are amenable to detection and quantification by automated processes—once all constraints have been specified. One can write fairly simple scripts for this purpose: several third-party tools will even take a list of constraints specified in a simple syntax and generate scripts.

Data that confirm to the constraints but are still erroneous (e.g., an incorrect address) are much harder to identify, requiring manual processes that are often prohibitively expensive. Therefore, rather than attempting to detect and fix every possible error *before* starting the integration effort, it is more feasible to estimate the proportion of erroneous records by manual checking of random samples, and then try to judge their impact on the quality of reports that would be run on the integrated data.

The presence of certain types of errors may indicate flawed processes or operational systems: new errors will continue to arise until these are fixed. A well-known retail pharmacy chain, prior to commencing an integration effort, found that the common drug acetaminophen was entered into their production systems with 20 different spellings (and 20 different unique identifiers): poorly educated retail clerks who were creating inventory would mistype it during data entry: when the drug name did not match, rather than suggesting possible candidates with similar spellings, the inventory software simply allowed them to create a new drug. Thus a feature originally intended to prevent hold-ups in workflow (because new drugs are periodically introduced) became abused because it was incorrectly implemented. Similar lax processes in medical workflows have resulted in the creation of "uncontrolled vocabularies."

Errors can be fixed at two locations: in the original source or in the integrated system. The former is always desirable when possible, because they are fixed once and for all: in cases where physical integration is employed. Difficulties arise with poorly understood legacy systems: here, it may be simpler to bulk-update their outputs (using programs that replace specific incorrect or meaningless values with correct/feasible ones) during transformation, even if such updates must be performed every time. Knowledge Management, discussed shortly, may prevent or mitigate such situations in theory: as we shall see, there may be practical hurdles in implementation that have nothing to do with technology.

2.5.4 Documenting Data Sources and Processes: Metadata

The insights and knowledge that have been laboriously acquired in the previous steps can be easily lost unless they are documented: like skilled IT staff everywhere, integration teams have higher-than-normal turnover.

Detailed documentation mitigates risk: it has the goal of making implicit knowledge explicit.

The term *metadata* is used to describe information that describes data. Such information is classified by Kimball [31] into two kinds: narrative-text descriptions intended to be read by humans (*descriptive* metadata) and more structured information intended to be utilized primarily by software (*technical* or "process-related" metadata), though the latter may also be human-browsable if presented through a well-designed graphical user interface.

Examples of technical metadata are:

1. Structured documentation of each data source, the tables in each source, the columns in each table, inter-table relationships, and the permissible values of columns (enumerations). The structure (the *data dictionary*) is typically in a form of a relational design: sources, tables, columns (each succeeding element related many-to-one to the previous). Enumerations are related many-to-many to columns because the same enumeration may be used for more than one column. Data dictionary information can be extracted from RDBMSs by a wide variety of free and commercial query tools.

2. Constraints and rules, as described earlier. These are ideally specified using the syntax of an interpreted language (e.g., VBScript, JavaScript, Perl, or Ruby) that allows execution of syntactically correct text as though it were code. There are also commercial "business rule engines" [32,33] that facilitate both organized documentation as well as rule execution (by interoperation with other systems): many large-scale Enterprise Resource Planning (ERP) packages, such as SAP, incorporate rule engines.

3. Especially in logical integration (but also in physical integration efforts), metadata are used to record *mappings* between global and local data elements at the level of tables, columns, enumerations, and relationships. The paper by Marenco et al. [25] provides a detailed description of metadata design for a federation.

    In logical integration, metadata can exist at two levels. This is necessary when the schemas of local sources change. To minimize the challenge of manually coordinating every change with a remotely based integration team, the maintainers of a local source may maintain metadata that can be queried by the mediator software and used to update the unified model (which is best stored centrally). Structured documentation (point 1, above), for example, may be stored at each source.

Descriptive metadata are complementary to technical metadata: prose (e.g., descriptions about the purpose of particular tables or columns, or the rationale of a constraint or rule) can capture nuances in a way that structured information cannot. One important descriptive-metadata component, which is borrowed from the world of terminologies, is a *Glossary*. This comprises, at the minimum, a table of *Concepts* related to the problem domain, and a table of *Synonyms* ("*terms*") for these concepts. These tables should be related many-to-many, since the same term or phrase may sometimes refer to more than one concept. This situation is extremely common in biomedicine: the phrase "cold" may refer to rhinitis or to low temperature, for example. The UMLS records such information, but it is by no means complete. Every concept should be accompanied by a textual *definition*: in this context, one UMLS weakness is that many of its source vocabularies lack such definitions. The NIH-supported National Center for Biomedical Ontology is another useful ontology/terminology aggregator: its content can be accessed at http://bioportal.bioontology.org/.

Metadata are involved in all stages of an integration effort, including ongoing operations. For example, during the transformation process, metadata help to maintain a "breadcrumb trail" to record the exact steps involved. This is important because transformation of data from the original source to the final structure often involves numerous steps, which are often developed through a trial-and-error process. Once a sequence of steps has been worked out, it is desirable to document them, in detail so that one or more steps can be safely altered if anything (e.g., source-data formats or business requirements) changes.

Production systems, too, must evolve to meet changing needs, and detailed descriptions of the operational system facilitate change while minimizing the risk of introducing bugs. Kimball et al. [31] describe the various categories of metadata in physical integration efforts—source system descriptions, ETL processes, finished system, query tools—and point out that metadata includes everything except the data.

Knowledge Management (KM) [34] refers to the employment of management processes and technology to capture, organize, and distribute descriptive metadata within an organization, including the insight and experience of skilled personnel. At the most mundane level, KM involves discovery of information from various individuals about how they function, and documenting it as the basis for developing effective processes as well as reducing the dependence on individual people should they leave or become unavailable. While KM has been somewhat blighted by hype and occasional spectacular failures [35,36], its core principles are reasonable, and would apply to data integration as well: an important technological component of KM is ontologies, which are now discussed.

2.5.4.1 *Ontologies*

The term *ontology* [37] is gaining increasing prominence in computer science and biomedicine, and we introduce it here because of its relation to metadata. An "ontology" refers to a collection of metadata with both technical and descriptive components that tries to capture information about a problem domain using a fairly standard conceptual design. (While ontology researchers like to state that ontologies capture "knowledge," we believe that "information" is more accurate and less pretentious.)

Ontologies are used in the context of terminologies, where they deal with descriptions of concepts in the domain, as well as in non-terminology contexts, where they describe "objects." The term "object" is a more general term than "concept": it could refer to anything described by a row in a database table, for example. We will therefore use the word "object" in this section: you can mentally substitute "concept" when we are dealing with terminology issues.

The conceptual design of ontologies includes the following components:

- *Names* and *descriptions/definitions* of Objects, Synonyms of objects, and inter-object Relationships, both hierarchical and non-hierarchical.
- Object categories or *Classes*: Every object is a "member" of at least one Class. Classes themselves may be organized into a quasi-hierarchy (or directed graph), in that general/specific relationships may exist between classes (e.g., the category "Serum Electrolyte Tests" is a specific instance of "Clinical Chemistry Tests," in turn a specific instance of "Laboratory Tests").
- *Object Attributes* (also called *properties*): These vary with the object/concept class. Thus, for concepts belonging to the ancestral class "Lab tests," the properties of an individual laboratory test include the substance that is being measured, the measurement method, the time of measurement, measurement units, and the normal range.
- *Executable components*: Constraints, rules, and other forms of code.
- Any other (domain-specific) information appropriate to the ontology's purpose. For instance, Pardillo and Mazon [38] propose that an ontology intended to support an integration effort should also record system requirements, schema diagrams of existing systems, mappings, and so on.

The employment of ontology-based approaches does not dictate any particular technology. For example, Web Ontology Language (OWL) [39], an XML dialect, has gained popularity for ontology content interchange: however, it is not recommended for native (i.e., internal) information representation, because it does not scale to the millions of concepts that exist in large domains like biomedicine. Further, OWL does not address human-readable components of metadata, where significant volumes of prose must be indexed for rapid search, and non-textual components such as diagrams exist. Here, alternative approaches (e.g., relational designs) are more appropriate.

Ontologies are useful, but in data integration efforts, they are not a panacea or a replacement for sound management practices: their quality is determined by the usefulness of their contents rather than their design. One of the circumstances where KM itself has failed is in organizations where management has breached the social contract with employees through practices such as arbitrary layoffs or bonuses to top management while the rank-and-file is called upon to tighten their belts. In such organizations, there may be little incentive for individual employees to volunteer information that might result in new processes that might make the employees redundant.

2.6 **DATA TRANSFORMATION AND RESTRUCTURING**

Data transformation is necessary for physical integration. Minimal transformation is required even in the highly exceptional situation of identical schemas across all data sources. This may occur if multiple caregiver institutions coincidentally use the same version of the same EHR software, or when resellers happen to deploy identical autonomously running systems at each distribution/retail-sales site. Even here, at least one transformation is usually required: adding a column in most tables that specifies the source where a particular row of data originated.

The extent of transformation depends on the objective of transformation, and how the integrated data will be queried or analyzed.

- The most well-known transformation, intended to greatly improve query performance, is the "star schema," popularized by the work of Kimball. This design is so called because multiple "lookup" or "dimension" tables are linked to a central "detail" or "fact" table like the spokes of a star. Both the fact table and the lookup tables are *denormalized*, that is, they deliberately violate E.F. Codd's principles of table normalization, and may combine information from multiple tables. For example, in a star schema for hospital billing, the bill header table (which records the patient being billed and details such as the insurance provider, etc.) and the line items (which deal with individual services) are merged into a single detail table. Similarly, a lookup table such as medication details (if the service involved medication) may merge multiple tables, such as generic component information, dosage forms, batch and manufacturer details. (If the lookup table consists of a cluster of tables that retains a normalized structure, this variation is called a "snowflake" schema, because the main spokes of the star have smaller branches, like the tips of a snowflake.)

Kimball [40] provides an excellent step-by-step guide to transformation: one point that they emphasize is the recording of detail data at the most atomic level feasible. (For the business aspects of healthcare, this would imply recording individual transactions: at the clinical level, every observation would be recorded.) The rationale behind this dictum is that it is always possible to aggregate data into larger reporting units (e.g., at the patient, or medication, or department levels), but it is not possible to ask for detail if details were never recorded.

- It is important to note that the "star schema" is an optimization that greatly speeds up certain common queries (at the cost of extra space), but by no means all of them. Inmon [41] persuasively emphasizes that it is not appropriate for all situations. He refers to two classes of users, "explorers" and "farmers." Farmers, who execute well-defined queries on specific schedules, are best served by star schemas. However, explorers, who correspond mostly to business analysts and statisticians, have a rough idea of where they want to go, but the exact route is not defined, and their goals may change frequently. Explorers are best served by a normalized schema very similar to the ones used by the operational systems.

- *Homogenization*: Homogenization is a transformation that is performed when individual source systems deal with the same broad objective, but have totally different and incompatible designs. We have mentioned homogenization in the context of UMLS and Entity-Attribute-Value modeling. The integrated structure that results from the merged data has a simpler structure, so that differences that are unimportant to the integration effort's purpose are hidden. Homogenization greatly simplifies the creation of browsing interfaces to the integrated data, but does not necessarily simplify data query: complex Boolean queries focused on attributes may be considerably slower [42] as well as harder to formulate, as well as harder to focus on the quirks of individual sources if this is necessary. Greenfield [43] also points out that homogenization can occasionally be carried too far in business contexts: to use his words, an organization selling lines of dog food as well as auto tires might not be well served by homogenizing if these two businesses use separate logical and physical models and processes.

2.7 INTEGRATION EFFORTS IN BIOMEDICAL RESEARCH

Integration efforts in biomedical research follow the pattern of efforts elsewhere. That is, intra-institutional efforts are primarily physical, while trans-institutional efforts tend to be logical. The efforts are too numerous to list: many have not survived after the initial funding period, and so we will mention approaches that are, in our opinion, likely to have longevity.

Among HIEs, the most mature system, as well as the largest in terms of the number of patients and stakeholders, is currently the Indiana Health Information Exchange (http://www.ihie.com/). This effort initially began on a smaller scale in 1995 within the greater Indianapolis area as the Indianapolis Network for Patient Care and Research, as described by Overhage et al. [44] and was subsequently scaled up to operate throughout the state. In regard to the paramount importance of setting aside differences to work toward a common goal, it is worth noting that political turf battles have sunk at least one HIE effort, the California Regional Health Information Organization, which ceased to operate in 2010 [45].

Data warehouses have been deployed at numerous organizations. One of the first efforts to have a significant clinical focus was by the Intermountain Health Care group [46]. The most well-known data mart design for clinical research data (in part because of the open-source nature of its accompanying toolset) is the Informatics for Integrating Biology and the Bedside (i2b2) schema design that is becoming popular for clinical data warehouses is the i2b2 model, originally designed by Shawn Murphy and colleagues [47–49]. This combines aspects of Entity-Attribute-Value modeling with the star-schema design. Describing its details is beyond the scope of this chapter: the original reference is extremely accessible. Like all star-schema designs, i2b2 represents an optimization—specifically, support for determining patient sample sizes based on arbitrary clinical criteria as part of the clinical research proposal process. In many cases, such analyses may be performed without requiring Institutional Review Board approval, because they can be carried out without directly accessing personal health information (PHI). In the i2b2 design, patients are identified by machine-generated identifiers: the PHI is segregated securely from the clinical data to limit access, while almost anyone is permitted to perform sample-size analyses, which return only counts.

The field of neuroinformatics has several ongoing logical integration efforts. The Biomedical Informatics Research Network (BIRN) has developed open-source mediator software that facilitates connection to a variety of data sources [50]: the success of deployments by groups beyond consortium members is not clear. The Neuroscience Information Framework (NIF) [51] uses a hybrid design that employs the "unobtrusive pull" strategy described earlier. Elements of the QIS technology developed by Marenco et al. [25] are used here.

The National Cancer Institute's Cancer BioInformatics Grid (CaBIG) is an ambitious effort to support distributed computing and data integration across cancer centers in the USA. This has recently run into trouble: the reasons are beyond the scope of this article, but have been summarized by Foley [52].

The NIH Environmental Health Data Integration Network (www.nh.gov/epht/ehdin/) is a web portal designed to assist federal, state, and local agencies in distributing information about environmental hazards and disease trends: such information is intended to advance environmental-disease research, and guide the development of policies and public health measures to prevent such problems.

While the data integrated through health information exchanges can theoretically provide resources for research simply by being sources of aggregate data, such data are generally coarse-grained and not aggregated at the level of individual clinical observations (other than laboratory tests and diagnoses). In general, conclusions that are drawn from the analysis of such data (which were not originally collected for research purposes) are, at best, in the nature of hypothesis generation: confirmation needs to be done through prospective study designs.

2.8 IMPLEMENTATION TIPS

The single most informative article we have read in the physical integration field is Larry Greenfield's freely accessible article, "Data Warehouse Gotchas" [43], which elegantly summarizes the challenges in warehouse implementation. We have touched upon some of the issues, such as the effort required to understand the source systems, cleansing and validating data, and occasionally modifying the source systems, and the pitfalls of homogenization. We will now provide practical pointers relating to implementation.

2.8.1 Query Tools: Caveats

As stated earlier, it is easier to build (or purchase) query tools for a physically integrated store compared to a logically integrated one simply because, with the former, one does not have to address the problem of having to access a variety of vendor data-store engines (or proprietary non-standard designs). With warehouses, front-end tools are provided by a variety of vendors, including warehouse-engine providers, and many of the tools are reasonably easy to use for professionals who understand the data. However, there are several caveats:

- Never underestimate end-user inertia in terms of learning such tools, or even retaining such learning after you have imparted training. The fact is that understanding data requires significant effort, and the majority of "farmers," who have day jobs of a different nature, simply want to run stored queries on a regularly scheduled basis: they would rather have you develop the query for them rather than do it themselves. Thus Greenfield points out that the effort you spend developing reports may actually increase.
- Clinical data pose additional challenge because of EAV-modeling. As has been previously pointed out [53], querying such data can get tedious and error-prone even for trained analysts, and it is desirable to create a framework to ease query development. Consider yourself fortunate, however, if such a framework reduces the user's effort by 80%: trying to do a 95% job may require an unreasonable amount of effort.
- We do not know of any commercial tools that are currently EAV-aware. Further, there are several tools, notably those based on the "universal database" model [54], that we would consider almost unusable in medical context, because their setup would require a prohibitive amount of effort. This has been detailed elsewhere [55].

2.8.2 **The Importance of Iterative Processes**

It is important to emphasize that the integration effort should not follow a "waterfall" or "big bang" model, where the steps of planning, design, implementation, and testing follow sequentially. "Big bang" has been discredited for most types of software development, and integration efforts are no exception. The preferred approach is initial planning at a reasonably broad (but not excessively detailed) level, followed by incremental delivery of individual parts of the solution. The components delivered earliest are those that will get maximum user buy-in (based on prior ascertainment of their pressing needs) and/or address a technically risky aspect of the project. The benefits of such an approach (described as "top-down planning, bottom-up delivery") are:

- Early successes generate user and management enthusiasm, as opposed to their waiting forever before they can access the system. The experience of early implementation and testing generates feedback that results in revisions of both designs and plans. By contrast, excessively detailed planning and design before such testing is premature and likely to lead to wasted effort.

- At the start of the project, there are too many unknowns. An iterative process addresses risks such as technology hurdles, performance bottlenecks, and user issues (acceptance, learning curve) early in the game. If the project has significant risk of failure, one can ascertain this at a relatively modest cost by failing early: if, however, a technically challenging subgoal succeeds, one can guarantee that simpler aspects of the projects will also be addressed successfully.

2.9 **CONCLUSION: FINAL WARNINGS**

Physical-integration technology is quite mature, and today's hardware is more than capable of handling the typical medical-data integration effort. Yet failures still occur regularly (like IT efforts in general), and do so primarily for non-technological reasons. The commonest reasons for failure are:

- Political infighting subverting the stated objective of the integration effort.
- Failure to use an iterative process. Closely related to this is failure to involve users sufficiently in all phases of the integration process: most importantly, accepting their early (and continued) feedback, however humbling it may be, and fixing the perceived flaws.
- Failure to understand the tools and theory of integration (especially ETL, schema designs, database optimizations).
- Failure to determine user requirements and refine these iteratively as the system evolves. Greenfield points out in integration efforts, one starts with data and ends with requirements. That is, as users get a taste of what they can do with integrated data, their expectations rise, and they demand more. At this point, it is possible to snatch defeat from the jaws of victory by failing to anticipate the need for system enhancements and maintenance, and budgeting for inadequate resources to the same.
- "Silver-bullet syndrome"—a belief that the latest technological toy will solve your problem and save you the trouble of having to think the problem through.

While an integration effort may occasionally resemble climbing Mt. Everest in terms of its occasionally disheartening challenges, the possibility of significant benefits from the end-results justifies the investment in resources.

REFERENCES

[1] Overhage J, Evans L, Marchibroda J. Communities' readiness for health information exchange: the national landscape in 2004. J Am Med Inform Assoc 2005;12(2):107–12.

[2] Lindberg DAB, Humphreys BL, McCray AT. The unified medical language system. Meth Inform Med 1993;32:281–91.

[3] Inmon WH. Building the data warehouse. New York, NY: John Wiley; 1996.

[4] Inmon B. Data warehouse mart does not equal data. Inform Manage 1999;120.

[5] Greenfield L. The data warehousing information center; 2002 [updated 2002; cited]. Available from: <http://www.dwinfocenter.org>.

[6] Date CJ. An introduction to database systems. 8th ed. Reading, MA: Addison-Wesley; 2003.

[7] Date CJ. Selected database readings 1985–1989. 7th ed. Reading, MA: Addison-Wesley; 1990.

[8] Cormen TH, Leiserson CE, Rivest RL. Introduction to algorithms. 2nd ed. New York: McGraw-Hill; 2001.

[9] Parent C, Spaccapietra S. Database integration: the key to data interoperability. In: Papazoglou MP, , Spaccapietra S, Tari Z, editors. Advances in object-oriented data modeling. Cambridge, MA: MIT Press; 2000.

[10] Health Level Seven Inc. HL7 standard V2.3.1. Health Level Seven Inc., Ann Arbor, MI 48104; 2000.

[11] Smith B.HL7 Watch. 2012 [updated 2012; cited 6/2/2012]. Available from hl7-watch.blogspot.com.

[12] Epic Systems Corporation. Analytical warehouse: clarity enterprise reporting; 2002 [updated 2002; cited 10/1/2002]. Available from: <http://www.epicsystems.com/software/anware.php>.

[13] Kaye D. Loosely coupled: the missing pieces of web services. RDS Press; 2003.

[14] Kay R. QuickStudy: Representational State Transfer (REST). ComputerWorld; 2007 [updated 2007; cited 11/2/10]. Available from: <http://www.computerworld.com/s/article/297424/RepresentationalStateTransferREST>.

[15] Martin R. Web services: hope or hype? 2004 [updated 2004; cited 4/6/2010]. Available from: <http://www.cs.rutgers.edu/~rmartin/talks/WS-comrise.pdf>.

[16] Francia S. SOAP vs. REST; 2011 [updated 2011; cited 6/20/2012]. Available from: <http://spf13.com/post/soap-vs-rest>.

[17] Wikipedia. Hash table; 2012 [updated 2012; cited 3/2/2012]. Available from: <http://en.wikipedia.org/wiki/hash_table>.

[18] Wikipedia. Bitmap index; 2010 [updated 2010; cited 3/2/2010]. Available from: <http://en.wikipedia.org/wiki/Bitmap_index>.

[19] O'Neil P, Graefe G. Multi-table joins through bitmapped join indices. SIGMOD Record 1995;24(3).

[20] Bontempo CJ, Saracco CM. Accelarated indexing techniques. Database Program Design 1996;9(July):36–43.

[21] Greenfield L. Data warehousing: political issues; 2012 [updated 2012; cited 5/18/2012]. Available from: <http://www.dwinfocenter.org/politics.html>.

[22] Demarest M. The politics of data warehousing; 1997 [updated 1997; cited 5/18/2012]. Available from: <http://www.noumenal.com/marc/dwpoly.html>.

[23] Kimball R, Caserta J. The Data warehouse ETL toolkit. New York: Wiley Computer Publishing; 2008.

[24] Marenco L, Wang R, Nadkarni P. Automated database mediation using ontological metadata mappings. J Am Med Inform Assoc 2009;16(5):723–37.

[25] Marenco L, Wang T, Shepherd G, Miller P, Nadkarni P. QIS: a framework for bio-medical database federation. J Am Med Inform Assoc 2004;11(6):523–34.

[26] Friedl JEF. Mastering regular expressions. Sebastopol, CA: O'Reilly & Associates, Inc.; 1997.

[27] Kim W, Seo J. Classifying schematic and data heterogeneity in multidatabase systems. IEEE Comput 1991;24(12):12–18.

[28] International Health Terminology Standards Development Organization. SNOMED Clinical Terms (SNOMED CT); 2012 [updated 2012; cited 2/1/02]. Available from: <www.snomed.org>.

[29] Nadkarni PM, Brandt C, Frawley S, Sayward F, Einbinder R, Zelterman D, et al. Managing attribute-value clinical trials data using the ACT/DB client-server database system. J Am Med Inform Assoc 1998;5(2):139–51.

[30] Dinu V, Nadkarni P. Guidelines for the effective use of entity-attribute-value modeling for biomedical databases. Int J Med Inform 2007;76(11–12):769–79.

[31] Kimball R, Reeves L, Ross M, Thornthwaite W. The data warehouse lifecycle toolkit: expert methods for designing, developing, and deploying data warehouses. 2nd ed. New York, NY: John Wiley; 2008.

[32] Agosta L. Business rules meet the business user. Intell Enter Mag; 2005 [updated 2005; cited 11/2/2010]. Available from: <http://intelligent-enterprise.information-week.com/showArticle.jhtml;jsessionid=HYXHSZHIOSJOPQE1GHRSKHWATMY32JVN?articleID=167100318>.

[33] Ross R. Principles of the business rule approach. Boston: Pearson Education Inc; 2003.

[34] Maier R. Knowledge management systems: information and communication technologies for knowledge management. Springer-Verlag; 2002.

[35] Chua A, Lam W. Why KM projects fail: a multi-case analysis. J Knowl Manage 2005;9(3):6–17.

[36] Braganza A, Mollenkramer GJ. Anatomy of a failed knowledge management initiative: lessons from PharmaCorp's experiences. Knowl Process Manage 2002;9(1):23–33.

[37] Gruber T. Toward principles for the design of ontologies used for knowledge sharing. Int J Hum-Comput Stud 1995;43(5–6):907–28.

[38] Pardillo J, Mazon J. Using ontologies for the design of data warehouses. Int J Database Manage Syst 2011;3(2):73–87.

[39] World Wide Web Consortium. OWL 2 web ontology language document overview; 2009 [updated 2009; cited]. Available from: <http://www.w3.org/TR/owl2-overview/>.

[40] Kimball R. The data warehousing toolkit. New York, NY: John Wiley; 1997.

[41] Inmon W, Rudin K, Buss C, Sousa R. Data warehouse performance. New York: John Wiley & Sons; 1998.

[42] Chen RS, Nadkarni PM, Marenco L, Levin FW, Erdos J, Miller PL. Exploring performance issues for a clinical database organized using an entity-attribute-value representation. J Am Med Inform Assoc 2000;7(5):475–87.

[43] Greenfield L. Data warehouse gotchas; 2012 [updated 2012; cited 5/18/2012]. Available from: <http://www.dwinfocenter.org/gotchas.html>.

[44] Overhage JM, Tierney WM, McDonald CJ. Design and implementation of the Indianapolis network for patient care and research. Bull Med Libr Assoc 1995;83(1):48–56.

[45] Rauber C. CalRHIO closes, but board to help state on IT. San Francisco Business Times; 1/10/2010.

[46] Lau LM, Lam SH, Barlow S, Lyon C, Sanders D, editors. Enhancing an enterprise data warehouse with a data dictionary. In: Proceedings of the AMIA fall symposium; 2001.

[47] Murphy SN, Barnett GO, Chueh HC. Visual query tool for finding patient cohorts from a clinical data warehouse of the partners HealthCare system. Proc AMIA Symp. 2000:1174.

[48] Murphy SN, Chueh HC. A security architecture for query tools used to access large biomedical databases. Proc AMIA Symp 2002:552–6.

[49] Murphy SN, Gainer V, Chueh HC. A visual interface designed for novice users to find research patient cohorts in a large biomedical database. AMIA Annu Symp Proc 2003:489–93.

[50] Bioinformatics Research Network. BIRN mediator; 2012 [updated 2012; cited 6/1/2012]. Available from: <https://wiki.birncommunity.org/display/BIRNDOC/Mediator>.

[51] University of California San Diego. Neuroinformatics information framework; 2012 [updated 2012; cited 6/1/2012]. Available from: <www.neuinfo.org>.

[52] Foley J. Report blasts problem-plagued cancer research grid. InformationWeek; 04/08/2011.

[53] Nadkarni P, Brandt C. Data extraction and ad hoc query of an entity-attribute-value database. J Am Med Inform Assoc 1998;5(6):511–27.

[54] Maier D, Ullman J. Maximal objects and the semantics of universal relation databases. ACM Trans Database Syst 1983;8(1):1–14.

[55] Nadkarni PM. Chapter 15: Data retrieval for heterogeneous data models. In: Metadata-driven software systems in biomedicine. London UK: Springer; 2011.

Knowledge Representation

Mark A. Musen

Stanford Center for Biomedical Informatics Research, Stanford University, Stanford, CA, USA

3.1 KNOWLEDGE AND KNOWLEDGE REPRESENTATION

In biomedical informatics, our primary objective is the study of data, information, and knowledge—their structure, their communication, and their use. This goal is more than philosophical; our aim often is to capture knowledge in electronic *knowledge bases* that can enable computers to do intelligent things, such as providing decision support, integrating heterogeneous datasets, performing natural language processing, or aiding information retrieval. Attempting to understand the very essence of knowledge poses thorny problems that can keep us up all night. Indeed, philosophers have argued about the nature of knowledge for millennia. Scholars who study epistemology worry about the basis of how we know what we know, about belief, and about truth. Fortunately, in biomedical informatics, our approach to thinking about knowledge can be rather pragmatic.

Allen Newell, in making the case to the artificial intelligence (AI) community in 1980, suggested that we can understand knowledge in terms of the behavior of agents—either human or computational [1]. An agent has goals, and can select actions from a repertoire of things that it can do to bring the agent closer to its goals. In Newell's view, an agent has knowledge if it is perceived to select actions in a rational manner, such that it appears to perform actions that inexorably bring it closer to its goals. Newell made a careful distinction between *knowledge*—the "stuff" that causes an agent to act rationally—and *knowledge representation*—the use of symbols to write down the "stuff" that an agent knows. As a computer scientist originally trained in psychology, Newell felt comfortable ducking centuries of epistemological nuance and suggested that it was most helpful to define knowledge simply as the capacity "to do the right thing."

Newell argued that computational scientists should construe knowledge in terms of the goals that an intelligent agent might have, the actions of which the agent was capable, and the means by which the agent might select actions in order to achieve its goals. This understanding of knowledge—at what Newell referred to as the *knowledge level*—enables developers to characterize knowledge independent from how that knowledge might be encoded in any computer system [1]. At the knowledge level, knowledge is the foundation for intelligent behavior, the set of ingredients that allow an agent "to do the right thing." Although the means by which a system developer actually might achieve this kind of behavioral, knowledge-level understanding of an agent has itself led to decades of further discussions [2], Newell's distinction between *knowledge* (a capacity for intelligent behavior) and *knowledge representation* (a set of symbols for describing how that capacity might be achieved) has been instrumental in guiding the biomedical informatics community in the development of intelligent computer systems. More important, Newell's suggestion that knowledge itself can have structure independent of any particular encoding of that knowledge has reinforced the objectives of workers in biomedical informatics to attempt to model knowledge as a first-class entity. Indeed, research in biomedical informatics takes on a different emphasis from that in computer science because biomedical informatics typically stresses the modeling of content knowledge, in addition to the elucidation of new computational methods [3].

Computation, of course, is an essential element of work in biomedical informatics, and knowledge ultimately has to be rendered in some computational form to play a useful role within information systems. At what

Newell referred to as the *symbol level* [1], where we actually encode knowledge in some programmatic form, there are a variety of choices that developers can make. In this chapter, we discuss several methods for representing knowledge as symbols within computer systems, and some of the design considerations that may cause developers to favor one approach over another.

3.2 PROCEDURAL VS. DECLARATIVE REPRESENTATIONS

One of the first and, arguably, one of the most successful computer-based decision support systems was developed by Howard Bleich who was then at the Beth Israel Hospital in Boston in the 1960s [4]. Bleich's program was designed to diagnose abnormalities in clinical acid-base balance, and made recommendations to physicians regarding clinical disorders that could cause the blood to become too acidic or too alkaline. At the knowledge level [1], Bleich's program had a goal (diagnose and treat acid-base disorders), it had a set of actions that it could perform (ask questions about the patient's blood chemistry), and it had a mechanism to select among those actions (use hardcoded branching logic and the results of plugging certain values into pre-specified formulas to determine what to do next). Because everything that Bleich's program "knew" was written into the program code, we would say that Bleich's program used a *procedural* knowledge representation; the knowledge was represented as an algorithm to be followed. The computer was programmed to ask about the levels of sodium, potassium, and other electrolytes in the blood, to ask for the blood pH and for the patient's weight, and to follow a fixed pathway of calculations that ultimately would lead to a diagnosis. The program determined whether the patient's abnormalities were primarily the result of problems with kidney function or of problems with respiration, and offered possible treatments for the physician to consider depending on the underlying cause.

Procedural representations such as the one embodied by Bleich's program are extremely efficient. They ask just the right questions and get to the final answer as quickly as possible [5].

A decade later, across the river from Beth Israel Hospital at MIT, Ramesh Patil built a different program, known as ABEL, that also reasoned about **A**cid, **B**ase, and **EL**ectrolyte disorders [6]. Like Bleich's program, ABEL could determine whether a patient's acid-base disturbance was the result of kidney problems or respiratory problems. ABEL did so by reasoning about a causal network of relationships that was encoded as a data structure (Figure 3.1). ABEL did not adhere to a fixed algorithm, but instead followed the causal relationships in the network to reason about the patient's

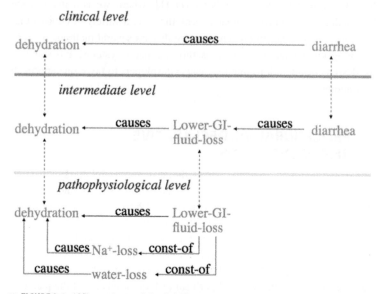

■ **FIGURE 3.1**   ABEL causal network. Patil's ABEL system used a representation of graph of causal relationships to drive its reasoning. The system could reason simultaneously at three different levels of abstraction (the level of clinical findings, the level of pathophysiological phenomena, and an intermediate level) to infer a patient's clinical state with regard to abnormalities in acid-base and electrolyte balance. Adapted from Patil [6].

problems. The program could reason about the patient situation at different levels of abstraction depending on what data were available and the nature of result that the user was expecting. Because the program's inference was driven by the causal network, it was possible for the user to pose "what if?" questions to the program and to ask the program for a justification of its reasoning that could be couched in terms of the underlying causal relationships. ABEL was much more versatile than Bleich's program was, but ABEL ran slowly and never was put into routine clinical use.

Whereas the Bleich program represented knowledge procedurally, ABEL used a *declarative* representation that encoded knowledge as a data structure that the program examined at run time. (As we shall see in Section 3.3.2, ABEL's knowledge of causal relationships is stored in a kind of declarative knowledge representation that we call a *semantic network*.) Procedural representations are optimized for one particular task and are very efficient at solving that task algorithmically. Declarative representations, on the other hand, have the potential to address a variety of tasks when a reasoning program is able to perform appropriate computations [5]. Thus, ABEL's causal network can be used to solve different tasks relating to acid-base disorders, depending on what the problem solver chooses to do with the information that it reads off the representation. A problem solver can use the network to diagnose a patient's current situation, to predict what might happen if some aspect of the current state were to change, or to suggest ways in which a patient could have developed current abnormalities. At the same time, if we wish to represent additional knowledge about acid, base, and electrolyte abnormalities, we can do so in ABEL by editing the causal network; to augment the knowledge in Bleich's acid-base program, on the other hand, we would have to modify the computer code.

3.3 REPRESENTING KNOWLEDGE DECLARATIVELY

In this chapter, we will focus on declarative knowledge representations. We do so because we are most interested in the encoding of knowledge in a manner that allows the knowledge representation to be inspectable and editable. Our approach is driven by Brian Smith's *knowledge representation hypothesis*: that any mechanical embodiment of an intelligent process comprises structural ingredients that: (a) provide to external observers an account of the knowledge that the process exhibits and (b) play a causal and essential role in engendering the behavior that manifests that knowledge [7]. Declarative representations thus serve the dual function of communicating to people what it is that a computer system knows and of enabling the system to use what it knows to behave in an appropriate manner.

3.3.1 Logics

For thousands of years, when people have wanted to write down what they know about the world, they have turned to logic. A *logic* is a system for expressing statements about the world as formal sentences, coupled with a means for reasoning about those sentences. Since Aristotle first proposed the system of logic that has formed the basis for much of Western philosophy, it has seemed natural to represent propositions about the world in terms of variables, constants, predicates, and quantifiers.

A logic provides a grammar for the construction of sentences about the world. The grammar assures that such sentences are *well-formed formulas* that abide by a particular syntax. Thus, if we want to indicate that "every paper published in the Journal of the American Medical Informatics Association (JAMIA) is indexed in PubMed," we can use a standardized knowledge representation system known as Common Logic to write down the following well formed formula:

```
(forall (?x)
        (implies (and (Paper ?x) (PublishedIn JAMIA ?x))
            (IndexedInPubMed ?x)))
```

The Common Logic syntax used here assumes a format similar to statements in the Lisp programming language, where clauses are nested using parentheses and predicates precede the variables to which they pertain. In Common Logic, variables are denoted by strings that begin with a question mark.

Suppose one were to assert the following proposition:

```
(exists (?y)
        (Paper ?y)
        (PublishedIn JAMIA ?y)
        (AuthorOfPaper ?y Sarkar))
```

Logical inference would allow the conclusion that Sarkar is the author of a paper indexed in PubMed.

Thus, given a standard syntax for a logic, a reasoning system can manipulate the symbols expressed in that syntax to perform inference.

There are many reasons that logic is appealing as a means for representing knowledge. The syntax is precise, and it offers a clear means for saying just about anything that someone would want to say about anything. There are well-known mechanisms for logical inference that have been studied for centuries. Not only is logic the *lingua franca* that philosophers use routinely for discussing knowledge, but also the International Standards Organization recently identified Common Logic as a standard means to represent logical sentences in computers [8].

In the 1950s, when work on Artificial Intelligence was first taking root, it was naturally assumed that logic would become the definitive means to represent knowledge for purposes of computation. Computer scientists got to work designing automated theorem-provers that would operate on knowledge bases represented as scores of logical sentences. The goal would be to represent goal propositions in logic, and to determine whether a theorem-prover could conclude that those propositions might be true by performing deduction on the knowledge base using rules of inference.

Although many computer systems use logic as the basis for knowledge representation, and a subset of first-order logic—known as *description logic* (Section 3.3.5)—has become particularly important for use on the World Wide Web, systems builders rarely use unadulterated logic by itself as the basis for constructing knowledge bases. Despite the clean syntax and semantics of logic, knowledge bases built up from logical sentences often are not practical. Theorem proving, in the worst case, is not computationally tractable. More important, knowledge bases that comprise a list of myriad logical sentences are very difficult to debug and to maintain. Tracing down errors and fixing problems is enormously hard when the knowledge base consists of a list of unstructured propositions. The relationship between one proposition and another may not be obvious simply by inspection. More important, intelligent systems often require knowledge to perform *tasks* (e.g., diagnosis or therapy planning), not simply to deduce whether a given proposition is true [9]. How a particular logical sentence in a knowledge base might relate to a given task may not be at all apparent when the knowledge base comprises a long enumeration of axioms in a uniform syntax.

That said, logic-based representations are important in biomedical informatics. The programming language Prolog provides the most convenient mechanism for building knowledge bases using logic. The result of the largest, most comprehensive, known knowledge-engineering initiative to date—the CYC knowledge base—contains more than 2 million propositions about more than 239,000 entities, all entered in logic known as CycL [10]. The developers of CYC have attempted to represent knowledge about all areas of human endeavor, and claim significant success in biomedicine, where CYC has been used as the basis of commercial systems developed for the pharmaceutical industry and in support of healthcare information technology.

3.3.2 **Semantic Networks**

Like the history of programming languages, the history of knowledge-representation systems has been dominated by an effort to find ways in which the content can be made more understandable to humans, and thus easier to debug. The goal has been to develop abstractions to reduce complexity, to encapsulate details to reduce "clutter," and to make knowledge representations more modular, to ease the focus of attention. Although the goals of encapsulation and modularity were hard to achieve in standard logic-based approaches to knowledge representation, computer scientists understood by the 1960s that knowledge representation would be easier for humans to understand if the paradigm could move from lists of logical sentences to graphs. Recognizing that the cognitive ability of system developers to comprehend the contents of a knowledge base is at least as important as the soundness of the underlying semantics, researchers turned their attention to graphs as a more humanly tractable form of knowledge representation [11].

Using the very general term *semantic network*, workers in AI explored the use of graphs to represent propositions about the world that a computer might be able to interpret. As we have already seen, the core of the ABEL system was a graph (Figure 3.1). The idea of a graph structure to represent knowledge was not new, however. In the early 20th century, philosopher Charles S. Pierce had suggested that logic could be represented in a diagrammatic fashion; thus, philosophers were debating the relative merits of graph-based logics long before computer scientists became interested in the problem [12]. By the 1960s, it had become clear that graph-based representations would be extremely useful for computational purposes when there was a need to emphasize what the entities in an application are and how those entities might be related to one another. Semantic networks that linked entities to one another and to information about those entities became increasingly popular (Figure 3.2).

Although the term *first-order* logic suggests a singular approach to knowledge representation, the term *semantic network* does not conjure up the notion of anything with such a clear, definitive semantics. There are many different kinds of semantic networks, each of which may make different assumptions about what the nodes and links in the graph might mean. In Figure 3.2, for example, an entity named Jim (an individual) has a Disease (an abstraction) with the diagnosis Mumps (another abstraction), which has a duration of 5 days (an integer value). The graph makes it clear to humans that we should be focusing on Jim, and that his diagnosis has elements such as duration. A computer can query the graph and answer questions such as "What is the duration of Jim's disease?" or "What is Jim's age?"

Although we call this data structure a "semantic network," it is not always clear what the semantics *are*. What exactly does it mean to "have" a disease? When we say that a disease has a "duration," when precisely does the clock start ticking? Is the relationship between Jim and "Person" really the same relationship as that between "Person" and "Mammal?" As we will

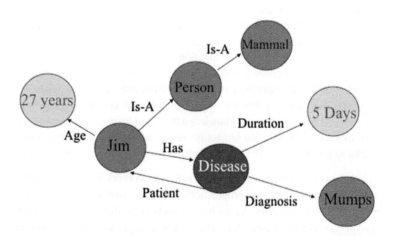

■ **FIGURE 3.2** A simple semantic network. In this example, we presume that Jim, a 27-year-old *person*, has a *disease* that carries the diagnosis *mumps*. Although humans may find the graph to be intuitive, computers may have a hard time processing the ad hoc relationships in the network.

discuss later in this chapter, the meaning of any element of a knowledge representation always is something that developers impose on the symbols that constitute the representation—not something intrinsic to the data structure itself. The intuitive graphs that underlie semantic networks, however, often offer the allure of a readily understandable set of symbols that, only with further reflection, can be seen to lack the clear semantics that observers may initially ascribe to them. Thus, relations such as "having a disease" or "having a duration" can take on clear semantics when the creator of the knowledge base and the user of the knowledge base share the same beliefs about the corresponding meanings. Unfortunately, it is easy to look at a semantic network and to draw false conclusions about the underlying semantics simply because the nodes and links have labels that appear to be so intuitive.

The lack of rigid semantics caused open-ended semantic-network formalisms to drift out of favor toward the end of the 1970s, and other knowledge-representation approaches soon replaced them in more contemporary architectures for intelligent computer systems. In the past decade, however, semantic networks have made a remarkable comeback, in the form of *linked data* on the Semantic Web [13].

Although the World Wide Web is generally viewed as an enormous collection of distributed hypermedia documents that are intended for access by people, almost from the beginning, the developers of the Web recognized the value of making information available in a globally distributed fashion for processing by *machines*. The result has been the emergence of the Semantic Web, work that makes available on the Internet both data and knowledge designed to be accessed, interpreted, and applied by computers [14].

A major component of the Semantic Web entails making data available in a uniform, machine processable form. The Resource Description Framework (RDF) is a language recommended by the World Wide Web Consortium for making data available on the Internet. RDF encodes data using sets of *triples*, where a triple can be viewed as a subject-predicate-object sentence, much like the entity-attribute-value triples used to model databases (as described in Chapter 2). Thus, we could use RDF to encode triples such as:

Jim *has-age* 27.
Jim *is-a* Person.
Person *is-a* Mammal.
Jim *has-a* Disease.

Although this list of triples looks rather linear at first blush, a computer can process the triples to enable their interpretation as a graph, much like the graph in Figure 3.2. In fact, the rigid triple structure makes it easy to construct the graph from these subject-predicate-object statements.

Suppose someone else in cyberspace were to have a list of triples, including statements such as:

Jim *has-sex* Male.
Jim *usually-votes* Republican.
Mammal *is-a* Vertebrate.

We could link the two sets of triples, rounding out our description of Jim. Furthermore, if we had knowledge that the *is-a* relation is transitive, the mash-up of the two sets of triples would allow us to conclude that Jim *is-a* Vertebrate, something that no one would have been able to conclude previously from the two sets of triples taken individually. The biomedical informatics community is currently in the midst of a major effort to publish data on the Web as triples, allowing datasets to be linked to one another, enabling the generation of new biomedical knowledge [15].

In the real world, when people use RDF, they are careful to note where the terms used in the triples might be defined, in order to provide clarity about their semantics. One group of developers, for example, may make different assumptions about the subtle meanings of "has" and "disease" than others do. Real users of RDF also use Uniform Resource Indicators that point to defined locations on the Web to identify the specific entities to which the terms refer. Otherwise, there would be no way of knowing that my "Jim" is also your "Jim."

The whole idea behind linked data is not to create a knowledge representation by top-down design, but rather to tag datasets with meaningful labels that will enable the explorations of serendipitous associations between the data collected for one purpose and those data collected for another. Thus, unlike the knowledge engineers of the 1970s who laboriously crafted semantic networks to encode explicit, fixed relationships among the entities in an application area about which a computer could reason (as was the case with ABEL; Figure 3.1), the communities of scientists who publish their data as RDF triples are hoping that opportunistic linkages among different datasets will lead computers to discover novel correspondences and to integrate the data in new ways. For example, the Bio2RDF Linked Data Network has described a mash-up between the HIV-1 Human Protein Interaction Database and databases of gene-expression results to discover a network of protein interactions that arises during the first hours of an HIV infection of human macrophages [16].

Graph-based representations for knowledge are an important component of Bayesian belief networks—graphs in which nodes, representing possible states of the world, are connected with links, representing probabilistic relationships among those states of the world [17]. The links in a belief network merely denote that there is some probabilistic relationship between the two nodes that they join together; there is no other semantics implied by the edges of the graph (for more details about Bayesian methods, see Chapter 8).

3.3.3 **Frames**

Although semantic-network representations demonstrate that graphs can offer more intuitive descriptions of knowledge than are possible using lists of logical sentences, the frequent lack of a uniform structure and precise semantics have always remained bothersome. In the mid-1970s, Marvin Minsky at MIT offered a more principled approach to modeling knowledge that is both cognitively accessible and yet clear in its semantics. At the root of Minky's approach was something that he called a *frame*, a data structure that served as a template for describing a recurring pattern in the world [18]. Frames describe some abstraction, with *slots* that enumerate the expected properties of that abstraction. Instances of the abstraction (*individuals*) are defined by the particular values that become assigned to the slots. In more modern parlance, we would refer to a frame as an *object*, as Minky's theory of frames has become the foundation of object-oriented analysis and programming in languages such as C++, Java, Python, and Ruby (for a primer on programming in Ruby, see Appendix 2). Thus, while Minksy's idea was a significant advance at the time, the obvious utility of the approach and the degree to which it was subsequently adopted now make it seem quite familiar to current-day workers in informatics.

In his classic paper [18], Minsky called out the notion of a child's birthday party as a familiar kind of abstraction that could be represented as a frame. He suggested that birthday parties have standard properties, such as a child who is being honored, some sort of cake, a collection of games that the children play, special decorations, and so on. What distinguishes one instance of a birthday party from another is a function of the particular child whose birthday it is, the particular cake that is eaten, and particular games that are played, and so on. More important, a birthday party is a kind of party in general; and birthday parties for toddlers entail different types of attributes than do birthday parties for teenagers. Minsky sought to represent knowledge by not using lists of logical sentences or graphs with arbitrary structure, but rather with hierarchies of *templates* (Figure 3.3). He suggested that these templates (frames) might be used to represent classes of entities in the world, and that individuals could be defined by assigning values to the

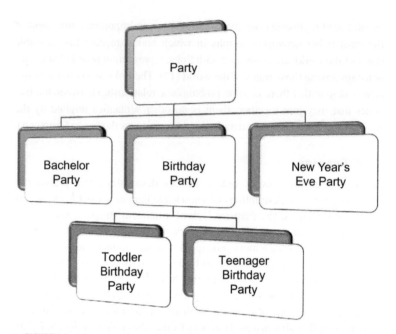

■ FIGURE 3.3 A hierarchy of frames. Minsky [18] proposed to define knowledge in terms of a hierarchy of templates, where each template would enumerate properties characteristic of the class of entity that it denotes. In the Figure, a *party* has properties that are inherited by subclasses such as *birthday party*. A *toddler birthday party* inherits properties of both *birthday party* and *party*. An instance of a *toddler birthday party* would be defined by assigning values to each of the properties of the corresponding frame.

slots of each frame—and that some of those values might actually be other frames or instances of those frames.

Unlike first-order logic, which allows a developer to say just about anything, the kinds of things that can be represented using frame systems are much more limited. Frames allow knowledge-base builders to enumerate abstractions (e.g., birthday parties; *classes*) in the world being modeled, and further abstractions (e.g., parties in general; *superclasses*) and specializations (e.g., toddler birthday parties; *subclasses*). The frames specify a hierarchy of classes and relationships among them. The *is-a* relationship (as in, a "birthday party" *is-a* kind of "party") receives special status, since the primary links among frames in the hierarchy are *is-a* relationships. If a subclass (e.g., toddler birthday party) is-a kind of a superclass (e.g., birthday party), then the slots of the class are inherited by the subclass (e.g., if a birthday party has a *cake* property, then a toddler birthday party inherits the *cake* property as well).

There are many different kinds of systems for encoding frame-based knowledge bases. They differ from one another mainly on the particular assumptions that they make about inheritance of properties among the frames. Nearly all frame systems assume that a subclass will inherit the slots (properties) of its superclasses (thus, all specializations of "birthday party" also will have a *cake* property). Many frame systems allow a value to be assigned to a slot so that, by default, that value also will apply to the slot when inherited by the frame's subclasses (thus, if the "birthday party" class has "crêpe paper streamers" for the value of its *décor* slot, then the subclass "toddler birthday party," by default, will inherit the value "crêpe paper streamers" for its *décor* slot as well). Some frame systems allow the computer to override inheritance in different ways. Some frame systems allow for classes to have more than one parent class, so that a "birthday party" can be both a kind of "party" and a kind of "family gathering." If a given class can have more than one parent class, then the frame system needs a mechanism to resolve conflicts when, for example, the default *décor* of a "party" is different from the default *décor* of a "family gathering," and the frame "birthday party" needs to inherit a single, consistent value from its parent classes. The manner by which such conflicts are handled depends on the particular frame system. Unlike logic, where the mechanisms for inference are well understood and are standardized, the manner in which frame systems support inferences, when developers get into the fine details, is much more idiosyncratic.

Despite the nuances of the semantics of particular frame systems, it is much easier to represent descriptions about the world as a hierarchy of frames than as a list of propositions in first-order logic. Frame hierarchies enable a clear depiction of abstraction relationships, and the individual frames offer a natural mechanism to encapsulate information about particular types of entities. The kind of inference supported by a frame system by itself is extremely limited, however. A frame system may be able to tell you that a "toddler birthday party" is a kind of "party," and it may be able to indicate the kind of cake that should be served by default, but such a representation in isolation cannot really help to plan a toddler birthday party or to suggest how to clean up from one. Whereas frames are good for supporting inheritance of properties and values, any reasoning beyond inheritance has to be supported by system elements external to the frames. Thus, it is quite common to mix frame systems either with procedural program code or with rule-based systems (described in the next section). CLIPS [19], a knowledge-representation system which was created by NASA to enable the engineering of intelligent computer systems for the International Space Station, is a good example of popular framework that supports the integration of both frames and rules.

In biomedicine, several classic knowledge-based systems turned to frames as the basis of knowledge representation. In Internist-1 [20] and in its successor program, QMR [21], descriptions of diseases were encoded as frames.

As already noted, modern object-oriented programming or scripting languages such as Java, have features that are inspired by frame systems. Such languages allow software engineers to create hierarchies of objects with inheritable properties. In object-oriented programming, developers typically create objects to facilitate specific program behaviors, rather than to encode a faithful representation of entities in the world about which their system might want to reason. Thus, many objects in conventional Java programs typically are designed to encapsulate methods that are components of some overall algorithm, not to represent knowledge in a declarative manner. Nevertheless, object-oriented languages such as Java provide a very natural mechanism to represent frame-like information. It is fairly common for developers to use object-oriented programming languages as if they were frame systems. Knowledge-representation systems such as Jess [22], in fact, assume that developers will rely on native Java objects as the mechanism for encoding frames. Like CLIPS, Jess assumes that knowledge that is not convenient to write down in terms of frames will be specified in terms of rules.

3.3.4 **Rules**

When people describe their knowledge, they invariably speak in rules. "Buy low, sell high." "Don't mix stripes with plaids." "$c^2 = a^2 + b^2$." From the beginning of work on knowledge-based technology, rules seemed to be a very natural mechanism for writing down knowledge and for reasoning about it.

The first well-described program to make use of rules to represent knowledge about clinical medicine, and perhaps the best example to date, is the MYCIN system [23]. Developed at Stanford University in the 1970s, MYCIN was a computer system that took as input information about a patient with presumed blood infection or meningitis, and that generated as output a list of microorganisms that might be causing the infection, as well as a plan for treating the patient with antibiotics. Although MYCIN was never used in a clinical setting, the developers imagined a scenario in which a clinician might enter into the computer a patient's age, risk factors for infection, laboratory-test results, and any data regarding microbiological smears or cultures that may have been taken. The computer program might ask for additional information, and then offer its conclusions and recommendations for treatment. At the heart of the system was an electronic knowledge base of several hundred rules, each of which could be translated into English in a form that appears in Figure 3.4.

RULE 579

If: 1) The infection that requires therapy is meningitis, and

2) The patient's chest x-ray is abnormal, and

3) Active-Tb is one of the diseases that the

patient's chest x-ray suggests

Then:

There is strongly suggestive evidence (.8) that

Mycobacterium-Tb is one of the organisms

(other than those seen on cultures or smears)

that might be causing the infection

■ **FIGURE 3.4**   A MYCIN rule. This rule from the MYCIN program has been translated into English. To establish whether the conclusion that appears on the right-hand side of the rule is true, the program evaluates the clauses in the left-hand side of the rule one by one. If MYCIN does not know the truth value of one of the clauses in the premise, it will see whether there are any rules in the knowledge base that can be invoked to make the necessary determination.

All of MYCIN's knowledge was encoded as rules with a *premise* consisting of a pattern of data that might be known to the system and a *conclusion* indicating what might be deduced from the pattern, if the pattern were known to be true. MYCIN had a rule interpreter—an *inference engine*— that would reason using the rules to reach conclusions about the patient's infection and, ultimately, its treatment. When the inference engine examined a rule (such as the rule in Figure 3.4), if all the clauses in the premise of a rule were known to be true, then the conclusion of the rule—in the case of the rule in Figure 3.4, that Mycobacterium-Tb might be causing the infection—would be added to a database of propositions that are known to be true (or false). More often than not, when evaluating the clauses in the premise of a rule, MYCIN would come upon a clause whose truth value is unknown. For example, when evaluating the rule in Figure 3.4, MYCIN might not know whether "the patient's chest x-ray is abnormal." To determine whether the infection might be Mycobacterium-Tb, however, the system needs to know the status of the chest x-ray. Thus, the inference engine would determine whether there are any other rules in the knowledge base that would enable it to conclude whether "the patient's chest x-ray is abnormal." If there are such rules, then those rules will be considered; they in turn might cause the inference engine to examine yet other rules in the knowledge base. Ultimately, if there is no rule that will allow the system to know whether "the patient's chest x-ray is abnormal," then MYCIN simply will ask the user for the information. If the chest x-ray is indeed abnormal, MYCIN will then consider the next clause of the premise of the rule shown in Figure 3.4, and it will determine whether "active-Tb is one of the diseases that the patient's chest x-ray suggests." Note that, if the inference engine fails to conclude that "the patient's chest x-ray is abnormal," there is no need to determine whether the chest x-ray suggests active Tb, as the rule will fail right then and there.

The pattern of rule execution in MYCIN is called *backward chaining*. The inference engine starts with a goal (e.g., "determine the antibiotics that should be prescribed for this patient") and then identifies rules that might allow it to conclude that goal. The inference engine next invokes those rules one by one. If a rule can reach a conclusion, then that conclusion is added to a database that stores all the results that the system has concluded so far. If, however, the rule requires additional information before it can reach its conclusion, then the inference engine examines any rules that can bear on that additional information, and so on. The process is recursive, and the system reasons *backward* from the goal statement to invoke whatever rules are required to enable MYCIN eventually to conclude a value for the goal.

Most contemporary rule-based systems do not use backward chaining from a goal. Instead, they use a reasoning method called *forward chaining*, where the actions of the inference engine are driven by the available data. Thus, as information becomes available to the program (e.g., "the patient's chest x-ray is abnormal"), the inference engine will ask, "Are there any rules that can make an inference on the basis of this new datum?" The program then might consider the rule in Figure 3.4 and, if other data are known to the system, it might be able to conclude that, "Mycobacterium-Tb is one of the organisms that might be causing the infection." On making this conclusion, the program would ask, "Are there any rules that can make an inference by knowing that 'Mycobacterium-Tb is one of the organisms that might be causing the infection'?" If so, then those rules might be invoked. The process is recursive, and the system reasons in a forward direction—from the conclusions of rules that fire when the new data become available, and from the conclusions of rules that then fire when the conclusions of the earlier rules become available, and so on.

There are several widely used development environments that enable system builders to encode rules that are designed to be used in a forward-chaining manner. CLIPS and Jess adopt a syntax similar to the one used in forward-chaining systems pioneered at Carnegie-Mellon University in the 1970s. Drools is a popular forward-chaining platform that has been developed by the JBOSS community for use in Web-based applications [24].

At first glance, a representation of knowledge based on if-then rules looks a lot like a logic. Rules represent implications between premises and conclusions, and thus capture the essence of logical inference. There are significant differences between rule-based representations and logic, however. Rule languages do not permit the arbitrary use of variables that we associate with logic. The rule in Figure 3.4, for example, has no unbound variables. More important, rules are inherently procedural [25]. Developers choose the order of the clauses in the premises of rules to control the execution of the inference engine. For example, when processing the rule in Figure 3.4, a backward-chaining inference engine first determines whether the chest x-ray is abnormal before seeking to determine whether the x-ray is suggestive of tuberculosis; the rule author has programmed the rule to be evaluated in this manner because there is no need to determine whether the chest x-ray shows evidence of tuberculosis if the x-ray already is known to show no evidence of any disease in the first place. The rule author also does not want MYCIN to look stupid to its user: if the user has already told the system that the chest x-ray has no abnormalities, it would not be appropriate for MYCIN then to ask whether the chest x-ray shows evidence of tuberculosis. The particular sequence of clauses used in the rule in Figure 3.4 thus makes MYCIN's reasoning more efficient, and prevents the program from asking impertinent questions when it already has all the information that it needs to reach a conclusion. A logic would not be concerned with these procedural considerations; a logic would seek to specify what is believed to be true about the world, not worrying about hacks to enhance reasoning performance or to avoid asking silly questions in the course of problem solving.

Although classic rule-based systems such as MYCIN reason about atomic, "flat" data that have no intrinsic structure (e.g., an isolated chest x-ray that is either normal or abnormal, a single blood culture that is either positive or negative), developers of modern intelligent systems have sought to model data that have more complexity and that can be described with varying degrees of abstraction. It therefore has become natural to integrate rule-based systems with frame-based systems—enabling the rules to operate over abstractions of the data, when appropriate, by taking frames as input, and to generate conclusions at different levels of specificity, adding information to the frames as the rules generate their conclusions. CLIPS comes with its own proprietary frame language. Jess and Drools allow their rules to operate on Java objects that the developer can treat as a frame system.

By far and away, rules form the most common form of knowledge representations in biomedical informatics. Rule-based systems routinely analyze and interpret electrocardiogram tracings, screen patients seeking insurance coverage for major procedures, and evaluate electronic health-record data for potential drug-drug interactions. Rule-based systems perform quality-assurance functions and alert clinicians when they may be administering inappropriate therapy.

Rules are important not only for encoding knowledge needed for decision-support applications, but also for enabling deductive database systems that ensure that data are internally consistent and that derive new conclusions to be added to the database whenever the database is updated (see Chapter 2). In this spirit, HL7 has defined a standard rule language, known as Arden syntax [26], that generates alerts for clinicians when the database of an electronic patient record is changed in a manner that indicates an abnormal test result, a potential drug-drug interaction, or other problems that demand the attention of healthcare personnel. Arden syntax rules (or *medical logic modules*; MLMs) typically do not "chain," but instead denote single associational relationships between data that may appear in the electronic patient record and problematic conditions that warrant reporting to clinical personnel. The approach works well to encode individual rules that alert healthcare workers to aberrancies in the data for particular patients. The use of Arden Syntax rules is not well suited for the encoding of knowledge related to the treatment of chronic disease or of conditions that unfold over time; instead, Arden Syntax rules are intended for encoding simple situation-action relationships. The primary goal of the representation is to offer a standard framework for encoding such situation-action rules so that clinical alerts and reminders can be disseminated and shared across institutions that may use different electronic health record systems and different patient databases [26].

Arden Syntax does not attempt to standardize the meaning of any of the data on which rules operate. Instead, rules written in Arden Syntax that are intended to be adopted by different institutions include statements enclosed in {curly braces} that denote places in the rule where a programmer should insert an actual query to the local patient database (Figure 3.5). These *ad hoc* database queries will then relate a symbol used in the logic of the Arden Syntax rule to the clinical data that actually populate the health information system where the rule will operate. Customizing a rule in Arden Syntax to run in a local system can be an arduous process, as a database query needs to be written for each symbol within curly braces. The HL7 community whimsically refers to the lack of standard semantics for the symbols manipulated by Arden Syntax rules as the "curly braces problem."

penicillin_order := event {medication_order where class = penicillin};

/* find allergies */

penicillin allergy := read last {allergy where agent_class = penicillin};

;;

evoke: penicillin_order ;;

logic: If exist (penicillin_allergy) then conclude true; endif; ;;

action: write

"Caution, the patient has the following allergy to penicillin

documented:" || penicillin_allergy ;;

■ **FIGURE 3.5** A rule in the Arden Syntax. This excerpt from a rule in the Arden Syntax is meant to generate an alert if a patient who is known to be allergic to penicillin is prescribed a drug in the penicillin class. The expressions that appear within curly braces are intended to be replaced with calls to the local patient database to provide values for the corresponding variables.

3.3.5 **Description Logic**

In the past decade, interest in the Semantic Web [14] has surged. As a result, the biomedical informatics community has placed considerable attention on methods for representing knowledge in a manner that may be useful to intelligent computational agents that operate on the Internet. The result has been renewed excitement about both rule systems and frame systems—but rethought in the context of the Web, with its vastness and with its chaos. The discussion regarding frame systems has gone beyond hierarchies of classes and their associated instances, and now emphasizes methods by which those classes can be defined in a formal logic, enabling intelligent agents to classify newly encountered objects in terms of the class definitions programmatically, and facilitating automated management of enormous class hierarchies. These capabilities are provided by description logics— knowledge-representation languages that can add rich semantics to the basic constructs found in frame systems [27].

Work on description logics dates from the 1970s, when investigators sought to develop knowledge representation systems that could encode not only hierarchies of frames, but also formal definitions of the frames themselves [28]. In a description logic, frame declarations are augmented with logical propositions that defined the necessary and sufficient conditions for an entity to belong to the class represented by the frame. Thus, pneumonia is *necessarily* a disease located in the lung; to diagnosis pneumonia, it is *sufficient* that there be inflammation in the lung; cough, however, is neither a necessary nor sufficient property of pneumonia. Thus, if a patient does not have lung disease, then that patient, by definition, does not have pneumonia; if a patient has pulmonary inflammation, however, then that patient, by definition, does have pneumonia. These logical properties make it possible for the computer automatically to establish the relationship between classes such as *lung disease* and *pneumonia*. They also make it possible to assign to individuals who have different properties the most specific classification entailed by their particular properties.

When frame hierarchies become large, the distinctions between the various classes may become lost in the background of all the detail. In this situation, description-logic definitions become an extremely attractive feature to help developers—and computer systems—to manage the complexity. When a developer creates a new class, such as *bacterial pneumonia*, the necessary and sufficient properties tell the system exactly where the class should go in the hierarchy. It is likely that *bacterial pneumonia* will be placed in the hierarchy as a subclass of *pneumonia*. It is also likely that *bacterial pneumonia* will be defined as a subclass of *bacterial infection* (Figure 3.6).

Description logics use a special reasoning system known as a *classifier* to identify the places in the hierarchy that each class should occupy. The classifier may indicate relationships among classes that might not be intuitive at

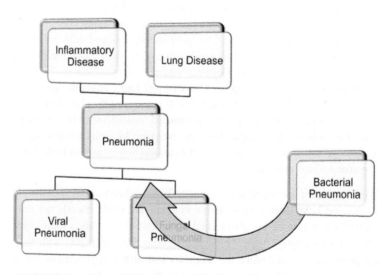

■ **FIGURE 3.6** Automatic classification in a description logic. A classifier uses the properties of the classes to assign classes to the correct location in the graph. The classifier already has reconfirmed that *pneumonia* is both a *lung disease* and an *inflammatory disease*. In the figure, the classifier is about to place *bacterial pneumonia* as a subclass of *pneumonia*, based on the properties of the various classes.

first glance, but that are a logical consequence of the description-logic definitions. Sometimes the classifier may suggest that a class should be placed in the hierarchy in a location that a developer considers to be patently incorrect. Such a "false" classification may occur because necessary or sufficient conditions have been inadvertently omitted from the definition, or because one or more definitions simply may be wrong. Classifiers thus have the useful property of helping system builders to debug a knowledge base in addition to providing novel insights into the relationships among classes when the definitions are known to be correct. A major attraction of description logics in general is that they enable classifiers to reason about potentially complex relationships among classes in a computationally efficient manner.

Although there have been many description-logic systems developed over the years, perhaps the only one that really matters for the construction of new knowledge bases is the Web Ontology Language (OWL), a knowledge-representation standard recommended by the World Wide Web Consortium since 2004 [29]. OWL is achieving increasing importance in both commercial and academic sectors because of its status as a knowledge-representation standard. OWL builds on both the syntax and semantics of RDF, and offers a logic for describing classes and properties of classes, as well as annotations that allow developers to comment on the logical formalisms. The OWL standard is now in its second version, OWL 2. There are three subsets (or *profiles*) of the OWL 2 language that optionally limit the kinds of things that developers can express in the language in different ways in order to maximize the computational efficiency of using the resulting knowledge bases for particular tasks. OWL 2 EL is a subset of the complete OWL standard that guarantees that classification can be performed in polynomial time, as only *existential quantification* of properties is allowed. OWL 2 QL is an OWL subset that is optimized for situations in which the knowledge base contains huge numbers of instances, and the emphasis is on *querying* the instances as if they comprised a database. OWL 2 RL is a profile that limits the expressivity of the language so that classification can be implemented using a simple *rule-based* reasoning engine. Developers are always free to use the entire OWL language, of course. By restricting themselves to the language constructs that occur in one of the three profiles, however, knowledge-base authors can be assured that their representation will display certain computationally favorable properties when they can anticipate that one of the three corresponding situations will pertain.

Like all description logics, OWL makes the open-world assumption. Thus, any instance of a class (i.e., any *individual*) potentially can be a member of any class in the knowledge base, unless the knowledge base declares explicitly that it cannot be. If there is a class *kidney*, and one subclass of *kidney* is *right kidney* and another subclass of *kidney* is *left kidney*, then an instance of *kidney* could be *both* a *left kidney* and a *right kidney*—unless the knowledge base happens to contain an axiom declaring that the subclass *right kidney* and the subclass *left kidney* are disjoint. Otherwise, any *right kidney* could also be a *left kidney,* unless the knowledge base explicitly states that this situation is impossible. OWL has been created with the World Wide Web in mind, and the Web is an environment where anyone can say anything about anything. In this situation, it seems reasonable for a knowledge representation to be able to assume anything until it is told otherwise. The open world of OWL, however, is very different from the closed world of frame languages. In frame systems, if something is not known, it is assumed to be false. Subclasses of frames are ordinarily mutually exclusive; an instance of *kidney* cannot be a *left kidney* if it is already known to be a *right kidney*. Although more limiting, the close-world assumption of frame systems often seems more natural to novice knowledge-base developers. (At a minimum, the closed-world assumption causes systems to behave in more predictable ways.) The open-world assumption of OWL and of other description logics can cause enormous confusion when the system infers bizarrely erroneous relationships that are, nevertheless, the logical consequence of the knowledge base—results that never would have been inferred had the developer added the "closure" axioms needed to instruct the system that, for example, *left* and *right* are disjoint concepts.

Although we often speak as if OWL is the only description logic that we care about, the biomedical informatics community has adopted other description logics in its work. The Open Biomedical and Biological Ontologies group, for example, manages a library of several dozen knowledge bases encoded in a description logic known as the OBO Format [30]. The International Health Terminology Standards Development Organization continues to develop SNOMED CT in a proprietary description logic that has properties similar to those of the OWL 2 EL profile.

3.4 WHAT DOES A REPRESENTATION MEAN?

The knowledge-representation hypothesis [7] suggests that a declarative knowledge representation is inspectable by humans who wish to understand what a computational system *knows*, and is the driving mechanism for engendering the consequences of that knowledge in the behavior of that system. Thus, we take it at face value that we can examine a knowledge representation and understand what it means; when we see symbols such as "(PublishedIn JAMIA ?x)", we take it for granted that we know intuitively what the predicate "PublishedIn" means and that we know what the object "JAMIA" refers to. The problem is, we don't.

Symbols have meaning because humans say they do. You may read this text and stumble upon the symbol *kidney*, and believe that you know what that symbol means. Earlier in this chapter we were distinguishing between right kidneys and left kidneys. It consequently is natural to assume that the symbol *kidney* refers to a paired organ found in vertebrates. As a reader, you are seeing this symbol on the page and second-guessing what I, as the author, mean by it. But *kidney* might also refer to a kind of bean. It might refer to a kind of meat. It might refer to a kind of swimming pool. It might refer to none of these things. When readers encounter the symbol *kidney*—or any symbol—they ascribe meaning to the term by inferring what the author must have meant when using that term. As discussed in detail in Chapter 6, natural language is inherently ambiguous, and readers must constantly conjecture what terms denote as they attempt to derive meaning from the symbols that compose sentences. The process of disambiguation is not impossible, however, because the readers can infer the intentions of the authors and, in the context of those intentions, ascribe meaning to each term that is read.

The same situation applies to computer programs [31]. Whenever we communicate with computers, we must ascribe meaning to the symbols that the computer presents to us by second-guessing the intention of the person who created the computer dialog. For example, when using our personal computers, when we select the command *save* from a file menu, we know that the term *save* has very precise semantics in the context of certain computer programs. We know that, when we select *save*, a fresh copy of our document will be written out to the disk. We know that the file will appear in whatever directory or folder we accessed last. We know that the most recent version of our work also will be erased in the process. We know all these things about the semantics of the symbol *save* because we and the software engineers who wrote our program share a common background that allows us to ascribe precise meaning to this symbol in the context of using our computers. (Users who do not share this common background notoriously are perplexed when they discover for the first time that the *save* command has the side effect of deleting their previous file.)

When the MYCIN program asks, "Does the patient's chest x-ray suggest Active-Tb?", the user can answer this question only if he or she shares the same background knowledge that the developers of MYCIN have, and thereby can ascribe the same semantics to the term *Active-Tb* that the developers do. Even a trained radiologist who is intimately familiar with the radiographic features of tuberculosis may answer MYCIN's question incorrectly if the physician cannot second-guess why the program is asking for this information and what the program intends to do with it. Is the program asking for the presence of subtle indications of tuberculosis? Should the user answer the question affirmatively if there are signs of tuberculosis on the radiograph but the overall pattern is suggestive of something else? Unless the user of the program can fathom what the developers of the program had in mind by having the computer pose the question, there is no way to know the semantics of a term such as *Active-Tb*.

Whenever we consider any knowledge representation that we might enter into a computer—whether we are using a logic, a semantic network, a frame language, or rules—we are constructing data structures using symbols. Like symbols such as *kidney*, *save*, or *Active-Tb*—and like the words on this page—the symbols in our knowledge bases have no intrinsic semantics; the symbols mean whatever the user legitimately can infer them to mean, which hopefully is the same thing that the knowledge-base author intended them to mean.

A representation such as:

        (exists (?y)
                (Paper ?y)
                (PublishedIn JAMIA ?y)
                (AuthorOfPaper ?y Sarkar))

has no innate meaning. It means precisely the same thing as:

        (exists (?y)
                (A ?y)
                (B C ?y)
                (D ?y E))

This situation causes obvious grief for adherents of the knowledge-representation hypothesis. How can anyone look at a knowledge representation and "know what the system knows" simply by inspection? How can we ever know what "(A ?y)" means? The short answer is, we can't.

The process of knowledge representation is possible only when knowledge-base authors can impose a strict meaning on each symbol in the knowledge base, and if the users of the system in turn will be able to apply the same strict meaning. Logicians use the term *model* to refer to a possible set of entities in the world such that the symbols in a knowledge base can denote those entities. Given such a model, it doesn't matter whether we use the symbol *Active-Tb*, or *tuberculosis*, or *A*, or *foo*, or *kidney*: a symbol means only what its mapping to the world being modeled says it means. To use any computer program being driven by such a knowledge base, the user must share the same model as that of the knowledge-base authors. As a result, the user and the knowledge-base authors necessarily will ascribe the same fixed semantics to the symbols in the knowledge base.

This perspective on knowledge representation does not make intelligent computer systems seem all that intelligent. The computers come across as machines that are very good at manipulating symbols in accordance with predefined rules—rules such as *modus ponens* when manipulating symbols in first-order logic, rules such as inheritance when manipulating symbols in a frame system, rules such as classification when manipulating symbols in a description logic. Computers process symbols; they don't "know" anything. What makes knowledge representations useful is that people understand how to ascribe meaning to the symbols in the representations, and that knowledge-base builders can communicate intelligently with the knowledge-base users through the representations in a knowledge base when everyone can share the same model.

When intelligent systems such as MYCIN were first described for the biomedical informatics community, however, there was awe at the prospect of a computer that could "know" so much about the diagnosis and treatment of infectious diseases. At the time, workers in our field thought of knowledge as a thing—as a commodity—that could be extracted from the heads of experts and represented in a knowledge base. It was only later that Newell's *knowledge-level perspective* forced us to view knowledge as a capacity for rational behavior, rather than as a set of physical symbols [1]. Winograd and Flores [31] refined the perspective further and made it clear that, when we represent knowledge declaratively in a computer, we are merely creating a symbol system that enables the computer to seem to act intelligently because the developers of the knowledge base ascribe meanings to the symbols that are shared with the users of the system. The behavior of a system such as MYCIN seems intelligent both because the behavior of the system appears to use available data and knowledge in a rational manner to achieve the system's goal (diagnosis and treatment on infection) and because the logical implications of manipulating the symbols in the knowledge base (in the case of MYCIN, invoking all the rules) are not at all obvious to the observer by simple inspection.

Knowledge representation is possible only when there is a shared semantics. If anyone in the system development chain or the users themselves begins to ascribe discordant meanings to any of the symbols, then the performance of the system will be affected. Indeed, the semantics of the symbols in a knowledge base can drift over time when new populations of developers, users, or cases enter the picture. DeDombal's famous Bayesian system for the diagnosis of the cause of abdominal pain performed fabulously at the institution where it was developed (the University of Leeds in the UK), but never did quite as well elsewhere. Although there is speculation that one reason its diagnoses were not as correct elsewhere may have been a matter of different prior probability of disease in different populations, another possible cause may be that descriptions of different kinds of abdominal signs and symptoms may take on different semantics in different locations [32]. Thus, terms such as *sharp pain*, *colic*, and *rebound tenderness* may not have invariant meanings among clinicians. Patients themselves may also describe their symptoms differently in different regions (with different amounts of emotion or stoicism), causing the clinicians using the system to choose terms to describe their cases that are different from the ones that would have been selected by the developers back in Leeds. In the end, the symbols in a knowledge base mean whatever the users and developers say they mean.

3.5 BUILDING KNOWLEDGE BASES IN PRACTICE

Although the theoretical characteristics of different knowledge-representation formalisms are well understood, the decision of which approach to use in the context of a given project generally involves other kinds of considerations. Fortunately, workers in biomedical informatics have many choices for building electronic knowledge bases. The options often depend on the computational complexity that the developers are willing to tolerate, the need to integrate with other software (such as database systems or Web-based applications), or the need to adhere to particular standards for a given project.

System builders who want to stay close to first-order logic often will choose a programming language such as Prolog to express propositions about the world that they are modeling. Prolog has the advantage of being extremely popular in the logic-programming community, and is enabled by a wide range of development environments, some of which are commercially supported platforms. Although Common Logic now carries the imprimatur of the International Standards Organization and has found considerable uptake in several niche communities, support for engineering systems in Common Logic still remains somewhat limited at this time. In general, developers choose logic-based representation systems when they see a need for developing a knowledge base that can express both complex and nuanced relationships among the entities being modeled, and where the users are willing to tolerate the long processing times that may be required to perform many kinds of inferences in the worst case.

For system builders seeking a more pragmatic approach to knowledge representation, the rule-based approach dominates current work in biomedical informatics. Simple situation-action rules for use in clinical systems frequently are represented in Arden Syntax. As discussed in Section 3.3.2, the symbols on which Arden Syntax rules operate do not have a standard semantics. Each time that an Arden Syntax rule is adopted for use within a local information system, a programmer needs to write the database queries that will relate the symbols in the rule to the information available in the patient database (see Figure 3.5). At the same time, Arden is not designed as an execution language for rules. Thus, rules written in Arden Syntax typically need to be compiled into a format that can be interpreted natively within the target information system.

For developers who do not need to adhere to HL7 standards, writing rules with widely used packages such as Jess or Drools is an extremely attractive option. Unlike Arden Syntax rules, Jess or Drools rules can use forward chaining in a very natural manner. Because the inference engines that interpret Jess and Drools are Java based, they integrate well into modern software architectures. In practice, rules constitute the dominant approach that developers choose for representing knowledge, even though the expressive power of rules is limited when compared with full first-order logic. The ease with which developers can express domain relationships using rules and the efficiency of rule-based inference engines often make the rule-based approach convenient for many practical knowledge-representation tasks.

Developers typically turn to frame-based systems or description logics such as OWL for representing hierarchies of terms and their relationships. These approaches have become widely used for encoding domain ontologies—representations of the entities that constitute an application area and the relationships among those entities [33]. The importance of these knowledge-representation formalisms—and of OWL in particular—has soared in recent years, as the informatics community has recognized the importance of making explicit the ontologies that underlie all software systems. The use of ontologies to add metadata to biomedical datasets, to encode the lexicons used by natural-language processing systems, and to form the basis of modern controlled terminologies (such as SNOMED CT and the International Classification of Diseases) has made knowledge representation using description logics particularly important for work in biomedical informatics.

As noted in Section 3.3.5, representation of knowledge using description logic can be complicated, given the considerable expressiveness of languages such as OWL and the confusion sometimes caused by the open-world assumption. Many developers therefore opt to use older frame-based languages, or to construct the equivalent of frame hierarchies out of RDF triples, rather than to commit to knowledge representation using OWL. Nevertheless, OWL is the language that the World Wide Web Consortium currently recommends for the construction of ontologies, and the existence of the standard by itself makes OWL an important foundation for this kind of work.

There are several ways in which developers can construct knowledge bases in OWL. The most widely used nonproprietary development environment for OWL is called Protégé (Figure 3.7), a Web-based editor that facilitates the construction of large hierarchies of classes with associated axioms and annotations [34]. Protégé has a plug-in architecture that has enabled third parties to construct scores of modular enhancements to the system—for example, plug-ins that support editing rules in Jess or in the Semantic Web Rule Language (SWRL) that can operate on data stored as OWL individuals [35]. This admixture of representing entities and relationships (and instances of those entities) in OWL and of representing decision logic in rules is a very common paradigm in the construction of contemporary knowledge bases.

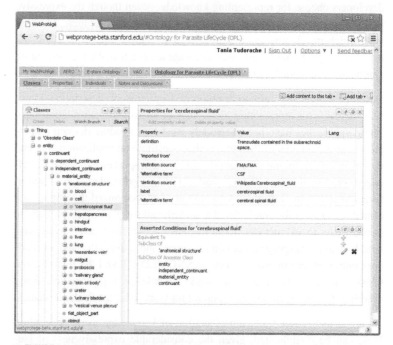

■ **FIGURE 3.7** WebProtégé. The Web-based version of the Protégé knowledge-editing system offers a convenient platform for authoring OWL classes and their properties. Here, the WebProtégé browser shows the Ontology for Parasitic Lifecycle.

3.6 **SUMMARY**

Although knowledge always can be programmed into a computer in a procedural way, there are significant advantages that ensue when a knowledge representation is declarative. A declarative representation makes it possible for a human developer to inspect the corresponding knowledge base to develop an understanding, at some level, of what the computer "knows." At the same time, a declarative representation ensures that the knowledge base has a direct role in driving the behavior of the computer system. As a result, a developer can modify the computational behavior by *editing* the knowledge base, without the need to reprogram the system.

We have discussed several approaches to representing knowledge in computers, including the use of first-order logic, semantic networks, frames, rules, and description logics. There are different trade-offs associated with using any of these approaches, although the dominant issue is often one of trading off minimizing the computational complexity of inference with maximizing the expressiveness of the language. Languages such as logics that allow the developer to say as much about the world as possible often have computationally poor performance in the worst case; simple languages such as rule-based systems often are guaranteed to perform with considerable computational efficiency. Such languages also may be easier for humans to use reliably for knowledge-base development. On the other hand, system builders may prefer to use a more cumbersome, less computationally efficient knowledge-representation framework when they know that their applications will require the encoding of complex or subtle relationships, or when their programs will need to explore deep implications of the propositions in the knowledge base.

The ascription of meaning to the symbols in a knowledge base is a tricky business, since symbols by themselves—regardless of the natural-language terms that we might use to label them—have no intrinsic meaning. The symbols in a knowledge base take on meaning only when we create some model of the world about which the computer system will use the knowledge base to perform inference—mapping in our minds the symbols in the knowledge base to the entities in our model. Knowledge bases do not contain knowledge intrinsically; computers don't know anything by themselves. Knowledge bases merely provide data structures that allow the knowledge-base authors to ascribe meaning to those data structures. The end users can acquiesce to these meanings, thus enabling the authors to communicate with the users through the behavior of the computer system that reasons about the particular knowledge base.

The process of modeling biomedical knowledge with sufficient precision to encode that knowledge in a knowledge base is at the heart of much of what we do in biomedical informatics. Indeed, the essence of biomedical informatics is the construction of computational models [3]. Not only do knowledge-representation systems provide workers in informatics with a medium for creating models of the manifold layered elements of biomedicine [36], but also they offer a practical vehicle for translating those models into information systems that can play pragmatic roles in the biomedical enterprise.

REFERENCES

[1] Newell A. The knowledge level. Artif Intell 1982;18:87–127.

[2] Steels L, McDermott J, editors. The knowledge level in expert systems. Boston: Academic Press; 1994.

[3] Musen MA. Medical informatics: Searching for underlying components. Method Inform Med 2002;41:12–9.

[4] Bleich HL. Computer evaluation of acid-base disorders. J Clin Invest 1969;48: 1689–96.

[5] Winograd T. Frames and the procedural-declarative controversy. In: Bobrow DG, Collins AM, editors. Representation and understanding: studies in cognitive science. New York: Academic Press; 1975.

[6] Patil R, Szolovits P, Schwartz W. Causal understanding of patient illness in medical diagnosis. In: Proceedings of the seventh joint international conference on artificial intelligence; 1981. p. 893–9.

[7] Smith BC. Reflection and semantics in a procedural language. Ph.D. thesis, technical report MIT/LCS/TR-272, MIT, Cambridge, MA; 1982.

[8] Common logic standard. <http://iso-commonlogic.org>. [accessed 26.05.13].

[9] Eriksson H, Shahar Y, Tu SW, Puerta AR, Musen MA. Task modeling with reusable problem-solving methods. Artif Intell 1995;79:293–326.

[10] Lenat DB, Guha RV. Building large knowledge-based systems: representation and inference in the cyc project. Boston: Addison-Wesley Longman; 1989.

[11] Sowa JF, Borgida A. Principles of semantic networks: explorations in the representation of knowledge. San Francisco: Morgan-Kaufmann; 1991.

[12] Sowa JF. Conceptual structures: information processing in mind and machine. Reading, MA: Addison-Wesley; 1984.

[13] Bizer C, Heath T, Berners-Lee T. Linked data—the story so far. Int J Semant Web Inform Syst 2009;5(3):1–22.

[14] Berners-Lee T, Hendler J, Lassila O. The Semantic Web. Sci Am 2001:29–37.

[15] Belleau F, Nolin M-A, Tourigny N, Rigault P, Morissette J. Bio2RDF: towards a mashup to build bioinformatics knowledge systems. J Biomed Inform 2008;41:706–16.

[16] Nolin M-A, Dumontier M, Belleau F, Corbeil J. Building an HIV data mashup using Bio2RDF. Brief Bioinform 2012;1:98–106.

[17] Koller D, Friedman N. Probabilistic graphic models: principles and techniques. Cambridge, MA: MIT Press; 2009.

[18] Minsky M. A framework for representing knowledge. In: Winston P, editor. The psychology of computer vision. New York: McGraw-Hill; 1975.

[19] CLIPS: a tool for building expert systems. <http://clipsrules.sourceforge.net>. [accessed 26.05.13].

[20] Miller RA, Pople HE, Myers JD. Internist-1: an experimental computer-based diagnostic consultant for general internal medicine. New Engl J Med 1982;307:468–76.

[21] Miller RA, Masarie FE. Use of the quick medical reference (QMR) program as a tool for medical education. Methods Inform Med 1989;28:340–5.

[22] Jess, the rule engine for the java platform. <http://www.jessrules.com>. [accessed 26.05.13].

[23] Buchanan BG, Shortliffe EH, editors. Rule-based expert systems: the MYCIN experiments of the Stanford heuristic programming project. Reading, MA: Addison-Wesley; 1984.

[24] Drools—The business logic integration platform. <http://www.jboss.org/Drools>. [accessed 26.05.13].

[25] Clancey WJ. The epistemology of a rule-based system: a framework for explanation. Artif Intell 1983;29:215–51.

[26] Samwald M, Fehre K, De Bruin J, Adlassnig K-P. The arden syntax standard for clinical decision support: experiences and directions. J Biomed Inform 2012;45:711–8.

[27] Baader F, Calvanese D, McGuinness D, Nardi D, Patel-Schneider P. The description logic handbook: theory, implementation, and applications. Cambridge, UK: Cambridge University Press; 2003.

[28] Brachman RJ, Schmolze J. An overview of the KL-ONE knowledge representation system. Cogn Sci 1985;9:171–216.

[29] OWL 2 web ontology language document overview, 2nd ed. <http://www.w3.org/TR/owl2-overview/>. [accessed 26.05.13].

[30] OBO flat file format 1.4 syntax and semantics [Working draft]. <http://oboformat.googlecode.com/svn/branches/2011-11-29/doc/obo-syntax.html>. [accessed 26.05.13].

[31] Winograd T, Flores F. Understanding computers and cognition: a new foundation for design. Norwood, NJ: Ablex; 1986.

[32] Staniland JR, Clamp SE, de Dombal FT, Solheim K, Hansen S, Rønsen K, et al. Presentation and diagnosis of patients with acute abdominal pain: comparisons between Leeds, U.K. and Akershus county, Norway. Ann Chir Gynaecol 1980;69:245–50.

[33] Shah NH, Musen MA. Ontologies for formal representation of biological systems. In: Studer R, Staab S, editors. Handbook on ontologies. New York: Springer; 2009. p. 445–61.

[34] Tudorache T, Nyulas C, Noy NF, Musen MA. WebProtégé: a collaborative ontology editor knowledge acquisition tool for the web. Semant Web 2013;4:89–99.

[35] O'Connor MJ, Das A, Musen MA. Using the semantic web rule language in the development of ontology-driven applications. In: Handbook of research on emerging rule-based languages and technologies: open solutions and approaches. Hershey: IGI Global; 2009. p. 525–39.

[36] Blois MS. Information in medicine: the nature of medical descriptions. Berkeley: University of California Press; 1984.

Hypothesis Generation from Heterogeneous Datasets

Yves A. Lussier[a,b,c] and Haiquan Li[a]

aDepartment of Medicine, University of Illinois at Chicago, Chicago, IL, USA
bDepartment of Bioengineering, University of Illinois at Chicago, Chicago, IL, USA
cCancer Center, University of Illinois, Chicago, IL, USA

4.1 INTRODUCTION

Despite a handful of biomedical studies based on general knowledge-driven approaches (e.g., the Human Genome Project [1], metagenomics [2], the Encyclopedia of DNA Elements (ENCODE) [3], and the Cancer Genome Atlas [4]), most biomedical studies are driven by explicit hypotheses.

Traditional hypotheses typically arise from the domain knowledge of a researcher's expertise. With rapidly accumulated large-scale data, hypothesis generation becomes an almost impossible mission without the assistance of computerized or information technology. Furthermore, recent years have witnessed an exponentially increased volume of heterogeneous data sources from the broad spectra of biomedical studies, such as biomedical literature, electronic health records and their underlying genomics data at multiple scales of measurements, from single nucleotide and DNA methylation to RNA expression and protein interactions levels. It has thus become critical for discovery science to automatically generate high-quality hypotheses for biomedical studies. However, multiple barriers hamper the integration of highly heterogeneous datasets in terms of data formats and variable types (ordinal, discrete, etc.), correspondence between distinct biological scales, and the combinatorial dimensionality that risk generating excess poor quality hypotheses (false positives).

The categorization of hypotheses generation methods depends on multiple facets, such as the number of data sources, the types of hypotheses, or the methodology foundations. Examples for the method of categorization based on types of hypotheses include: (i) hypotheses leading to the identification of one or multiple functional or structural characteristics of a biomedical concept, (ii) hypotheses generating associations between concepts, such as disease associations or identification of causative genes from the study of medical records and genetic data [5,6], (iii) hypotheses that provide contextual or conditional associations, and (iv) hypotheses for the discovery of patterns between biological modules such as complexes of multiple proteins required to interact with other biological modules. These hypotheses may relate biomedical entities or functions within the same biological scale or across biological scales, which compounds the complexity of the analyses.

This chapter focuses on common issues for hypothesis generation in mechanism-oriented biomedical studies and discusses related major methodologies in addition to illustrating their applications in the context of biomedical problems. Originally from corroborative methods specifically tailored for a few scales of data, recent methodologies tend to fuse highly heterogeneous data with distinct format and numeric scales within one uniform framework, employing theories from statistical, mathematical, and computational disciplines. These methods, targeting from disease-gene prioritization and disease mechanisms to biomarker discovery and outcome prediction, have been validated experimentally and have demonstrated fruitful applications in biomedicine and health care. This chapter is specifically focused on biomedical studies; hypothesis generation for purely biological problems [7] or clinical outcome prediction [8] is out of scope.

4.2 **PRELIMINARY BACKGROUND**

This section enumerates the prerequisite knowledge and skills required to conduct studies for hypothesis generation from heterogeneous datasets. We proceed from modeling biomedical information, to representing and formatting the data and knowledge utilized in these models and common skills for hypotheses generations using data from measurements each of which remains within a biological scale.

4.2.1 **Modeling Biological Structures and Their Interplay**

The scale of the structures of life is well understood ranging from single nucleotides (10^{-9} m) to the organism as a whole. Further, the interplay of these structures and their respective contextual function can be modeled. For example, Francis Crick articulated the first model of information flow across different scales of the molecules of life in 1958 [9,10], known as the "central dogma of molecular biology." In 1984, Marsden Blois codified a broader model that encompasses explicitly the biological structures, their functions, their interplay within as well as across biological scales, and the emergence of new properties from these interacting biomodules [11]. This latter model subsumes the former one and has shown utility in modeling biological ontologies hierarchically as well as explicitly formalizing experimental frameworks in biomedical informatics studies [12].

4.2.2 **Data and Knowledge Representation**

An essential feature of heterogeneous data sources is the difference in data formats due to their distinct nature. For instance, biomedical narratives are generally comprised of unstructured free text formats with some structured or semi-structured metadata (e.g., Medical Subject Headings [MeSH] descriptor and key words for literature or clinical abbreviations and medication codes in electronic health records). Genomic data comprise structured measurements and unstructured or missing context and phenotypes (e.g., experimental conditions and clinical/biological description of samples). As highlighted in Chapter 2, the various data representations are problematic for effective integration for heterogeneous hypothesis generation.

There is an obvious gap of representation and format as most computational algorithms require well-structured formats, such as tuples, vectors, matrix/tables, semi-structure format XML for trees, and graphs, which consist of a set of nodes for concepts and a set of edges for their linkage among the concepts.

4.2.3 **Data Format Conversion**

Distinct data formats can be converted to one another. For example, graphs and trees/XMLs can be converted into tables. However, free texts are extremely difficult to convert into simple formats and have to be processed before any hypothesis generation can occur. Natural Language Processing, a technique specifically tailored for this purpose, begins converting with entity recognition, followed by semantic analysis and relationship construction. It finally converts free texts into semi-structure formats such as XML or relational tables with some extent of information loss. Typical software packages for natural language processing of literatures or electronic medical records include MedLEE [13], MetaMap [14], and cTAKES [15]. For more details, refer to Chapter 6 and review papers [16].

4.2.4 **Text Mining for Knowledge Discovery**

Text mining is often a fundamental step for hypothesis generation because of the integration of free text. It extracts and discovers unknown knowledge such as novel associations between diseases and other phenotypes and between disease and genes. Novel associations may be discoverable by co-occurrence studies, network linkage, or vector-based semantic approaches. Please refer to Chapter 6 of this book and review papers [17] for details about text mining.

4.2.5 **Fundamental Statistical and Computational Methods**

Some statistics, such as correlation studies and enrichment statistics tests, are frequently applied in text mining and homogenous hypothesis generation, which also are the fundamental statistics for heterogeneous hypotheses. Correlations identify the co-occurrence of two concepts using either vector-based correlation studies or conditional dependency measurements. For enrichment studies, two factors are tested relative to a background condition, and the occurrences of the four possible combinations of the two factors are represented in a contingency table, by which the enrichment is tested using either a hyper-geometric test or the Fisher's exact test.

Machine-learning and graph algorithms are other fundamental techniques for text mining and genomic hypothesis generation. In machine learning, a model is built from multiple features of labeled training instances, and then tested on independent testing instances, using measures such as recall/sensitivity, precision, specificity, or AUC of ROC (Area Under the Curve of Receiver Operating Characteristic curve). For graph algorithms, linkage and neighborhood are often used to model related knowledge and

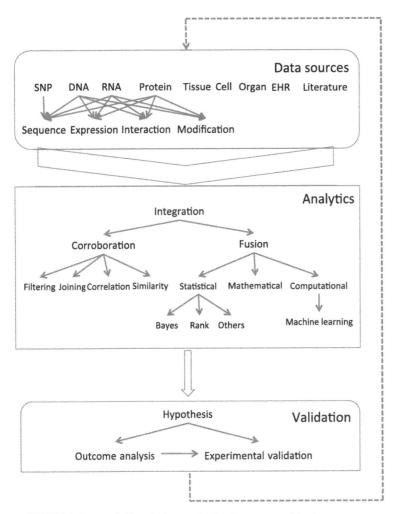

■ FIGURE 4.1 Framework of hypothesis generation from heterogeneous datasets.

their propagation. Graph patterns, such as shortest paths, spanning trees, or even subnet community structure like cliques, are essential for hypothesis generation.

4.3 **DESCRIPTION OF METHODS**

This section builds on the prerequisite for generating hypotheses using data from measurements that cross multiple biological scales and may require advanced integration. There is an art to designing computational biology experiments that can successfully solve a problem (Figure 4.1). First, a problem is identified as one that requires a large number of prioritized hypotheses to restrict and thus accelerate the discovery process (*why?*). Second, an information model serves as a high-level framework for hypothesis generation and its underpinning data integration (*what?*). Third, datasets are selected and may in part constrain the model—there is generally some iteration at this stage between availability of data and type of model that can be supported (*how?*). The specific integrative strategies are next followed by the analytics that address the problem (*how?*). Here, computational biologists refer to the analytics as analytical modeling or simply modeling. Of note, these analytical models further specify information models that we discussed earlier as the latter are generally cast at the level of representations in nomenclature, classifications, data formats, and their potential joint utilization in an analytical model. These models may also be formally represented using engineering principles, as described in Chapter 10. Finally, validation studies are conducted to confirm the hypotheses generated (e.g., synthetic datasets, cellular or biological models, and clinical trials). This section focuses on integration as well as approaches to mitigate the large number of hypotheses that can potentially be obtained, upstream via filtering, within the analytics themselves using simplifying hypotheses and finally downstream to sift through the results (e.g., false discovery rate).

4.3.1 Determination of Study Scales and Associated Simplifying Hypotheses

The first step for heterogeneous hypothesis generation is to select the right biomedical scales for an information model and its corresponding dataset integration. There are a number of such possible scales, as shown on the top of Figure 4.1: biomedical literature, electronic health records, genomic sequence at various levels (single nucleotide polymorphic, gene and protein level), genomic expression at various levels (DNA microarray, RNA-Seq, copy number variation, protein array, and proteomic mass spectral data), epigenetics such as DNA methylation and posttranslational modifications, organ images, among others that have not been fully developed.

There are several issues when modeling across scales. First, there is an integration problem addressed in Section 4.3.3. In summary, corroborative models are tailored for each combination of the scales of biology that they address (Section 4.3.3.1), while data fusion models are more scalable because they proceed with a uniform approach to integration regardless of the specific biological measurement being integrated (Section 4.3.3.2). The vast majority of corroborative studies are not designed to use more than one corroborative model and thus are limited to a few scales of biology that can be modeled within the same equation. Indeed, studies involving multiple corroborative models would be quite complex to empirically control as one model would feed into another, each consisting of multiple biological measurements at different scales.

A second issue is the combinatorial explosion of analyzing measurements across biological scales. For example, eQTL studies require the correlations between each of 1,000,000 single nucleotide polymorphisms (SNPs) and ~40,000 transcripts resulting in 4×10^{10} combinations [18]. In part, filtering can mitigate the number of combinations. SNPs that cannot be called "positive" on enough samples should be altogether disregarded. Similarly, mRNAs that have a low coefficient of variation (i.e., normalized variance) across all samples are unlikely to yield statistical significance for any group comparison and should be disregarded as well. Simplifying hypotheses can also reduce the dimensionality. For example, one gene can yield multiple distinct mRNAs and their translated proteins via alternate splicing (1➜ Many relationship). One commonly used simplification approach when dealing with this relationship across the genetic scale and the expression scales is to reduce the relationship to a 1➜ 1. The integration of expressed mRNAs from RNA-sequencing in meta-analysis studies with older experiments conducted over expression arrays exemplifies this approach: the former measures each exon or splicing variant, the latter measures the expressed genes [19].

4.3.2 Curse of Dimensionality, Classification, and Feature Selection

With the increase of integrated scales, the number of dimensions may increase exponentially. Indeed, if eQTL measures—that comprise statistics for each SNP and mRNA into one statistics (Section 4.3.1)—are paired with protein interactions, then the number of hypotheses that can be generated across protein interactions and eQTL can be as high as 10^{16} comparisons ([1,000,000 SNPs] × [25,000 mRNAs] × [500,000 protein interactions]) [20]. Obviously, these combinations could be limited by the lack of corresponding proteins (perhaps 7000 distinct proteins in interactions); however, that only reduces the problem by one order of magnitude. In Section 4.3.1, we suggested the use of eQTL derived from sufficiently powered SNPs and mRNA, which could further reduce the combinations by an order or two of magnitude. Nonetheless, the resulting combinations remain legion size. The curse of dimensionality, which refers to this issue [21], is particularly severe for any discovery hypothesis generation requiring a large number of biological scales, each of which contains genome-wide or legion-size datasets. Statistical power to find global patterns is reduced; however, feature selection and appropriate use of simplifying hypotheses can significantly reduce the considered combinations [22]. Another dimensionality reduction method consists of classification of elementary functions or structures into a higher-level function or structure. For example, genes can be classified into a KEGG pathway [23] or cellular processes in Gene Ontology [24] or as associated to a disease in OMIM [25]. Similarly, using an ontology such as SNOMED [26], diseases can be grouped by their anatomical location, organ, or clinical system affected, which significantly reduces the dimensions. Finally, various databases, ranging from biological to clinical ones, are useful sources to pick up the relevant data fields and narrow down the search space.

4.3.3 **Approaches of Integration**

Integrative methods for heterogeneous hypothesis generation can be categorized into two approaches: corroborative and fusion. Corroborative approaches handle each scale of data individually and then link them one by one, using specific and usually distinct methods. Corroborative methods are specific to the problem and do not apply easily to a different group of measurements at a different biological scale. In contrast, fusion approaches use a uniform mathematical, statistical, or computational framework to integrate all scales of data, and the methodology is smoothly extendable to more scales, and scalable in nature. We will take a closer look at the integrative approaches by these two categories accordingly (See Figure 4.1 for the categorization details).

4.3.3.1 *Corroborative Approaches*

4.3.3.1.1 **Logical Filtering Evidence From Multiple Scales**

Basic logical filtering, such as AND operations, is effective for the integration of multiple heterogeneous data. For instance, miRNA, assumed to be associated with diseases due to their deregulation, should be reinforced by corresponding deregulation of their target mRNAs, which may be from another data source [27]. Co-reported mechanisms with diseases, such as gene ontology terms, are expected to be consistent with the annotations of candidate genes that are prioritized separately [28]. In summary, basic logical operations could filter out many candidate hypotheses and improve the specificity of the final hypothesis.

4.3.3.1.2 **Information Joining From Multiple Datasets**

An extension of basic logical filtering is information joined from multiple datasets, which are often organized into relational models. These datasets consist of distinct information, some of which may overlap features and values; joining this information could lead to novel hypotheses. For instance, databases, such as VARIMED [29], catalog the associations between genetic variants and disease phenotypes; while NHANES (National Health and Nutrition Examination Survey) [30] collect environment exposures and their association to disease phenotypes. By joining these two datasets after mapping genetic variants to genes, hypotheses can be generated for interactions between environmental factors and genes that account for diseases [31]. These hypotheses can be further refined by checking existing gene-environment factor interactions reported in other databases, such as CTD (Comparative Toxicogenomics Database) [31]. While the previous example proceeds with joining a crisp variable with an explicit common data dictionary between the distinct datasets, an alternative approach consists of joining related variables by phylogeny [32], fuzzy variables [33], fuzzy ontology [34], or information theoretic similarity in ontologies [35] (Section 4.3.3.1.4).

4.3.3.1.3 Correlation Among Multiple Scales

Correlation assesses the numeric dependency between two factors for studies beyond value-based connections as those in logical operations and value joining. Factors from heterogeneous datasets can be combined and evaluated for their correlations, if they can be modeled numerically. For instance, gene expression profiles of drugs can be compared with those of diseases and used to reposition existing drugs from anti-correlations between the two types of expression profiles [6,36]. As another example, Korbel et al. aligned genomic and phenotypic occurrences in a common set of species: the occurrence of a gene was represented as a vector of either presence or absence in the species, while a phenotype via a MeSH descriptor was represented by its occurrence in the corresponding species according to literature abstracts in MEDLINE. The correlation between the two vectors hypothesized potential associations between genes and studied phenotypes [37].

4.3.3.1.4 Similarity Measurement Between Datasets

Similarity measurements can help link different heterogeneous datasets to conclude new hypotheses. Semantic similarity could be employed to evaluate the textual or descriptive information between two types of concepts [38], whereas correlation-like measures evaluate similarity between two numeric vector values [39]. Further, homology can also be used as an indicator of similarity of two sequences, which has proven to be effective in biology hypothesis generation. In biomedical studies, homology can discover additional genes based on those that have established linkage to a disease phenotype. For instance, high homology to a known disease gene has been combined with other companying evidence, such as co-occurrence between MeSH descriptors or Gene Ontology concepts and disease phenotypes in literature, to build disease gene associations from genomic and literature data sources, as seen in G2D (Genes to Diseases) tools [40,41].

4.3.3.2 *Fusion Approaches*

4.3.3.2.1 **Statistical Fusion**

The applications of statistical methods are theoretically advantageous to the integration of multiple heterogeneous data sources by providing a better understanding of the weight of each dataset as well as increasing the level of scalability. In these methods, each scale of data may be first normalized and then fed into a uniform statistical distribution. Optimal parameters of the statistical models are automatically learned from the observed datasets, as long as the considerable computational resources can be fulfilled.

The Bayesian model is the most frequently used statistical model in biomedical studies (see Chapter 8). It first estimates prior probabilities of a variable or a set of variables, such as a disease gene from each heterogeneous dataset, and then evaluates the posterior probabilities based on the prior probabilities and the weights among all datasets. Usually, it further defines the likelihood ratio of posterior probability and estimates its maximum value from the data. Simple *naïve* Bayesian integration has been exploited on eight genome-scale datasets and achieved best performance as compared to its alternatives, in which features of distinct heterogeneous datasets were assumed to be independent of one another for computational convenience. The prioritized genes were experimentally validated [42].

Aerts et al. demonstrated an interesting statistical approach for disease-gene prioritization [43]. In this approach, all evidence about candidate genes, no matter the type of sequence-based data (such as protein sequences, motifs, and domains), expression-based data (such as Expression Sequence Tags), functional annotations, interaction data, or literature-based evidence, were ranked independently within each scale. The rank of a candidate gene in each scale was then integrated and reordered by an order statistics, such as beta or gamma distribution, which inputs the individual ranks. The approach was applied for disease-gene prioritization with as many as 11 scales within this uniform, scalable framework; experimental validation confirmed the effectiveness of the approach [43].

Other statistical models have been applied to the integration of heterogeneous data and generation of hypotheses. For instance, a tri-modal Gaussian distribution has been used to model three different factors with respect to a disease phenotype: established associated factors, potential associated factors, and unassociated factors. The parameters of the tri-modal factors were derived from MeSH terms of literatures and expert knowledge. Of note, the model of potential associated factors was used to generate novel hypotheses [44].

4.3.3.2.2 **Mathematical Fusion**

Many mathematical methods can model multiple scales of data and generate hypotheses. The joint Non-negative Matrix Factorization (NMF), an ideal example, is a technique in which multiple heterogeneous data from the same sample are underlined by common factors, but possess different strengths. Mathematically, heterogeneous data are modeled as matrices with each matrix being projected onto a common space consisting of several orthogonal axes that correspond to the common factors among the multiple heterogeneous datasets. Consequently, various matrices are projected differently in the new factorized space and then naturally merged to allow pattern mining such as clustering analysis. Using this approach, heterogeneous modules/clusters were identified from cancer genomics data [45].

4.3.3.2.3 **Computational Fusion**

The most typical computational method in biomedical studies is machine learning, which includes classification and clustering. Kernel-based classification techniques, such as support vector machines, have been used for integrating heterogeneous data sources and predicting clinical outcome, potentially hypothesizing their most relevant features. In Kernel-based support vector machines, each dataset is studied separately to discover the optimal kernel. The kernels are then summed and optimized again as a whole by weighting each dataset [46,47].

Graphs and networks are sophisticated, computational data structures for knowledge presentation and discovery. Integration of all information from each heterogeneous data source into a uniform network opens a door for subsequent hypothesis generation based on the network topology. An integration approach between a protein-protein interaction network and known Alzheimer disease genes illustrated a straightforward and effective example for such an approach [48]. In this approach, candidate genes in the protein interaction network were ranked by their proximity to known disease genes; the more known genes a candidate was connected to, the more likely it was a novel candidate gene and thus was prioritized before others. Another example includes the integration of existing pharmacogenetic interactions with drug-target interactions and protein interactions to predict novel genes involved in the pharmacology of a target drug [49]. This generated a subnetwork for each candidate gene, which comprised all relevant interactions with respect to this gene: physical protein interactions; drugs targeting to the protein of the gene or its direct interacting proteins; and drugs whose pharmacology involved the protein or its direct interacting partners. The drug and all its treated indications were then compared to drugs and indications in this subnetwork for structure or topology similarities, resulting in the generation of four features for the candidate gene. Machine-learning methods were subsequently incorporated to measure the relevant genes based on the similarity features with a logistic regression model.

4.3.4 Multiple Comparison Adjustments, Empirical and Statistical Controls

After generating multiple hypotheses, the conventional way to address the multiplicity of comparisons is to conduct either *a posteriori* tests [50] or the more recent science of false discovery rate adjustments [51]. However, there is a concern with the type of statistic to use, either theoretical or empirical. Many theoretical statistics assume random or Gaussian distributions that are inherently anticonservative when considering biology or medicine. Indeed, a random pick of genes will find more protein interactions or more mRNA co-expression among them than expected by chance. We thus highly recommend empirical controls such as bootstraps or permutation resampling [52]. Often, when integrating multiple measurements at different scales, multiple empirical distributions are required to control a number of potential biases. Computational biology is converging with classical biology, as both require multiple controls. Sources of biases have to be conceptualized early on in the experimental design. For example, a gene may yield multiple proteins via alternate splicing. A protein interaction network may comprise these alternatively spliced variants of the genes as heterodimers of some protein complex. In other words, a single gene may create a bias in a sample of genes as it increases the probability of finding protein interactions between members of the sample. One has to address whether the biological significance of these complexes is required in the hypothesis generation. In the context of finding two proteins interacting in the same pathway among deregulated mRNAs, the above-mentioned protein complex is irrelevant and contributes to a statistical bias. In this case, the protein interaction could be represented as a gene interaction network, where single gene interactions are not allowed and adequately control the bias. The selection of appropriate controls may be essential, but it is not a straightforward task. For instance, with more accumulated electronic health records and cheaper sequencing technology, genome-wide association studies (GWAS) may be conducted automatically without manual selection of cases and controls as done in current fashion (see eMERGE project [6,53,54]).

4.4 APPLICATIONS IN MEDICINE AND PUBLIC HEALTH

Since the release of the human genome and the launch of microarray techniques in 2000, remarkable endeavors, focusing on *3% of the genomic sequences* that are protein coding, have identified disease genes for commonly occurring diseases, such as diabetes and cancer. Although single-scale studies led to validated hypotheses and discovery, numerous efforts were also reported for the integration of multiple scales of data for generating candidate disease genes, using either corroborative approaches for a small number of scales or in a fusion fashion extendable up to 11 scales [42,43]. In this decade, the publication of the ENCODE database that implicates *95% of the genomic sequences* in cellular processes [55] is expected to provide a paradigm shift beyond the protein coding focus and create more opportunities for integrative discovery for medicine than the last decade did.

With the emergence of genome-wide association studies (GWAS) for complex diseases in 2005, the pinpointing of disease loci was tackled with an unprecedented pace. Indeed, recent results from ENCODE projects show that approximately 80% of SNP variants identified by GWAS have a nearby functional element with high linkage disequilibrium, which profoundly facilitates a more concise location of the causing disease variants in the near future [56].

With the concurrent accumulation of electronic health records, GWAS can be conducted more efficiently through automatic generation of case and control cohorts from the large population size in voluminous repositories, which is currently under way by eMERGE consortium scientists [6,53,54]. This approach will prospectively increase the statistical power substantially while improving the population selection.

The physiology of complex diseases is not only an issue of polymorphism at a single nucleotide level but also with interplay of the variations. It comprises a cascade of perturbations as reflected in expression and interactions between variation elements in biological systems, along with modifications that are likely to be triggered from the environment. Investigation of a single scale only touches a facet of the complex system and therefore, requires highly demanding integrative studies. For instance, GWAS should be corroboratively studied with eQTLs (Expression Quantitative Trait Loci) to search for polymorphism with concordant expression variations [57]. Furthermore, other biological perturbations should be investigated, such as methylation [58]. The rapid accumulation of data from The Cancer Genome Atlas (TCGA) provides additional opportunities for identification of relevant biological elements simultaneously at multiple levels for cancer disorders and the capability to plot a comprehensive map of those interplayed elements that are often referred to as disease modules [45,59].

Even though the set of genes and their products associated to a disease may be unveiled, the underlying mechanisms often remain vague. Indeed, single gene diseases (Mendelian) are caused by a single gene defect and yet may have thousands of deregulated genes downstream involving multiple cell types, organs, and systems. Complex disease genes are obviously far more complicated. For example, little is known about the functions of the SNPs identified by GWAS at this point in time and there remains a heritability gap: the sum of the odds ratio remains low and explains a fraction of the disease's inheritance (often less than 5–10%) [60]. Integrative studies or hypotheses, such as extracting relevant pathways and biological and clinic features from literatures, are still necessary to reveal the mechanisms of the complex biological system, which underline the physiology of complex diseases.

Apart from disease causing genes and biological mechanisms, the identification of biomarkers for disease's early diagnosis, prognosis, and response to therapy is also an integrative mission [61]. Over the last decade, clinical outcome classifiers derived from genomic assays proceeded from single biological scale measurements to corroboration and then fusion of multiple measurements from distinct biological scales involving heterogeneous datasets [8]. Alternative multiscale analyses were developed to discover single molecule biomarkers (e.g., SNP, DNA expression, and proteomics) [61]. Meanwhile, the pharmacogenetics studies have deepened the understanding of drug metabolism and shed light on the discovery of new biomarkers for response to therapy [49]. Again, this is not an easy, efficient task without overseeing multiple relevant scales of data.

Integrative hypothesis generation from large-scale data and effective experimental validation will accelerate the pursuit of personalized, predictive, preventive, and participatory medicine (P4 medicine [62]; see Chapter 11) in the next few decades. By exploiting multiple scales of biology and their interactions, the most relevant polymorphisms, including personalized rare variants [63], are to be identified as the keys of drug responser for the best medicine with optimal outcome. Furthermore, through (i) the investigation of the biological mechanisms, (ii) the interplay among multiple scales [64,65], (iii) the interactions with environments, and (iv) the perturbation of biological polymorphisms on each level, the risk of particular diseases is anticipated to be accurately predicted and managed with preventive medicine or changing of lifestyles. Finally, the integration of electronic health records and biological repositories with the collaborative efforts between health care providers and patients will facilitate the goal of preventive and participatory medicine. Taken together, integration of multiple heterogeneous information for a comprehensive roadmap is essential for the implementation of P4 medicine.

4.5 SUMMARY

This chapter reviewed the requirements of conducting discovery science across legion-size datasets spanning many biological scales. The revolution of high-throughput biotechniques and the opportunities for translational research resulting from these developments and data-driven projects have fostered the strong demand for integration of heterogenous data and generation of hypotheses, as well as big data processing approaches. We proceed by dividing this problem into representation and integration of heterogeneous datasets. We also describe *modeling* approaches to limit the consequent geometric explosion of hypotheses: simplifying hypotheses, ontological classification, and filtering of undiscriminating features (e.g., underpowered or low quality measurements, machine-learning feature reduction, and relevance testing). In brief, the integration of these data sources experienced an era of disease-gene/loci prioritization, disease module and mechanism pinpointing, and biomarker discovery for outcome analysis. The underlying methodologies range from corroborative analysis of a few scales to seamlessly fusion of a large number of scales, covering almost the entire spectra of biological and biomedical data. A salient problem associated with discovery science is the reproducibility of experiments. In this chapter, we have provided an explicit framework to systematically implement computational experiments that prioritize hypotheses across heterogeneous datasets with the hope that with better formalisms, documentation, and implementation, these can be more easily and rapidly reproduced (e.g., in a cloud virtual environment).

ACKNOWLEDGMENTS

The authors appreciate critical comments from Dr. Ikbel Achour and Ms. Colleen Kenost.

REFERENCES

[1] International Human Genome Sequencing Consortium. Initial sequencing and analysis of the human genome. Nature 2001;409:860–921.

[2] Turnbaugh PJ, Ley RE, Hamady M, Fraser-Liggett CM, Knight R, Gordon JI. The human microbiome project. Nature 2007;449:804–10.

[3] The ENCODE Project Consortium. An integrated encyclopedia of DNA elements in the human genome. Nature 2012;489:57–74.

[4] The International Cancer Genome Consortium. International network of cancer genome projects. Nature 2010;464:993–8.

[5] Giallourakis C, Henson C, Reich M, Xie X, Mootha VK. Disease gene discovery through integrative genomics. Ann Rev Genomics Hum Genetics 2005;6:381–406.

[6] Kho AN, Pacheco JA, Peissig PL, Rasmussen L, Newton KM, Weston N, et al. Electronic medical records for genetic research: results of the eMERGE consortium. Sci Trans Med 2011;3.79re1.

[7] Hawkins RD, Hon GC, Ren B. Next-generation genomics: an integrative approach. Nat Rev Genet 2010;11:476–86.

[8] Lussier YA, Li H. Breakthroughs in genomics data integration for predicting clinical outcome. J Biomed Inform 2012;45:1199–201.

[9] Crick FH. On protein synthesis. Symp Soc Exper Biol 1958;12:138–63.

[10] Crick F. Central dogma of molecular biology. Nature 1970;227:561-3.

[11] Blois MS. Information and medicine: the nature of medical descriptions. University of California Press; 1984.

[12] Lussier YA, Chen JL. The emergence of genome-based drug repositioning. Sci Trans Med 2011;3.96ps35.

[13] Friedman C, Shagina L, Lussier Y, Hripcsak G. Automated encoding of clinical documents based on natural language processing. J Am Med Inform Assoc 2004;11:392–402.

[14] Aronson AR. Effective mapping of biomedical text to the UMLS Metathesaurus: the MetaMap program. AMIA Annu Symp Proc 2001:17–21.

[15] Savova GK, Masanz JJ, Ogren PV, Zheng J, Sohn S, Kipper-Schuler KC, et al. Mayo clinical text analysis and knowledge extraction system (cTAKES): architecture, component evaluation and applications. J Am Med Inform Assoc 2010;17:507–13.

[16] Jensen PB, Jensen LJ, Brunak S. Mining electronic health records: towards better research applications and clinical care. Nat Rev Genet 2012;13:395–405.

[17] Jensen LJ, Saric J, Bork P. Literature mining for the biologist: from information retrieval to biological discovery. Nat Rev Genet 2006;7:119–29.

[18] Zhang W, Duan S, Kistner EO, Bleibel WK, Huang RS, Clark TA, et al. Evaluation of genetic variation contributing to differences in gene expression between populations. Am J Hum Genet 2008;82:631–40.

[19] Perez-Rathke A, Li H , Lussier YA. Interpreting personal transcriptomes: personalized mechanism-scale profiling of RNA-Seq data. Pacific symposium of biocomputing, Hawaii; 2013. p. 159–70.

[20] Zhu J, Sova P, Xu Q, Dombek KM, Xu EY, Vu H, et al. Stitching together multiple data dimensions reveals interacting metabolomic and transcriptomic networks that modulate cell regulation. PLoS Biol 2012;10:e1001301.

[21] Beyer K, Goldstein J, Ramakrishnan R, Shaft U. When is nearest neighbor meaningful? Database Theory ICDT'99 1999:217–35.

[22] Saeys Y, Inza I, Larrañaga P. A review of feature selection techniques in bioinformatics. Bioinformatics 2007;23:2507–17.

[23] Liu Y, Li J, Sam L, Goh C-S, Gerstein M, Lussier YA. An integrative genomic approach to uncover molecular mechanisms of prokaryotic traits. PLoS Comput Biol 2006;2:e159.

[24] Tao Y, Sam L, Li J, Friedman C, Lussier YA. Information theory applied to the sparse gene ontology annotation network to predict novel gene function. Bioinformatics 2007;23:i529–38.

[25] Cantor MN, Sarkar IN, Bodenreider O, Lussier YA. Genestrace: phenomic knowledge discovery via structured terminology. Pac Symp Biocomput. NIH Public Access; 2005. p. 103.

[26] Lussier YA, Rothwell DJ, Côté RA. The SNOMED model: a knowledge source for the controlled terminology of the computerized patient record. Method inform med 1998;37:161–4.

[27] Wang Y-P, Li K-B. Correlation of expression profiles between microRNAs and mRNA targets using NCI-60 data. BMC Genomics 2009;10:218.

[28] Tiffin N, Kelso JF, Powell AR, Pan H, Bajic VB, Hide WA. Integration of text- and data-mining using ontologies successfully selects disease gene candidates. Nucleic Acids Res 2005;33:1544–52.

[29] Chen R, Davydov EV, Sirota M, Butte AJ. non-synonymous and synonymous coding SNPs show similar likelihood and effect size of human disease association. PLoS ONE 2010;5:e13574.

[30] CDC, National health and nutrition examination survey. In: (CDC) CfDCaP, editor. Atlanta, GA; 2009.

[31] Patel CJ, Chen R, Butte AJ. Data-driven integration of epidemiological and toxicological data to select candidate interacting genes and environmental factors in association with disease. Bioinformatics 2012;28:i121–6.

[32] Goh C-S, Gianoulis T, Liu Y, Li J, Paccanaro A, Lussier Y, et al. Integration of curated databases to identify genotype-phenotype associations. BMC Genomics 2006;7:257.

[33] Perfilieva I, Močkoč J. Mathematical principles of fuzzy logic. Springer; 1999.

[34] Yaguinuma CA, Afonso GF, Ferraz V, Borges S, Santos MTP. A fuzzy ontology-based semantic data integration system. J Inform Knowl Manag 2011;10:285–99.

[35] Lee Y, Li J, Gamazon E, Chen JL, Tikhomirov A, Cox NJ, et al. Biomolecular systems of disease buried across multiple GWAS unveiled by information theory and ontology. AMIA Summits Transl Sci Proc 2010;2010:31.

[36] Sirota M, Dudley JT, Kim J, Chiang AP, Morgan AA, Sweet-Cordero A, et al. Discovery and preclinical validation of drug indications using compendia of public gene expression data. Sci Transl Med 2011;3.96ra77.

[37] Korbel JO, Doerks T, Jensen LJ, Perez-Iratxeta C, Kaczanowski S, Hooper SD, et al. Systematic association of genes to phenotypes by genome and literature mining. PLoS Biol 2005;3:e134.

[38] Li H, Lee Y, Chen JL, Rebman E, Li J, Lussier YA. Complex-disease networks of trait-associated single-nucleotide polymorphisms (SNPs) unveiled by information theory. J Am Med Inform Assoc 2012;19:295–305.

[39] Suthram S, Dudley JT, Chiang AP, Chen R, Hastie TJ, Butte AJ. network-based elucidation of human disease similarities reveals common functional modules enriched for pluripotent drug targets. PLoS Comput Biol 2010;6:e1000662.

[40] Perez-Iratxeta C, Wjst M, Bork P, Andrade M. G2D: a tool for mining genes associated with disease. BMC Genetics 2005;6:45.

[41] Perez-Iratxeta C, Bork P, Andrade MA. Association of genes to genetically inherited diseases using data mining. Nat Genet 2002;31:316–9.

[42] Calvo S, Jain M, Xie X, Sheth SA, Chang B, Goldberger OA, et al. Systematic identification of human mitochondrial disease genes through integrative genomics. Nat Genet 2006;38:576–82.

[43] Aerts S, Lambrechts D, Maity S, Van Loo P, Coessens B, De Smet F, et al. Gene prioritization through genomic data fusion. Nat Biotech 2006;24:537–44.

[44] Abedi V, Zand R, Yeasin M, Faisal F. An automated framework for hypotheses generation using literature. BioData Mining 2012;5:13.

[45] Zhang S, Liu C-C, Li W, Shen H, Laird PW, Zhou XJ. Discovery of multi-dimensional modules by integrative analysis of cancer genomic data. Nucleic Acids Res 2012;40:9379–91.

[46] Lanckriet GRG, De Bie T, Cristianini N, Jordan MI, Noble WS. A statistical framework for genomic data fusion. Bioinformatics 2004;20:2626–35.

[47] Daemen A, Gevaert O, Ojeda F, Debucquoy A, Suykens J, Sempoux C, et al. A kernel-based integration of genome-wide data for clinical decision support. Genome Med 2009;1:39.

[48] Krauthammer M, Kaufmann CA, Gilliam TC, Rzhetsky A. Molecular triangulation: Bridging linkage and molecular-network information for identifying candidate genes in Alzheimer's disease. Proc Natl Acad Sci USA 2004;101:15148–53.

[49] Hansen NT, Brunak S, Altman RB. Generating genome-scale candidate gene lists for pharmacogenomics. Clin Pharmacol Ther 2009;86:183–9.

[50] Sokal RR, Rohlf FJ. Biometry: the principles and practice of statistics in biological research. New York: WH Freeman; 1995. p. 887.

[51] Benjamini Y, Yekutieli D. The control of the false discovery rate in multiple testing under dependency. Ann Stat 2001:1165–88.

[52] Westfall PH, Young SS. Resampling-based multiple testing: examples and methods for p-value adjustment. Wiley-Interscience; 1993.

[53] Ritchie MD, Denny JC, Crawford DC, Ramirez AH, Weiner JB, Pulley JM, et al. Robust replication of genotype-phenotype associations across multiple diseases in an electronic medical record. Am J Hum Genet 2010;86:560–72.

[54] Denny JC, Ritchie MD, Basford MA, Pulley JM, Bastarache L, Brown-Gentry K, et al. PheWAS: demonstrating the feasibility of a phenome-wide scan to discover gene-disease associations. Bioinformatics 2010;26:1205–10.

[55] Khatun J. An integrated encyclopedia of DNA elements in the human genome. Nature 2012.

[56] Schaub MA, Boyle AP, Kundaje A, Batzoglou S, Snyder M. Linking disease associations with regulatory information in the human genome. Genome Res 2012;22:1748–59.

[57] Boyle AP, Hong EL, Hariharan M, Cheng Y, Schaub MA, Kasowski M, et al. Annotation of functional variation in personal genomes using RegulomeDB. Genome Res 2012;22:1790–7.

[58] Baranzini SE, Mudge J, van Velkinburgh JC, Khankhanian P, Khrebtukova I, Miller NA, et al. Genome, epigenome and RNA sequences of monozygotic twins discordant for multiple sclerosis. Nature 2010;464:1351–6.

[59] Kristensen VN, Vaske CJ, Ursini-Siegel J, Van Loo P, Nordgard SH, Sachidanandam R, et al. Integrated molecular profiles of invasive breast tumors and ductal carcinoma in situ (DCIS) reveal differential vascular and interleukin signaling. Proc Natl Acad Sci 2012;109:2802–7.

[60] Quigley E. Epigenetics: filling in the 'heritability gap' and identifying gene-environment interactions in ulcerative colitis. Genome Med 2012;4:72.

[61] Kulasingam V, Pavlou MP, Diamandis EP. Integrating high-throughput technologies in the quest for effective biomarkers for ovarian cancer. Nat Rev Cancer 2010;10:371–8.

[62] Hood L, Friend SH. Predictive, personalized, preventive, participatory (P4) cancer medicine. Nat Rev Clin Oncol 2011;8:184–7.

[63] Regan K, Wang K, Doughty E, Li H, Li J, Lee Y, et al. Translating Mendelian and complex inheritance of Alzheimer's disease genes for predicting unique personal genome variants. J Am Med Inform Assoc 2012;19:306–16.

[64] Lee Y, Li H, Li J, Rebman E, Achour I, Regan KE, et al. Network models of genome-wide association studies uncover the topological centrality of protein interactions in complex diseases. J Am Med Inform Assoc 2013.

[65] Wang X, Wei X, Thijssen B, Das J, Lipkin SM, Yu H. Three-dimensional reconstruction of protein networks provides insight into human genetic disease. Nat Biotech 2012;30:159–64.

Geometric Representations in Biomedical Informatics: Applications in Automated Text Analysis

Trevor Cohen[a] and Dominic Widdows[b]

[a]*University of Texas School of Biomedical Informatics at Houston. Houston, TX, USA*
[b]*Microsoft Bing, Serendipity, Palo Alto, CA, USA*

CHAPTER OUTLINE

5.1 INTRODUCTION

In this chapter, we discuss ways in which biomedical data can be represented in high-dimensional space, for the purpose of information retrieval, exploration, or classification. Representations of this nature provide natural ways to measure similarity, or relatedness, between entities of interest in an efficient manner. Once two entities are represented in geometric space, their relatedness can be measured using distance metrics, without the need to consider their individual components.

The mathematical basis for these ideas has developed gradually over the past two centuries: as well as the development of metric spaces in the abstract [1], concepts in analytic coordinate geometry have been represented more succinctly in algebraic geometry (in which surfaces are defined as sets of points that are solutions of algebraic equations), and in topology (which considers properties that remain the same whatever coordinate systems are used) [2, Chapter 28]. Such methods are appealing in cognitive science for theoretical reasons: there is now a rich body of work documenting the role of similarity judgments in human cognition [3], and the proposal has been raised that geometric representations mediate fundamental mechanisms of thought such as the categorization of concepts [4]. The ability to measure similarity holistically, without the need for decomposition to compare the number of common features explicitly, is also desirable for practical reasons, as relatedness can be measured efficiently and directly.

As well as similarity (or relevance), geometric representations have been used successfully to model logical connectives like OR and NOT [5], conditionals and implication [6], and eventually any well-defined semantic relationship [7].

5.2 THE NATURE OF GEOMETRIC REPRESENTATIONS

Search engines using geometric models came to the forefront as early as the 1970s [8], and by the 1990s the "vector space model" had become one of the three standard models for information retrieval, alongside Boolean and probabilistic models [9]. Vector space representations make it easy to measure and rank similarities between terms and documents, and use superposition (that is, coordinatewise addition) to combine individual term-vectors into query statements that can be used to retrieve documents quickly and reliably from a large collection.

5.2.1 **Vectors and Vector Spaces**

Vectors can be thought of as an approach to storing different sorts of information that relates to the same concept or object. For example, a patient with the patient identifier 011539; a Hemoglobin (Hb) of 9 g/dl and a Mean Corpuscular Volume (MCV) of 64 fL could be represented by concisely as the following vector:

011539	9	64

Each value in the vector corresponds to one of the test results. However, this vector also has a geometric interpretation, illustrated in Figure 5.1, in which the vector representing patient 011539 is plotted against a set of axes representing each of the categories of values in the vector. Interpreting the vector this way suggests regions of the resulting vector space that correspond to particular physiological conditions. For example, we would anticipate the vicinity of the vector represented being occupied by vectors of patients afflicted with types of anemia that are characterized by a decrease in the size of red blood cells, such as iron deficiency anemia. While we have elected to represent this patient as a vector, we could as easily have plotted this patient as a point in space, the point at the tip of the arrow representing this vector. Representations of this sort, albeit at higher dimensionality, have been used as a means to represent large volumes of physiological data that are measured in ICU settings (see for example [10]).

Note that this vector is the sum of its component vectors in each axis. The Hb value alone would be represented as the vector (9,0), and similarly the MCV vector would be (0,64). Vector addition is accomplished by adding the values in each dimension, and has a physical interpretation that corresponds to a journey in the plane across each of the component vectors in succession, as illustrated in Figure 5.2.

This simple process of addition, which is a form of superposition, is commonly applied as a method of vector composition, such that composite

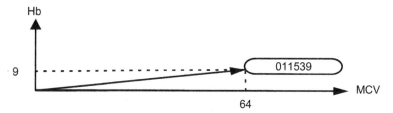

■ **FIGURE 5.1** A patient vector in a two-dimensional physiological space.

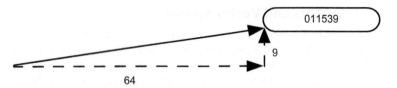

■ **FIGURE 5.2**   Generation of the vector for patient 011539 by adding its component vectors.

representations can be built up from atomic data points. For example, physiologically based vector representations of patients with a particular clinical condition could be superposed to generate a summary representation of patients with that condition. Once generated, this composite representation could be used to measure the similarity between the physiological state of a new patient, and summary representations for clinical conditions of interest, in an attempt to infer the diagnosis of this patient.

5.2.2 **Distance Metrics**

In order to draw useful inferences from geometric representations, it is necessary to define a distance metric that can be used to measure the relatedness between them. Commonly used approaches include the measurement of the distance between coordinate representations using the Euclidean or city block distance metrics, and the measurement of the distance between vector representations using the cosine distance.

The city block metric measures the sum of the absolute differences between the values of two points on each of the coordinate axes in the space. This metric is also known as the "Manhattan distance," on account of the grid-like layout of much of New York City. For example to get from the corner of 24th Street and 8th Avenue to the corner of 11th Street and 7th Avenue requires walking a distance of 14 city blocks (13 streets and 1 avenue)—it is only possible to travel along the north-south or the east-west lines as the areas in between the streets and avenues are occupied by buildings. Represented symbolically in two dimensions, $D_{cityblock} = abs(X_1 - X_2) + abs(Y_1 - Y_2)$. This formula can be extended to accommodate any number of dimensions, as is the case with all of the formulae we introduce in this chapter. Coordinate geometry was developed to represent intuitive spatial concepts in up to three dimensions. Going beyond three, we lose the correspondence between coordinate representations and intuitive physical experience, but for the basic processes of coordinatewise addition and multiplication that underlie these formulae, this does not matter.

Euclidean distance measures the length of a line drawn between two points in space, and as such corresponds to the intuitive notion of the shortest distance between these two points. The calculation of the Euclidean distance between two points in a geometric space is based on Pythagoras' theorem, which states that in a right-angled triangle the square of the length of the hypotenuse is equal to the sum of the squares of the lengths of the other two sides. In two dimensions, the length of the line joining two points in space is equal to the square root of the sum of the squares of the distances between their x and y coordinates (as depicted in Figure 5.3), so $D_{euclidean} = \sqrt{(Y_1 - Y_2)^2 + (X_1 - X_2)^2}$. As was the case with the city block metric, this formula can be extended to accommodate vectors of more than two dimensions.

The cosine metric is commonly employed as a measure of the similarity between two vectors. It is called the cosine metric as it calculates the cosine of the angle between the two vectors concerned. However, it is not necessary to explicitly measure this angle in order to calculate the cosine metric. Rather, this is calculated based on the proportion of one vector that can be projected on another. This is illustrated geometrically in Figure 5.3, and is relatively straightforward to calculate algebraically as it corresponds to the scalar product between two normalized vectors (i.e., vectors of unit length). So, calculating the cosine metric requires the normalization of the vectors concerned, which is accomplished by dividing every dimension of a vector by the length (or norm) of this vector. Subsequently, rather than representing an absolute value, each dimension represents its proportional contribution to the total length of the original vector, and as this procedure is applied to both vectors they can be compared with one another on the basis of their orientation without taking their magnitude into account. The norm (or length) of a vector V_1, $|V_1|$, is the Euclidean distance traveled from the origin to its tip. In two dimensions this would be $\sqrt{Y^2 + X^2}$. The scalar (or dot) product of two vectors V and W, $V \cdot W$, is calculated

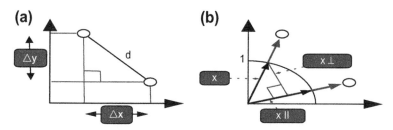

■ **FIGURE 5.3** Illustrations of the Euclidean/city block (a) and cosine (b) distance metrics.

by multiplying their values in each dimension, and summing together the results. The formulae we have discussed so far are presented in their general (n-dimensional) form below:

$$cityblock(V, W) = \sum_{i=1}^{n} abs(V_i - W_i) \qquad (5.1)$$

$$euclidean(V, W) = \sqrt{\sum_{i=1}^{n} (V_i - W_i)^2} \qquad (5.2)$$

$$V \cdot W = \sum_{i=1}^{n} V_i \times W_i \qquad (5.3)$$

$$|V| = \sqrt{\sum_{i=1}^{n} V_i^2} \qquad (5.4)$$

$$cosine(V, W) = \frac{V \cdot W}{|V||W|} \qquad (5.5)$$

Figure 5.3a illustrates the application of the city block and Euclidean distance metrics to measure the distance between two points in space. The city block distance is the sum of the differences between the coordinate values of the two points on each axis ($\Delta y + \Delta x$). The Euclidean distance is the length of the line "d" that joins the two points, which is the square root of the sum of the squares of these differences, $\sqrt{\Delta y^2 + \Delta x^2}$.

Figure 5.3b illustrates the application of the cosine metric to measure the similarity between vector representations of these two points. This metric uses the cosine of the angle between two vectors as a measure of their relatedness. The cosine metric is calculated based on normalized vectors of unit length, as illustrated in the figure, where the vectors have been truncated at the perimeter of the unit circle. In the figure, the vector x is decomposed into two component vectors, one parallel to ($x \parallel$), and one perpendicular to ($x \perp$) the other vector in the figure. By definition, the cosine of an angle is the ratio of the length of the adjacent side to the length of the hypotenuse. So one way to think about this metric is that it measures the proportion of one vector that is represented by its projection on another ($\frac{x\parallel}{x}$).

If we are willing to accept the conjecture that aspects of the meaning of a term, concept, query, or document can be captured by a vector representation; then it follows that the cosine metric measures the proportion of the "meaning" of one of these items that is represented by another.

5.2.3 Examples: Term, Concept, and Document Vectors

For example, consider the small document collection below:

- Document 1:   {diabetes mellitus}
- Document 2:   {diabetes insipidus}

These documents concern two clinical conditions, both of which contain the term "diabetes" in their name. The first of these, "diabetes mellitus," describes a set of conditions in which a defect in insulin metabolism results in elevated blood glucose. In contrast, "diabetes insipidus" describes a condition in which the kidneys are unable to conserve water. The term "diabetes" refers to the excessive output of urine that is a characteristic symptom of all of these disorders.

There are three unique terms in this document set. A common approach to representing the documents in a set with respect to the terms they contain is to construct a document-by-term matrix, in which each row represents a document, and each column represents a term, with each cell in the matrix representing the number of times a particular term occurs in a particular document, or some statistical transformation thereof. In our case, the document-by-term matrix is constructed as shown in Table 5.1.

From a geometric perspective, each column of the matrix can be considered as an independent axis, such that the documents can be represented as coordinates (Figure 5.4 left), or vectors (Figure 5.4 right) in a "term space" with x (diabetes), y (mellitus), and z (insipidus) axes. Representing documents in this manner enables us to use the distance between them as a measure of the relatedness between documents. Furthermore, given a user query, such as "diabetes," it is possible to measure the relatedness between this query

Table 5.1   Document-by-term matrix.

	Diabetes	Mellitus	Insipidus
Document 1	1	1	0
Document 2	1	0	1

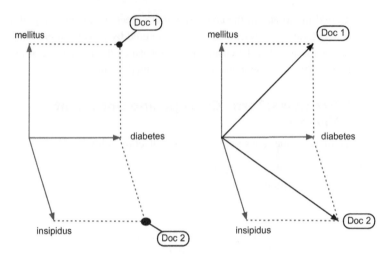

■ **FIGURE 5.4** Coordinate (left) and vector (right) representations of the two documents in term space.

and the documents in a collection to facilitate retrieval of those documents composed of similar terms to the query. These representations of documents and queries underlie the widely used "vector space model" of information retrieval [8].

Similarly, it is possible to represent the terms in a document collection in "document space," in which position is determined by the frequency with which these terms occur in each document in the collection (Figure 5.5). Consequently, terms that occur in the same contexts will have similar vector representations. The derivation of estimates of the relatedness between terms from the contexts in which they occur across a large set of documents is a fundamental concern of the field of *distributional semantics* [11,12], and the estimates so derived have been shown to correspond to human performance on a number of cognitive tasks [13,14].

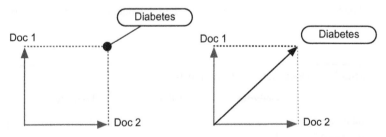

■ **FIGURE 5.5** (left) and (right) vector representations of the term "diabetes" in document space.

The definition of what constitutes a context varies from model to model. For example, in some approaches (for example [14,15]), individual documents are considered as contextual units, while in others (for example [13,16]), terms that co-occur within a fixed distance from the term of interest are considered to represent context. Models of this nature are generated by moving a sliding window through the corpus concerned. Sliding-window based models tend to emphasize synonymy (particularly with narrow windows), while term-document based models are less constrained with respect to the type of relatedness they measure [17]. This difference is illustrated in Table 5.2, which shows the nearest neighboring terms to a set of cue terms in a pair of distributional models derived from MEDLINE. With the narrow sliding-window model, the terms tend to be of the same class as the cue term. For example, the neighbors of the term "haloperidol," an antipsychotic agent, are also antipsychotic agents with the exception of domperidone, which acts by antagonizing the action of dopamine, a mechanism shared by many antipsychotic agents. While the neighbors of "haloperidol" in the term-document space do include the antipsychotic agent olanzapine (and the term "antipsychotic"), terms that are more generally related to haloperidol such as schizophrenia (a disease it is used to treat) are also included.

A similar approach can be applied to measure the relatedness between concepts defined in a controlled vocabulary, as illustrated in Figure 5.6, which shows the nearest neighboring concept vectors to the concept vector for

Table 5.2 Nearest neighbors of terms in sliding-window and term-document spaces derived from MEDLINE using Random Indexing.

Cue Term	Sliding Window	Term Document
Diabetes	Diabete; iddm; niddm; diabets; iidm	Mellitus; diabetic; nhv; glycemic; nondiabetic
Haloperidol	Sulpiride; pimozide; domperidone; amperozide; butaclamol	Schizophrenia; olanzapine; dopamine; antipsychotic; gsti
Streptococcus	Diplococcus; klebsiella; streptoccocus; streptococus; prsp	Pneumoniae; mutans; pyogenes; sanguis; mitis
Appendectomy	Appendicectomy; cholecystectomy; appendectomies; cholecystectomies; refunoplication	Appendicitis; appendectomies; appendix; methoxypolyethyleneglycol; adsom
Obesity	Dyslipidimeias; dyslipedima; dyslipemias; dyslipemia	Obese; bmi; overweight; waist; dyslipidemia

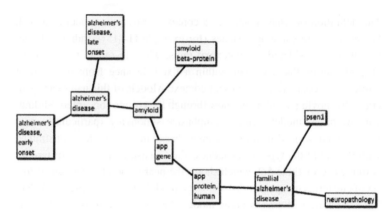

■ **FIGURE 5.6** Nearest neighboring concept vectors to the concept vector for "Alzheimer's disease," arranged using Pathfinder network scaling [22] and the Prefuse Flare visualization library [23].

the concept vector representing Alzheimer's disease. In this case, distributional information concerning concepts from the Unified Medical Language System [18], extracted from MEDLINE citations using MetaMap [19,20], was used to build the model. As was the case with the examples in Table 5.2, concept vectors were generated using a variant of Random Indexing [21], an approach we will discuss in detail later in the chapter.

5.2.4 **Term-Weighting**

There are many variants of these approaches to term and document representation. For example, in the generation of document vectors it is common to use a statistical approach to weight the contribution of each term to the document vector, in an attempt to capture the effect of differences in local term frequency (*local weighting*) and attempt to emphasize the contribution of more meaningful terms by favoring those that occur focally in the corpus (*global weighting*). This is an important consideration, as not all terms are equal with respect to the meaning they carry. Consider, for example, the set of terms {if, then, and, but}. These terms occur ubiquitously in language, but don't contribute much in the way of searchable content to the contexts in which they occur. There are two fundamental approaches to this problem. The first is a stopword list, a list of terms that should be ignored for indexing purposes. For example, PubMed uses a stopword list for word-based indexing of MEDLINE articles. The second involves weighting words, such that words that are more informative contribute more to the representation of the meaning of a document. One commonly used weighting metric is the TF-IDF approach, which stands for Term Frequency - Inverse Document Frequency. This approach has two components: a local weighting (term frequency) and a global weighting (inverse document frequency). Local weighting (TF) attempts to capture the extent to which a particular term contributes to the meaning of a particular document, and in this case is simply the count of the number of times this term occurs in the document. Global weighting (IDF) represents the extent to which a particular term can be used to distinguish between the meaning of documents in a large set. For example, near-ubiquitous terms such as "if" and "but" should have a lower global weight than infrequent terms such as "platypus." The IDF of a term is calculated as follows:

$$\text{IDF}(\text{term}) = \log \left(\frac{\text{number of documents in corpus}}{\text{number of documents containing term}} \right)$$

(5.6)

Consider the IDF weights and term frequencies of the terms in Table 5.3, which are derived from the widely studied OHSUMED corpus [24] of around 350,000 titles and abstracts extracted from MEDLINE, a large database of citations from the biomedical literature. Terms that occur infrequently, such as "insipidus," are weighted more heavily than terms that occur relatively frequently, such as "diabetes." Consequently, the geometric representation of the second document in our set would be positioned closer to the axis representing "insipidus" than to the axis representing "diabetes."

5.2.5 Example: Literature-Based Discovery

The field of literature-based discovery (LBD) originated with the serendipitous discovery by information scientist Don Swanson of a therapeutic association between Raynaud's phenomenon (poor circulation in the peripheries) and fish oils [25,26]. This discovery was made on the basis of an implicit association between fish oils and Raynaud's: no publication existed at the time in which these concepts appeared together, but

Table 5.3 Document-by-term matrix. Doc Freq = number of documents term occurs in. Tot Freq = total number of occurrences of term (which may occur multiple times in a given document).

Term	Doc Freq	Total Freq	IDF
The	257,644	2,030,747	0.13
Patient	37,269	52,989	0.97
Diabetes	4692	8780	1.87
Mellitus	2241	2804	2.19
Insipidus	164	259	3.33

they both appeared with certain *bridging concepts*, such as *blood viscosity* and *platelet function*. As geometric models of the meaning of terms aim to identify implicit connections between terms that occur in the context of similar other terms, they are a natural fit for this problem and several authors have attempted to use models of this sort to facilitate LBD [27–29]. It is possible to reproduce aspects of Swanson's initial discovery using such methods.

For example, Table 5.4 below shows the *nearest indirect neighbors* of the term "Raynaud," those terms with vector representations most similar to this term in the pool of terms that do not co-occur with it directly, in a geometric space derived from a set of around 190,000 MEDLINE titles from core clinical journals from the same time period as the set of titles Swanson used for his seminal discovery (1980–1985). The model was generated using Random Indexing, a technique that we will subsequently discuss, using a narrow sliding window with a stoplist and IDF weighting. The term "eicosapentaenoic," which represents eicosapentaenoic acid, the active ingredient of fish oils, is the fourth nearest indirect neighbor of the term "Raynaud." While subtle variations in the results of Random Indexing experiments are anticipated across runs on account of the stochastic nature of this technique, "eicosapentaenoic" reliably occurs in the top five neighbors when these parameters are used [28]. However, there is no guarantee that the parameters that reproduce this discovery will necessarily be the best parameters to use in another situation. What is by now clear is that geometric models are able to derive meaningful implicit associations between terms and concepts, but that these associations do not necessarily indicate potential discoveries. Consequently, recent work in LBD has leveraged advances in Natural Language Processing to identify the nature of the relationships between concepts to selectively identify plausible therapeutic and explanatory hypotheses [30–33].

Table 5.4 Nearest indirect neighbors of term "Raynaud." The term "eicosapentaenoic" represents eicosapentaenoic acid, the active ingredient of fish oils.

Rank	Term	Cosine
1	Terminals	0.39
2	Preeclamptic	0.33
3	Prinzmetal	0.28
4	Eicosapentaenoic	0.26
5	Hydralazine	0.25

5.2.6 **Summary and Implications**

In this section, we discussed ways in which data points can be projected into a geometric space, to enable the relatedness between these data points to be measured on the basis of the similarity between their vector representations. Once derived, these measures of relatedness can be applied for other purposes. For example, a meaningful measure of the relatedness between data points can mediate the classification of these data points. A relatively straightforward approach to classification is the *k-nearest neighbor* approach (discussed further in Section 5.4.1), in which a new data point is assigned labels that have been applied previously to its nearest neighbors in geometric space. This simple approach has been use to accomplish automated indexing of biomedical text [34,35] and automated grading of content-based essays [14], and presents a robust baseline for comparison against more sophisticated methods (for example [36]). While we have provided examples to do with text processing, the methods concerned are applicable to any dataset that can be numerically represented. For example, vector representations of diseases based on genomic sequence information concerning associated genes have been used to identify disease-disease relationships [37], and vector representations of protein sequences based on their functional properties have been used to predict their cellular location [38].

5.3 **DIMENSION REDUCTION**

As mentioned previously, once we move into spaces of higher dimensionality, we lose the intuitive correspondence between the human perceptual experience of existence in a three-dimensional world, while retaining a set of abstract mathematical operations that can be applied in spaces of any dimensionality. However, spaces of higher dimensionality carry computational consequences. A self-evident consequence of larger spaces is that they will require more disk space. Oftentimes it is desirable to retain all of the vectors in RAM so as to facilitate rapid search, which places a far more severe constraint on the number of dimensions that can be stored. Furthermore, the computational cost of comparing vectors to one another is proportional to the dimensionality of the space, as the distance metrics we have discussed involve pairwise comparisons across all dimension of the space.

On account of these computational concerns, it is often desirable to generate a reduced-dimensional approximation of a geometric space for convenient search and storage. In addition, with certain methods of dimension reduction, the approximation of the original space is constructed in such a way that it preserves as much of the variance (a concept we will introduce shortly) of the original dataset as possible, revealing patterns of association between data points that may otherwise be difficult to detect. Thus, while some of the *computational* improvements can be made using relatively simple sparse-matrix representations, dimension reduction techniques are also popular because they provide *semantic* improvements in some applications. For this reason, distributional models built using dimension reduction techniques have been applied to several language-related tasks that are of interest to biomedical informatics, including word learning and synonym detection [14,21], word sense discrimination [39,40], document summarization and segmentation, and cross-lingual search [41].

Given the range of techniques and applications, this area has become an enormous topic since the 1990s. Here we will give a necessarily brief overview of three main variants: Latent Semantic Analysis [42] (a name for methods that use Singular Value Decomposition [43]), Topic Models (a name for methods that use Latent Dirichlet Allocation) [44–46], and Random Indexing [47,21], which originates from Random Projection [48–50]. Many of these methods for generating a reduced-dimensional approximation are themselves computationally expensive, making them applicable mainly for smaller datasets and datasets that change relatively infrequently. In general, when choosing an approach, researchers and developers should consider several tradeoffs between semantic accuracy and computational cost over the lifetime of the system in question.

5.3.1 Approaches—Latent Semantic Analysis Using SVD

Singular Value Decomposition is an example of a relatively computationally demanding approach that optimally preserves variance. Consider the three sets of axes and coordinates in Figure 5.7. *Variance* is a measure of spread. This can be calculated for each axis, as the sum of the squared distance of the coordinate value of each point on this axis to the mean value on this axis. In Figure 5.7a, the y axis captures more of the variance than the x axis in

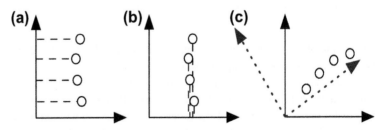

■ **FIGURE 5.7** Reducing a plane to a line: some axes capture more variance than others.

Figure 5.7b. So if we were to take a simple approach to dimension reduction by simply eliminating one of these axes, it would be preferable to preserve the y axis, as less information that is pertinent to distinguishing between the points in this space would be lost. The space depicted in Figure 5.7a and b was conveniently constructed such that most of the variance was captured by one axis. However, this is unlikely to be the case with real-world high-dimensional data. So if we are to generate a reduced-dimensional approximation by retaining a smaller set of axes that best preserve the variance in the space, it may be necessary to find a different set of axes than those that were used to construct the space originally, as depicted in Figure 5.7c, where an alternative set of axes is shown with a dashed line.

The challenge of finding the optimal set of k axes that captures as much of the variance as possible in a high-dimensional dataset can be solved using a technique called Singular Value Decomposition (SVD) [43,51, Chapter 4]. Any $m \times n$ matrix A can be factorized as the product of three matrices $U\Sigma V$, where the columns of U are orthonormal, V is an orthonormal matrix, and $\hat{\Sigma}$ is a diagonal matrix (see Figure 5.8).

The diagonal entries of Σ are called the *singular values*, and they can be arranged in nonincreasing order so that the biggest are at the top. If we only use the first k singular values and treat the rest as zero, the product $U\Sigma V$ uses only the left-hand k columns of U and the top k rows of V. Each m-dimensional row vector A can thus be mapped to a k-dimensional "reduced vector" in the k-dimensional subspace spanned by the top k rows of V.

5.3.2 **Approaches—Topic Models Using Latent Dirichlet Allocation**

It is easy to see that the application of Singular Value Decomposition to human language makes some questionable assumptions. Eigenvalue decompositions of matrices arose in the field of mechanics, initially through Euler's work on axes of rotation (during the late 1700s), and more recently in the analysis of self-adjoint operators in quantum mechanics. Key physical operators, starting with the moment of inertia tensor, were correctly represented

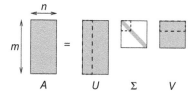

■ **FIGURE 5.8** Singular Value Decomposition.

by symmetric real matrices, from which it follows that the principal axes of rotation of any rigid object are mutually orthogonal—a conclusion that it is easy to demonstrate by throwing any object in the air and closely observing the way it spins. Other conventions follow from this: for example, it is natural to define a coordinate system whose origin is the center of gravity of the rotating object, and whose coordinate axes are the principal axes of rotation, so immediately, vectors with negative coordinates are not only intuitive but obviously necessary to describe the whole space.

The application of Eigenvalue decompositions to human language has no such *a priori* motivation, and thus the initial motivation—reducing the number of dimensions involved in a model and condensing similar information together—has led other researchers to try different techniques. In particular, probabilistic models have seen great success in many language-modeling tasks over recent decades, and it is no surprise that probabilistic techniques have been applied with increasing success to semantic modeling as well. One of the first such methods was called "Probabilistic Latent Semantic Analysis" or PLSA [52]. PLSA uses a non-negative matrix factorization technique to decompose matrices, and once the numbers in the decomposition are all non-negative and suitably normalized, they can be interpreted as probabilities.

Topic Models are a generalization of PLSA to use a variety of statistical techniques, the most popular of these being Latent Dirichlet Allocation [44,45]. Dirichlet distributions are defined over a *simplex*. In general terms, a simplex is the convex region in an n-dimensional vector space bounded by straight lines drawn between $n+1$ corner points or vertices (so in two dimensions, a simplex is a triangle, in three dimensions, a simplex is a tetrahedron, etc.). In probabilistic theories, it is common to use simplexes whose vertices are the origin and the unit vectors along each coordinate axis, which is the portion of the vector space in which all of the coordinates are non-negative, and their sum is not greater than 1. (Such a simplex in two dimensions would be a right-angled triangle whose corners are the points (0, 0), (1, 0), and (0, 1)). Latent Dirichlet Allocation is a method for estimating the parameters of such a distribution from training data. In natural language applications, the dimensions are called *topics*, and the training process determines a probability distribution for each word as a mixture of these topics. Documents are also modeled as a mixture of these topics, which can lead to a theoretical model for document generation, whereby the "authors" of documents choose a mixture of topics for the document, and then pick words randomly according to the distribution of these topics.

An appealing feature of Topic Models is that the probabilistic mixtures of terms that define topics are often intuitively interpretable. For example, Table 5.5 shows the most probable terms for selected topics from a 50-topic decomposition of a set of 190,000 MEDLINE titles from core clinical journals. The terms in Topic 11 suggest oncology; Topic 4 suggests cardiology; Topic 14 suggests obstetrics; and Topic 17 is suggestive of immunology.

5.3.3 Approaches: Random Indexing

For both SVD and LDA, the training process can be computationally intensive, sometimes prohibitively so for large datasets. Promising work has been devoted to solving these problems, to create both distributed implementations (that can use several machines in parallel) [54,55], and incremental versions (in which new documents can be added without retraining the whole model) [56]. Nonetheless, the methods remain quite complex and intensive, and in today's quest to apply methods to bigger and bigger data sets, the appearance of alternatives that are simpler and more scalable is not at all surprising.

Random Indexing (RI) [21,47] has recently emerged as precisely a simpler more scalable alternative to these approaches. While RI does not maximally preserve variance (as with SVD), or result in a set of interpretable topics (as with LDA), it provides an efficient approach to generating a reduced-dimensional approximation of a space that preserves the distance between

Table 5.5 Examples of interpretable topics from a 50-topic decomposition of a set of 190,000 MEDLINE titles from core clinical journals created using Gregor Heinrich's open source implementation of LDA [53]. Each column shows the 10 most probable terms for the topic concerned.

Topic 11	Topic 4	Topic 14	Topic 17
Primary	Heart	Fetal	Antibodies
Malignant	Chronic	Pregnancy	Antibody
Tumor	Failure	Fluid	Immune
Tumors	Disease	During	Monoclonal
Melanoma	Effects	Neonatal	Mice
Biliary	Severe	Maternal	Anti
Benign	Hemodynamic	Time	Antigens
Secondary	Renal	Rate	Antigen
Cutaneous	Congestive	Ultrasound	Specific
Cirrhosis	Ischemic	Outcome	i

points in this space. This is accomplished without the need to explicitly represent the full term-document matrix, and allows for the addition of new information incrementally, without the need to recompute the entire matrix, as would be the case with SVD and LDA. This is achieved by projecting information directly into a reduced-dimensional space, using close-to-orthogonal random index vectors, which we will refer to as *elemental vectors*, to approximate the orthogonal dimensions of the unreduced space.

For example, geometric approaches are frequently employed as a means to model distributional semantics by generating vector representations of terms that are similar to one another if the terms concerned have similar distributions across a large text corpus. One way of generating such representations is to consider as a starting point the distribution of terms across documents. With SVD or LSA this is achieved by first generating a term-by-document matrix, and subsequently reducing the dimensionality of this matrix. If new documents are added, the matrix must be regenerated, and the reduced-dimensional approximation recomputed.[1] RI is able to generate a reduced-dimensional approximation of the original matrix directly, using the following procedure:

1. An *elemental vector* is assigned to every document in the corpus. Elemental vectors are randomly constructed such that they have a high probability of being orthogonal, or close-to-orthogonal to one another. The dimensionality of these elemental vectors is predetermined, and much lower than the number of documents in the corpus.
2. A *semantic vector* is assigned to every term in the corpus. These semantic vectors are of the same dimensionality as the elemental vectors and are initially zero vectors. Semantic vectors can be thought of as repositories for information contained in elemental vectors.
3. Training of the semantic vector for a term is accomplished by adding the elemental vectors for all of the documents it occurs in.

Consequently each term is represented by a trained semantic vector that encodes, albeit approximately, the vector representations of the documents it has occurred in. As elemental vectors are constructed such that they have a high probability of being orthogonal, or close-to-orthogonal to one another, it is also highly probable that terms that occur in the same documents will have vector representations that are more similar than those of terms that do

---

[1] Variants of SVD that allow for the "folding in" of new information exist, but the resulting matrix no longer optimally preserves the dimensionality of the entire set.

not co-occur. A commonly used approach for the construction of elemental vectors involves the generation of sparsely populated high-dimensional vectors ($d \geq 1000$), in which a small number (commonly 10) of dimensions are initialized at random to either $+1$ or -1. There is a high probability of such vectors being orthogonal or close-to-orthogonal, as there is a relatively low probability of significant numbers of their nonzero dimensions aligning with one another (for a detailed analysis of the probability of orthogonality with different parameters, we refer the interested reader to [57]).

This approach offers further computational advantages, as storage of elemental vectors requires retaining the index and value of the non-zero dimensions only, and vector addition during training can be accomplished by considering these values only. Information from additional documents can be incorporated by generating new random vectors and adding these to the semantic vectors of the terms concerned. Despite its simplicity, RI has shown performance comparable to that of LSA on some evaluations, and is able to derive meaningful measures of semantic relatedness from large corpora such as the MEDLINE corpus of abstracts. This ability is illustrated in Figure 5.9, which displays the nearest neighboring terms to the term

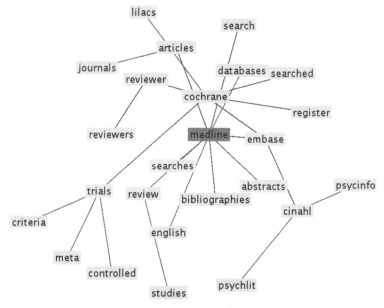

■ **FIGURE 5.9** Nearest neighbors of the term "medline" in a RI space derived from the MEDLINE corpus. Further details of the construction of the space concerned can be found in [58]. The image was generated using Pathfinder network scaling [22] and the Prefuse visualization library [59].

"medline" in a 2000-dimensional RI space derived from all of the abstracts in the MEDLINE corpus. The terms retrieved all relate to MEDLINE, and include other bibliographic databases (e.g., "embase," "lilacs," "psycinfo"); content indexed in MEDLINE ("journals," "articles") and purposes for which it is used ("search," "review").

Many variants of this approach exist. For example, Sahlgren and colleagues have shown that sliding-window based variants of RI tend to emphasize synonymy, and retrieve terms of the same part of speech [17]. Reflective Random Indexing is an iterative variant of RI that better captures implicit associations between terms that do not co-occur together directly [28]. The ease with which it is possible to incrementally add new information to a RI model has led to the generation of models that measure changes in relatedness between terms over time [60,61], and RI has been adapted to derive measures of semantic relatedness between nodes of graphs derived from Resource Description Framework triples [62]. As we will describe later in the chapter, further adaptations of RI have employed reversible vector transformations to encode additional information, such as the relative position of terms [63], structural relationships derived from dependency parses [64], and the type of relationship that links the concepts in a concept-relationship-concept triple [65].

5.3.4 **Summary and Implications**

In this section, we discussed ways in which reduced-dimensional approximations of geometric representations can be generated. These reduced-dimensional representations offer computational advantages when computing similarity, and save storage space in RAM and on disk. With some models, reducing dimensionality also leads to improved performance on certain tasks. However, the process of dimension reduction can be computationally demanding with established methods such as LDA and SVD. Consequently, we introduced RI, which has recently emerged as a computationally convenient alternative to these approaches.

One of the weaknesses that has long been recognized with all of these models is that many parts of language structure are ignored. For example, the very important factor of how the words are arranged within a particular document is typically neglected, and for this reason these techniques are often referred to as "bag-of-words" methods. The use of sliding-window based approaches is a first attempt to go beyond the bag-of-words assumption, and as we shall see later in the chapter, there are others: in recent years there has been rapid progress in this area. Still, any attempt to use these models in practice for document generation, for example, demonstrates how far we are from reproducing human language skills! However, in all informatics disciplines including the biomedical domain, there are many practical problems that are much less ambitious than full human-level natural language competence, but still extremely useful and increasingly necessary in professions where managing large collections of complex information is a day-to-day requirement. We will review a sample of such applications in the following sections.

5.4 **CLASSIFICATION**

A common application of geometric representations involves assigning a category to some hitherto unseen entity on the basis of the categories assigned to entities occupying similar regions of geometric space. In this section we will discuss two approaches to this problem.

5.4.1 *k*-Nearest Neighbor

The first, known as *k-nearest neighbor* classification, involves retrieving the nearest neighboring entities to a new entity and assigning a category, or set of categories, to this new entity based on those already assigned to other entities in the space. For example, Figure 5.10 illustrates the application of the *k*-nearest neighbor approach (with $k = 3$) as a means to assign a category to an unseen entity ("?") based on the categories assigned to its nearest neighbors. This is accomplished by assigning scores to the possible categories. In this case, there are only two possible categories, "gray" and "white." The score for the "gray" category is the sum of the similarity scores assigned to all entities of this type within the neighbors retrieved, which is calculated as $a + b$, where a and b are estimates of the similarity between

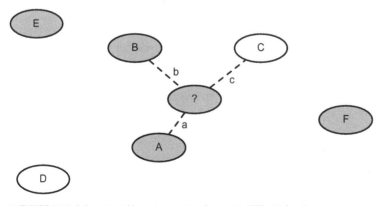

■ **FIGURE 5.10** *k*-Nearest neighbor categorization of new entity ("?") with $k = 3$.

the new entity and entities A and B respectively. As this score is greater than that assigned to the "white" category, the category "gray" is assigned to the new entity. While this method is relatively simple, it only considers categories assigned to the closest entities in the space, and all entities in the space must be considered in order to determine which of them is closest to the new entity. Therefore, the use of reduced-dimensional geometric representations is desirable as a means to prevent this search process from being prohibitively time consuming with larger datasets. For more details about k-Nearest neighbor, see Chapter 7.

5.4.2 Example: MEDLINE Indexing

The Medical Subject Headings (MeSH) vocabulary that is used to index MEDLINE and other databases were originally used in the Index Medicus, and "celebrated" their 50th anniversary of publication in 2010. As the conceptual territory of the biomedical literature has expanded, so too has the number of MeSH terms used for indexing: the 2010 edition contained more than 25,000 subject headings, considerably more than the approximately 4400 in the original set introduced in 1960. These subject headings are organized into an eleven-level hierarchy, as well as 83 subheadings. The vocabulary can be explored using the online MeSH browser provided by the US National Library of Medicine (NLM), at [66]. For example, the psychiatric disorder schizophrenia is assigned the MeSH term "Schizophrenia" and organized into the hierarchy as follows:

- Psychiatry and Psychology.
- Mental Disorders.
- Schizophrenia and Disorders with Psychotic Features.
- Schizophrenia.

In addition to this hierarchically structured set of canonical terms, the MeSH vocabulary also contains a vast number of entry terms, which are intended to be synonyms of the canonical heading terms. For example, the MeSH term Schizophrenia also contains the entry terms Dementia Praecox (a name for psychotic spectrum disorders popularized by influential German psychiatrist Emil Kraepelin in the late 1800s) and Schizophrenic Disorders. MeSH also contains other features such as conceptual relations, which we will not discuss here, but rather refer the interested reader to Hersh's comprehensive textbook on biomedical information retrieval [67] or the MeSH website [68] for further details.

Manual indexing of bibliographic content involves a human indexer assigning indexing terms to this content based on their impression of it. A large volume of references are constantly added to MEDLINE, and there are a limited number of human indexers available to manage these. So, the NLM has supported research on semi-automated indexing, in which a computer-based system provides recommendations for MeSH terms that provide suggestions to human annotators to speed the annotation process. One such system, the Medical Text Indexer (MTI), developed at the NLM is used by the NLM to support their in-house indexing [69]. k-Nearest neighbor classification has also been used to assign index terms to MEDLINE documents [34,35]. The procedure to do so is straightforward. Vector representations of biomedical abstracts contained in the MEDLINE database are generated. When RI is used to facilitate dimension reduction, this is accomplished by adding together *elemental term vectors* representing those terms contained in the document. Steps are taken to exclude terms that are likely to be uninformative (for example with a stoplist or frequency threshold), and selectively emphasize those terms that are likely to be more informative (for example with TF-IDF weighting). MEDLINE contains around twenty million citations that have been assigned MeSH terms by human annotators, and around ten million of these include abstracts. The k-nearest neighbor approach is used to retrieve a small set of abstracts with vector representations most similar to that of a cue document from a test set of abstracts. The MeSH terms assigned to abstracts in this set are then scored, and those with the highest score are applied to the test case, and compared to the MeSH terms assigned by human raters for the purpose of evaluation.

For example, consider the results shown in Table 5.6. This table depicts the five nearest neighbors of a cue article (PMID=15360816) to do with automated indexing. The MeSH terms for, and title of this article are shown in the second row of the table, and the five nearest neighbors of this article in a 1000-dimensional RI space are shown in subsequent rows. All but one of the indexing terms assigned to the cue article have also been assigned to one of the five nearest neighbors, and many of these indexing terms have been assigned to more than one of these neighboring documents.

Despite its simplicity, the k-nearest neighbor approach remains a strong baseline for comparison against, and an important component of, more sophisticated methods that utilize additional information in addition to that provided by the MeSH terms assigned to the nearest neighboring documents [70].

5.4.3 **SVMs**

Support Vector Machines (SVMs) [71,72] provide an alternative approach to the categorization of geometrically represented entities and have been used extensively for the purpose of text classification [73]. Unlike the k-nearest neighbor approach, in which every entity in the training set must

Table 5.6 Example of Nearest Neighbor Search using RI. MeSH terms shared with the cue article (15360816) are shown in bold. "*" denotes an indexing term selected by indexers as indicative of the major topic for the article concerned.

PMID	Cosine	Title	MeSH Terms
15360816 (the cue)	1.0	**The NLM Indexing Initiative's Medical Text Indexer**	**Abstracting and Indexing as Topic/methods*; MEDLINE; Medical Subject Headings*; National Library of Medicine (US); Natural Language Processing* Unified Medical Language System; United States**
18694044	0.503	Visualization of semantic indexing similarity over MeSH	**Abstracting and Indexing as Topic*/methods**; Audiovisual Aids; Computer Graphics*; Evaluation Studies as Topic; **MEDLINE; Medical Subject Headings*; Natural Language Processing**; Semantics
15360820	0.50	Application of a Medical Text Indexer to an online dermatology atlas.	**Abstracting and Indexing as Topic*/methods**; Anatomy, Artistic*; Dermatology*; Humans; Medical Illustration*; **Medical Subject Headings*; National Library of Medicine (US); Natural Language Processing***; Online Systems; Pilot Projects; Skin Diseases/diagnosis; **United States**
16779044	0.43	Semi-automatic indexing of full text biomedical articles.	**Abstracting and Indexing as Topic/methods***; Algorithms; Libraries, Digital; **MEDLINE; Medical Subject Headings*; National Library of Medicine (US); Natural Language Processing***; Periodicals as Topic; **United States**
17238409	0.41	Besides precision and recall: exploring alternative approaches to evaluating an automatic indexing tool for MEDLINE.	**Abstracting and Indexing as Topic/methods***; Evaluation Studies as Topic*; **MEDLINE; Medical Subject Headings*; Natural Language Processing***; Semantics
14728459	0.40	Automated indexing of the Hazardous Substances Data Bank (HSDB).	**Abstracting and Indexing as Topic/methods***; Automatic Data Processing*; Databases, Factual*; Hazardous Substances*; **Medical Subject Headings; National Library of Medicine (US); United States**

be considered every time a new example is to be categorized, SVMs use the training set to generate a classifier, which can be used to categorize new examples without comparing these to the training set directly. As training of a SVM necessitates solving a quadratic optimization problem, the training process can be computationally demanding, but a number of optimization procedures exist that aim to enable SVMs to scale to larger datasets (see for example [73], chapters 8 and 9). However, a classifier must be generated for each binary decision task, which makes this approach an unlikely fit for problems such as automated indexing, in which more than 25,000 possible categories must be considered.

The training process results in the derivation of a *decision surface* (Figure 5.11), a hyperplane that separates the positive and negative examples

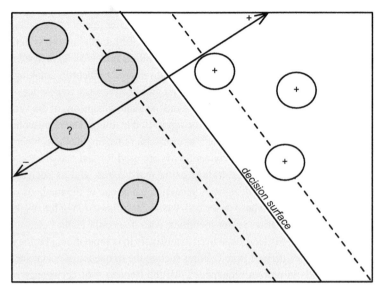

■ **FIGURE 5.11** SVM neighbor categorization of new entity ("?").

in space. This hyperplane optimally separates the positive and negative examples, which is to say that it is the hyperplane that falls midway between the negative and positive examples that are closest to it. So the distance from the hyperplane to these examples, which is referred to as the *margin*, is maximal. New examples are then classified on the basis of their position relative to the hyperplane. Those that fall "above" the hyperplane, in the unshaded region containing the positive ("+") examples, will be categorized as positive. Those that fall "below" the hyperplane, in the shaded region containing the negative ("−") examples, will be categorized as negative, as would occur with the new entity ("?") in the figure. Note that while the simple example in the figure depicts a set of positive and negative examples that can be perfectly separated by a line (which would be replaced by a hyperplane if we had depicted more than two dimensions), these characteristics of the training set are not requirements. So-called "soft margin" SVMs allow for, but aim to minimize, categorization errors during training [71]; and a standard approach to training sets that are not linearly separable involves mapping the geometric representations of the examples in this training set into an alternative geometric space in which linear separation is possible [74].

Support vector machines are by now well established as a method of text categorization [73]. To cite a biomedical example, in the 2006 i2b2 evaluation challenge, which compared the ability of various language processing systems and categorization tools to determine the smoking status of patients based on the content of their Electronic Health Record, many of the teams employed SVMs as a component of their system [75], including the system that performed best on this competitive evaluation task [76]. This system used a rule-based natural language extraction engine to identify smoking-related phrases in biomedical narrative, and used the presence or absence of these phrases as features, represented as independent dimensions of the vector to be learned from or classified, for supervised learning. The representation of selected linguistic units, such as terms, bigrams, or phrases as binary features, is a common practice when SVMs are used for text classification. However, SVMs can also be trained using real vectors, and as such are applicable to vector representations generated using one of the methods of dimension reduction we have described, where each dimension of the resulting vector representation is not identified with a specific feature (see for example [77]). SVMs have been used extensively in computational biology, to classify vectors derived from features such as the frequency of occurrence of amino acids in protein sequences [78]; the frequency of occurrence of substrings of these amino acids [79]; functional attributes such as hydrophobicity and polarity [78] and the presence or absence of a particular protein in the genomes of different species [80] (for a review see [81]). Additional details about SVMs are given in Chapter 7.

5.4.4 Clustering

When class labels are not known beforehand, automated clustering methods can be applied to geometric representations to facilitate exploratory data analysis. One widely-used approach, k-means clustering, divides the set into k clusters by partitioning the geometric space based on distance between each point and a set of k "centroids," each representing the midpoint between all data points assigned to a particular class. Centroids are originally randomly assigned, but as the algorithm proceeds iteratively both centroids and class labels are reassigned to reach a solution in which the clusters conform to the spatial configuration of the data points concerned.

Clustering is often used in practice to "see the wood for the trees"—there may be lots of individual data points, and clustering enables us to group the similar ones together so that we can understand large groups and trends in the data, not just individual datapoints. Clustering has been applied to many problems in natural language, search, and semantic computing generally.

5.4.5 Example: Word Sense Discrimination

Determining what a word means when it is used in context is an important challenge in any form of textual informatics: "ACL" might mean

"Association for Computational Linguistics," "Anterior cruciate ligament," "Access control list," several other current meanings, and in the next few years we can be relatively certain that new meanings will be coined. This leads to the challenge of "word sense discrimination," which has in practice been addressed by distributional models using clustering.

The problem is well known in natural language processing (See Chapter 6): "word sense disambiguation" means choosing the right meaning for a word in context, when several possible meanings are available. The further challenge of "word sense discrimination" is to infer the available senses purely from corpus data, instead of having them supplied to the system from external resources such as dictionaries. Sense discrimination is becoming increasingly important, because of the rapid invention of new technical terms, acronyms, person names, company names, and a host of other neologisms. Many of these have existing dictionary definitions (e.g., "bush," "apple," "gates," "rim") which are genuinely misleading to a literal-minded computer! Geometric methods have been particularly effective and robust at distinguishing these different uses: much of this is because when the model of meaning is learned entirely from corpus data, the model naturally reflects the fact that word usage is in practice often different from the meanings recorded in dictionaries.

Schütze pioneered the use of geometric models for word sense discrimination [83], demonstrating in the process that clustering of word vectors can be used to give word meanings. The basic intuition is that, for each occurrence of a word, the vectors of the neighboring words can be summed to give a "context vector" for that particular occurence: thus, for each word, we can collect context vectors for its occurrences, perform clustering on these context vectors, and discover different word senses.

Several applications of vector models and clustering for analyzing word senses have descended from this work. One attraction is that the approach can also be applied across languages, to bilingual vector spaces. (This chapter does not discuss bilingual models at length: for an introduction, see [5, Section 6.6].) For example, Figure 5.12 shows a visualization built from translated pairs of German and English medical abstracts. We examine the neighbors of the English word "drug," and discover that it is closely related to two German words, "drogen" (roughly corresponding to "illicit drugs") and "medikamente" (roughly corresponding to "medical drugs").

In this way, clustering and visualization tools can be used to explore distributional models, and this can be a powerful way to enable users to see a "bigger picture" that is not revealed by a single list of search results. Methods like this have been used to map and explore entire collections of scientific documents [84].

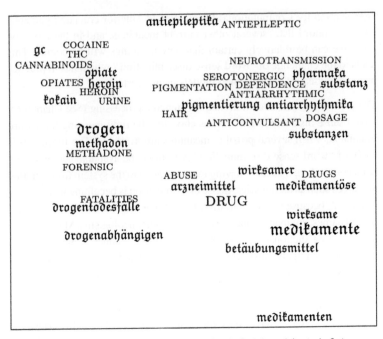

■ **FIGURE 5.12** ENGLISH and 𝔊erman terms related to the English word *drug* in the Springer medical abstracts.

5.4.6 **Summary and Implications**

In this section, we discussed the use of geometric representations as a basis for the classification or clustering of data points, with examples of algorithmic approaches to these ends. The approaches discussed are geometrically motivated: points nearby to one another in space are likely to form a part of the same cluster, and points in the same region of space are likely to be similarly classified. Consequently these methods depend upon the application of distance metrics to geometric representations of these data points, which may be composed from vector representations of their component parts (for example, vector representations of larger units of text may be composed from a set of existing term vectors). However, the mathematical properties of geometric spaces can mediate more sophisticated compositional operators than vector addition, providing the means to encode additional layers of meaning into vector space.

5.5 **BEYOND DISTANCE**

Up to this point, we have discussed the use of geometric representations as a means to derive a convenient measure of the relatedness between entities. While these estimates are useful for many purposes, they are clearly not enough to represent the meaning of natural language sentences and documents. The most common words demonstrate this most clearly: "if," "but," "not," "of," "the," and "is," are words that can occur in almost any context, so their meaning will certainly not be modeled by comparing the contexts in which the words do and don't occur. These are the words that are normally treated as stopwords by search engines, that is, those words that are ignored entirely and not included in the search index at all; and ironically, they are the words that language cannot do without.

Mathematically speaking, these words behave more like operators or functions than like elements of a set. For many years, distributional methods had relatively little to say about these basic function words, taking an unordered "bag-of-words" approach. But more recently, emerging methods have provided the means to use high-dimensional vector representations as a basis for computational operations that have traditionally been accomplished using symbolic representations. In the section that follows we will discuss ways in which vector transformations can be used to generate vector space equivalents of formal operators such as connectives and implication, and the encoding of additional information such as semantic relations.

5.5.1 **Boolean Connectives**

The Boolean connectives are the AND, OR, and NOT functions in logic, named after their inventor George Boole (1815–1864). Boolean connectives have become the cornerstones of modern mathematical logic. (By contrast, implication and negation are the initial building blocks of Aristotelian logic. This can become confusing especially because Boolean logic, from the Victorian period, is referred to as "classical" in this context.)

AND and OR are different ways of combining meanings together: AND makes outcomes more restrictive or specific, while OR makes them more permissive or general. Both operators are commutative, meaning that the order in which the arguments are placed does not matter. Traditionally, vector model search engines combine vectors by adding them together, which can be thought of as a cross between AND and OR. Varying the norm functions used for computing product vectors was used in the 1980s to give some distinction between more general and more specific products [85].

Negation (the NOT operator) is quite different: it removes rather than contributes meanings, and "*A* NOT *B*" means something quite different from "*B* NOT *A*." For many years, the lack of a negation operator in vector search engines was a sharp criticism of the model when compared with Boolean retrieval models. However, it turns out that vector negation is quite possible and very simple: it can be modeled by subtracting some part of the vector you want to negate. The question is "how much to subtract?" and this depends on the nature of the similarity score being used. If the similarity between two unrelated concepts is zero, then the answer is theoretically very nice: two concepts have zero similarity between them if their vectors are orthogonal to one another, in which case, a statement like "A NOT B" is modeled by projecting the vector for A so that it is orthogonal to B. In geometry, this is sometimes written as $A \perp B$, and it is computed by the formula $A - (A \cdot B)B$. This process can sometimes be used to remove unwanted meanings from the vectors for ambiguous words: for example, Table 5.7 shows an example of how this was used to remove the "legal" meaning of the word "suit," leaving the "clothing" meaning [86].

It turns out to be a small step from using orthogonal negation in vector spaces to recognizing a full logic including AND and OR operators as well. For two vectors A and B, A OR B is modeled as the plane generated by A and B, and in this way, subspaces of various dimensions become incorporated into the model. Similarly, for two subspaces A, B, the combination A AND

Table 5.7 Neighbors of the vectors for "suit" and "suit NOT lawsuit" in a distributional model built from New York Times data [86].

Suit		Suit NOT Lawsuit	
Suit	1.000000	Pants	0.810573
Lawsuit	0.868791	Shirt	0.807780
Suits	0.807798	Jacket	0.795674
Plaintiff	0.717156	Silk	0.781623
Sued	0.706158	Dress	0.778841
Plaintiffs	0.697506	Trousers	0.771312
Suing	0.674661	Sweater	0.765677
Lawsuits	0.664649	Wearing	0.764283
Damages	0.660513	Satin	0.761530
Filed	0.655072	Plaid	0.755880
Behalf	0.650374	Lace	0.755510
Appeal	0.608732	Worn	0.755260
Action	0.605764	Velvet	0.754183
Court	0.604445	Wool	0.741714
Infringement	0.598975	Hair	0.739573
Trademark	0.592759	Wore	0.737148
Litigation	0.591104	Wears	0.733652
Settlement	0.585363	Skirt	0.730711
Alleges	0.585051	Dressed	0.726150
Alleging	0.568169	Gown	0.723920

B can be modeled by taking their intersection, which is also a subspace. Historically, this is exactly the same logic that was used by Birkhoff and von Neumann to model the relationships between states in quantum mechanics, and for this reason the system is called *quantum logic* (see [87,88]).

The quantum logical operators demonstrated considerable effectiveness on concept-removal tasks in retrieval experiments [86], because instead of removing one word at a time (as with Boolean negation), an appropriate combination of the vector NOT and OR operators removes whole areas of meaning. However, there are also clear conceptual flaws in the system: for example, with the vector OR operation, three nearby vectors would generate as large a space as three very different vectors (provided the vectors are linearly independent, which is a very weak condition).

An intuitive example helps to make this clearer. If we said we saw a car traveling at "25 or 30 miles an hour," we would expect that an actual value of 27 miles an hour is consistent or included in this statement. However, we would not expect that 200 miles an hour fits this description because it is in the extended linear span of 25 and 30! Possibly the convex span of vectors would be a better model, as suggested also by Gärdenfors in the cognitive science literature [89].

5.5.2 **Conditionals and Implication**

The investigation of the logical OR operator leads naturally to the topic of "How do we generalize?" or "How do we extrapolate?" A core part of intelligent behavior is to use evidence from individual observations, and form a generalized rule or concept that can be applied to new situations, including those outside the original examples or training set.

In mathematics, the topic of generalization is related to the notion of implication, because both are modeled using *ordered sets* [5, Chapter 8]. In more common terms, "mammal" is a generalization of "horse" because being a horse implies being a mammal. This connection between biology and logic is no accident: both sciences were pioneered by Aristotle, and his logical writings are full of biological examples of this nature. Implication is itself related to the study of conditionals, because "A implies B" and "if A then B" are regarded as logically synonymous.

For a thorough description of the formal operators available in vector spaces to model conditionals, see [6, Chapter 5]. A key question for geometric approaches to informatics is "what shape should a generalized concept take?" The quantum disjunction or vector span operator in one example, but as said in the previous section, this space may often be too large (or to put it in different terms, unrealistically general). For a deeper discussion of the appropriate logic for such generalization in the context of quantum structures, see [90].

An intriguing answer to the question "what shape should a generalized concept take?" is that it's just like any other concept: a single point or vector. This is the path suggested by Kanerva [91], using the argument that when there are lots of dimensions, one point can be similar to many "ingredient" points, even if those ingredients are distant from one another. Perhaps surprisingly, this method has given extremely good results in analogical reasoning, answering questions of the form "A is to B, as C is to what?" To understand how relations like "A is to B" can be modeled, see Section 5.5.3. In this section, the important point is that we can take *many* such relations, superpose them together, and get a new representation that performs extremely well at recognizing new examples of this relation: better than any one of the training examples could perform alone [92]. This has further interest from the point of view of quantum structures: when new representations are created superposing many product states, but the new representation cannot be obtained as the product of any two individual elements, this product state is described as *entangled*.

5.5.3 **Typed Relations**

As we have seen, new vector methods have been discovered and applied that are able to represent more varied operations than simple addition, and more subtle relationships than just similarity. In this section, we will generalize this process even further and describe a method for modeling any kind of relationship between two elements in a vector representation.

Over the past two decades, models have emerged that enable the encoding of additional information into geometric representations using reversible vector transformations. These models, collectively known as Vector Symbolic Architectures (VSAs) [93], expand both the representational richness and the functional capacity of geometric approaches, by enabling a form of computation that has been termed *hyperdimensional computing* [91]. These models were originally developed within the cognitive science community, and as such have been used as the means to simulate performance on constrained cognitive tasks. However, many of these models scale comfortably to large datasets, and recent work has leveraged the additional representational richness they offer to enhance geometric representations of large datasets for the purpose of distributional semantics [94,63,64], text categorization [95] and literature-based discovery [33].

VSAs permit the encoding of additional information into a vector representation using an operator referred to as *binding* [93]. It is important that this operator be invertible, so that the information encoded into a bound product can be recovered. The way in which binding is accomplished varies from VSA to VSA, as does the underlying vector representation, as shown for selected VSAs in Table 5.8.

While a detailed discussion of each of these architectures is beyond the scope of this chapter, we provide here a description of the use of permutations to encode additional information to illustrate the ease with which it is possible to enrich geometric models in this way. Consider the Random Indexing model we described in Section 5.3.3, in which sparse high-dimensional elemental vectors are constructed to represent contextual information. As discussed previously, most of the dimensions in these vectors are zero, with a small number of nonzero dimensions initialized as either $+1$ or -1. This allows for elemental vectors to be represented economically, by keeping track of the index values of the nonzero dimensions only. For example, a 1000-dimensional elemental vector for the term diabetes, E(diabetes), with four non-zero values could be represented as follows:

diabetes	$+99$	$+503$	-79	-999

The absolute value in this representation denotes the dimension of the index vector that is non-zero (numbered from 0 to 999), and the sign denotes whether this dimension is occupied by a $+1$ or a -1. As the phrase "diabetes mellitus" occurs frequently, we would anticipate the term "mellitus" occurring in the same sliding window as the term "diabetes," an occurrence that a sliding-window based RI model would encode by adding the elemental vector for the term "diabetes" to the semantic vector for the term "mellitus." However, following the approach proposed by Sahlgren and his colleagues [63], we would

Table 5.8   Selected VSA vector representations and binding operators.

Model	Vector Representation	Binding Operator
Binary spatter code [96]	Binary vectors	Pairwise exclusive OR (XOR)
Holographic reduced representations [97]	Real vectors	Circular convolution
Circular holographic reduced representations [97]	Complex vectors with each dimension representing a point on the perimeter of the unit circle	Circular convolution implemented through pairwise multiplication
Vector permutation [63]	Real vectors, permutations	Permute elements of vector

like to encode information about the relative position of these terms, namely the fact that the term "diabetes" occurs *one position to the left* of the term "mellitus," into the model also. We accomplish this with a simple permutation operation, π^{-1}, by shifting all of the elements of the elemental vector for "diabetes" *one position to the left* to generate the following representation:

π^{-1} **(diabetes)**	+98	+502	−78	−998

This vector is then added to the semantic vector for the term "mellitus." So applying the reverse of this permutation, π^{+1}, to the semantic vector for the term "mellitus" will produce a vector that is similar to the elemental vector for "diabetes." Using this approach, it is possible to recover terms that tend to occur in particular positions relative to a target term, as demonstrated in Table 5.9. Note the difference in cosine across the retrieved terms. The lower cosine value for the term "bipolar" reflects the fact that several other terms also occurred repeatedly one position to the left of the term "disorder": other near neighbors of π^{+1}(disorder) included the terms "personality," "depressive," "panic," and "eating."

This approach can be used to encode other information aside from the relative position of terms. Knowledge is increasingly available in the form of concept-relation-concept triples. For example, over 50 million such triples extracted from the biomedical literature by the SemRep system [98] have been publicly released in the SemMedDB database [99]. Rather than assigning permutations to relative positions, it is possible to assign these permutations to specific relationship types. If we assign π^{-1} to the relationship type "TREATS," we can encode the fact that "insulin TREATS diabetes mellitus" into the semantic vector for insulin, S(insulin) by adding a permuted version of the relevant elemental vector, E(diabetes mellitus), with the operation S(diabetes mellitus) $+= \pi^{-1}E$(insulin). We can then recover an approximation of E(insulin) by reversing this permutation: $\pi^{+1}S$(diabetes mellitus) $\approx E$(insulin). This approach has been used to the generate of a vector space that can "answer" simple clinical questions, such as "what treats diabetes?"

Table 5.9 Nearest elemental vector to permuted semantic vectors in permutation-based RI model of MEDLINE.

Cue Term	Cosine: Neighbor
π^{+1} (mellitus)	0.996: diabetes
π^{-1}(diabetes)	0.978: mellitus
π^{+1}(disorder)	0.350: bipolar
π^{-1}(streptococcus)	0.876: pneumoniae

[65], and encode grammatical relations produced by a dependency parser into a distributional model of meaning [64]. With other VSAs, both concepts (or terms) and relationship types are assigned vector representations. For example, to encode the predication "insulin TREATS diabetes mellitus" into the semantic vector for insulin, the elemental vector for diabetes mellitus would be bound to an elemental vector representing the "TREATS" relationship, and added to E(insulin) [33,100].

5.5.4 **Summary and Implications**

In this section, we have introduced emerging approaches through which geometric representations can be used to accomplish computational procedures similar to those that have traditionally been associated with symbolic methods. These include use of geometric equivalents of logical connectives to eliminate unwanted components from vector representations in order to more precisely specify search queries, and the use of reversible vector transformations to encode the nature of the relationship between contexts. The latter approach originated in the cognitive science community, motivated by the desire to develop biologically inspired computational models of cognition. However, as is the case with many geometric models related to Random Indexing, it scales comfortably to large datasets, providing a layer of representational richness that cannot be obtained through the use of models based on co-occurrence alone. In the section that follows, we will introduce the Semantic Vectors package [101,102], which supports the generation of a variety of geometric models from large corpora of electronic text.

5.6 **BUILDING GEOMETRIC MODELS WITH THE SEMANTIC VECTORS PACKAGE**

In this section we will introduce the Semantic Vectors package [101,102], which was used to generate many of the examples used in chapter. The package provides the means to generate a range of distributional models including LSA, sliding-window and term-document based models, permutation-based models [102], and other Vector Symbolic models based on binary and complex vector representations [103].

Several of the algorithms and features described in this chapter are provided in Semantic Vectors, including tools for building bilingual models, quantum NOT and OR operators, a basic k-means clustering routine, and a two-dimensional plotter for visualization.

Semantic Vectors was developed initially by the University of Pittsburgh in collaboration with MAYA Design, and is now maintained by a small development community including both of the current authors. It is hosted by the Google Code website [104], and is also available for free download under a

BSD license. The software is written entirely in Java which, though somewhat slower than C, has made the package very easily portable, and so far no platform-specific problems have been encountered. The package depends on the Apache Lucene text search engine (also freely available and open-source) for basic tokenization, parsing, term-indexing, and optimized I/O.

Aside from the LSA implementation, random projection is used for dimension reduction, which has enabled the software to scale comfortably to large corpora such as MEDLINE within the limits of computational resources available to most researchers. The package has been downloaded over 10,000 times at the time of this writing, and is actively maintained with new features and tests, support for bilingual models, clustering, visualization, incorporating word-order information, a variety of logical and compositional operators, and considerable flexibility in tunable parameters, memory models, and I/O formats.

5.7 SUMMARY AND CONCLUSION

Geometric representations in biomedical informatics began as a model for keyword search engines. Since then, they have been successfully applied to many other challenges, including literature-based discovery, word-sense disambiguation, generalization and classification, and even relation discovery. Many techniques are available for building and exploring such representations, and have been developed over the years so that stable, scalable solutions are available for a wide range of situations. The best solutions for a given challenge will in many cases depend on the intended application, the amount of available language data, how rapidly these data change, and the computational resources available.

These techniques can be used to build entire solutions for biomedical informatics problems such as search, discovery, visualization, and even reasoning. However, some of the most successful applications have combined information from many sources, including more traditional symbolic and statistical systems.

Geometric representations are growing in their reliability, sophistication, and usefulness, and are likely to play an increasingly important and intertwined set of roles in biomedical informatics.

REFERENCES

[1] Hausdorff F. Grundzüge der Mengenlehre. Germany: von Veit; 1914. Republished as Set theory. 2nd ed. New York: Chelsea; 1962.
[2] Boyer CB, Merzbach UC. A history of mathematics. 2nd ed. Wiley; 1991.

[3] Gentner G, Medin DL, Goldstone RL. Respects for similarity. Psychol Rev 1993;100:254–78.

[4] Gärdenfors P. Conceptual spaces: the geometry of thought. Mit Pr; 2000.

[5] Widdows D. Geometry and meaning. CSLI Publications; 2004.

[6] van Rijsbergen K. The geometry of information retrieval. Cambridge University Press; 2004.

[7] Cohen T, Widdows D, Schvaneveldt R, Rindflesch TR. Logical leaps and quantum connectives: Forging paths through predication space. In: Proceedings of the AAAI Fall Symposium on Quantum Informatics for Cognitive, Social, and Semantic Processes (QI 2010); 2010.

[8] Salton G, McGill M. Introduction to modern information retrieval. New York, NY: McGraw-Hill; 1983.

[9] Baeza-Yates R, Ribiero-Neto B. Modern information retrieval. Addison Wesley: ACM Press; 1999.

[10] Abdala OT, Saeed M. Estimation of missing values in clinical laboratory measurements of ICU patients using a weighted K-nearest neighbors algorithm. Comput Cardiol 2004:693–6.

[11] Cohen T, Widdows D. Empirical distributional semantics: methods and biomedical applications. J Biomed Inform 2009;42(2):390–405.

[12] Turney PD, Pantel P. From frequency to meaning: vector space models of semantics. J Artif Intell Res 2010;37(1):141–88.

[13] Burgess C, Livesay K, Lund K. Explorations in context space: words, sentences, discourse. Discourse Process 1998.

[14] Landauer TK, Dumais ST. A solution to plato's problem: the latent semantic analysis theory of acquisition, induction, and representation of knowledge. Psychol Rev 1997;104:211–40.

[15] Kanerva P, Kristofersson J, Holst A. Random indexing of text samples for latent semantic analysis. In: Proceedings of the 22nd annual conference of the cognitive science society, vol. 1036; 2000.

[16] Karlgren J, Sahlgren M. From words to understanding. Found Real-World Intell 2001:294–308.

[17] Sahlgren M. The word-space model. Ph.D. dissertation. Stockholm University; 2006.

[18] Bodenreider O. The unified medical language system (UMLS): integrating biomedical terminology. Nucleic Acids Res 2004;32(Database Issue):D267.

[19] Aronson AR, Lang F. An overview of MetaMap: historical perspective and recent advances. J Am Med Inform Assoc 2010;17:229–36.

[20] Aronson AR. Effective mapping of biomedical text to the UMLS metathesaurus: the metamap program. AMIA Annu Symp Proc 2001;17:17–21.

[21] Kanerva P, Kristofersson J, Holst A. Random indexing of text samples for latent semantic analysis. In: Proceedings of the 22nd annual conference of the cognitive science society, vol. 1036; 2000.

[22] Schvaneveldt RW. Pathfinder associative networks: studies in knowledge organization. Norwood, NJ, USA: Ablex Publishing Corp.; 1990.

[23] Flare visualization library. <http://flare.prefuse.org>.

[24] Hersh W, Buckley C, Leone TJ, Hickam D. OHSUMED: an interactive retrieval evaluation and new large test collection for research. In: Proceedings of the 17th

annual international ACMSIGIR conference on research and development in information retrieval; 1994. p. 192–201.

[25] Swanson DR. Fish oil, Raynaud's syndrome, and undiscovered public knowledge. Perspect Biol Med 1986;30(1):7–18.

[26] DiGiacomo RA, Kremer JM, Shah DM. Fish-oil dietary supplementation in patients with raynaud's phenomenon: a double-blind, controlled, prospective study. Am J Med 1989;86:158–64.

[27] Cole R, Bruza P. A bare bones approach to literature-based discovery: an analysis of the Raynaud's/fish-oil and migraine-magnesium discoveries in semantic space. In: Disc Sci; 2005. p. 84–98.

[28] Cohen T, Schvaneveldt R, Widdows D. Reflective random indexing and indirect inference: a scalable method for discovery of implicit connections. J Biomed Inform 2010;43(2):240–56.

[29] Gordon MD, Dumais S. Using latent semantic indexing for literature based discovery. J Am Soc Inform Sci 1998;49:674–85.

[30] Hristovski D, Friedman C, Rindflesch TC, Peterlin B. Exploiting semantic relations for literature-based discovery. AMIA Annu Symp Proc 2006:349–53.

[31] Wilkowski B, Fiszman M, Miller CM, Hristovski D, Arabandi S, Rosemblat G, Rindflesch TC. Graph-based methods for discovery browsing with semantic predications. AMIA Annu Symp Proc 2011;2011:1514–23.

[32] Cameron D, Bodenreider O, Yalamanchili H, Danh T, Vallabhaneni S, Thirunarayan K, Sheth AP, Rindflesch TC. A graph-based recovery and decomposition of swanson's hypothesis using semantic predications. J Biomed Inform 2012.

[33] Cohen T, Widdows D, Schvaneveldt R, Davies P, Rindflesch T. Discovering discovery patterns with predication-based semantic indexing [under review].

[34] Yang Y, Chute CG. An application of expert network to clinical classification and MEDLINE indexing. In: Proceedings of the annual symposium on computer application [sic] in medical care; 1994. p. 157–61.

[35] Vasuki V, Cohen T. Reflective random indexing for semi-automated indexing of MEDLINE abstracts. J Biomed Inform 2010;43(5):694–700.

[36] Huang M, Névéol A, Lu Z. Recommending MeSH terms for annotating biomedical articles. J Am Med Inform Assoc 2011;18(5):660–7.

[37] Sarkar IN. A vector space model approach to identify genetically related diseases. J Am Med Inform Assoc 2012;19(2):249–54.

[38] Ganapathiraju M, Balakrishnan N, Reddy R, Klein-Seetharaman J. Transmembrane helix prediction using amino acid property features and latent semantic analysis. BMC Bioinform 2008;9(Suppl. 1):S4.

[39] Schutze H. Automatic word sense discrimination. Comput Linguist 1998;24:97–123.

[40] Schutze H. Word space. Adv Neural Inform Process Syst 1993;5:895–902.

[41] Widdows D, Dorow B, Chan CK. Using parallel corpora to enrich multilingual lexical resources. In: Third international conference on language resources and evaluation; 2002. p. 240–5.

[42] Deerwester S, Dumais S, Furnas G, Landauer T, Harshman R. Indexing by latent semantic analysis. J Am Soc Inform Sci 1990;41(6):391–407.

[43] Golub GH, Reinsch C. Singular value decomposition and least squares solutions. Numer Math 1970;14:403–20.

[44] Blei DM, Ng AY, Jordan MI, Lafferty J. Latent dirichlet allocation. J Mach Learn Res 2003;3.

[45] Blei DM. Probabilistic topic models. Commun ACM 2012;55(4):77–84. http://dx.doi.org/10.1145/2133806.2133826.. [online]

[46] Steyvers M, Griffiths T. Probabilistic topic models. Handbook of latent semantic analysis; 2007.

[47] Sahlgren M. An introduction to random indexing. In: Methods and applications of semantic indexing workshop at the 7th international conference on terminology and knowledge engineering, TKE 2005; 2005.

[48] Papadimitriou CH, Tamaki H, Raghavan P, Vempala S. Latent semantic indexing: A probabilistic analysis. In: Proceedings of the seventeenth ACM SIGACT-SIGMOD-SIGART symposium on principles of database systems; 1998. p. 159–68.

[49] Bingham E, Mannila H. Random projection in dimensionality reduction: applications to image and text data; 2001. p. 245–250

[50] Vempala SS. The random projection method. Am Math Soc 2004.

[51] Trefethen LN, Bau D. Numer Linear Algebr. SIAM; 1997.

[52] Hofmann T. Probabilistic latent semantic analysis. In: Proceedings of the Fifteenth conference on Uncertainty in artificial intelligence (UAI'99), Stockholm, Sweden; Morgan Kaufmann Publishers Inc. Burlington, Mass. 1999 p. 289–96.

[53] Heinrich G. Ldagibbssampler.java. <http://www.arbylon.net/projects/LdaGibbsSampler.java>.

[54] Berry MW, Mezher D, Philippe B, Sameh A. Parallel computation of the singular value decomposition. In: Kontoghiorghes E, editors. Handbook on parallel computing and statistics; 2003. p. 117–64.

[55] Newman D, Asuncion A, Smyth P, Welling M. Distributed algorithms for topic models. J Mach Learn Res 2009;10:1801–28.

[56] Brand M. Incremental singular value decomposition of uncertain data with missing values. In: Comput vision—ECCV 2002; 2002. p. 707–20.

[57] Sandin F, Emruli B, Sahlgren M. Incremental dimension reduction of tensors with random index; 2011. Available from: <arXiv:1103.3585> [preprint].

[58] Cohen TA. Exploring MEDLINE space with random indexing and pathfinder networks. AMIA Annu Symp Proc 2008:126–30.

[59] Heer J, Card SK, Landay JA. Prefuse: a toolkit for interactive information visualization. In: Conference on human factors in computing systems; 2005. p. 421–30.

[60] Jurgens D, Stevens K. Event detection in blogs using temporal random indexing. In: Proceedings of the workshop on events in emerging text types; 2009. p. 9–16.

[61] Cohen T, Schvaneveldt RW. The trajectory of scientific discovery: concept co-occurrence and converging semantic distance. Studies Health Technol Inform 2010;160(Pt 1):661–5.

[62] Damljanovic D, Petrak J, Lupu M, Cunningham H, Carlsson M, Engstrom G, et al. Random indexing for finding similar nodes within large RDF graphs. In: The semantic web: ESWC 2011 workshops; 2012. p. 156–71.

[63] Sahlgren M, Holst A, Kanerva P. Permutations as a means to encode order in word space. In: Proceedings of the 30th annual meeting of the cognitive science society (CogSci'08), July 23–26, Washington DC, USA; 2008.

[64] Basile P, Caputo P. Encoding syntactic dependencies using random indexing and wikipedia as a corpus. In: Amati G, Carpineto C, Semeraro G, editors, Proceedings of the 3rd Italian Information Retrieval (IIR) Workshop, Bari, Italy, January 26–27, 2012, vol. 835 of CEUR Workshop Proceedings; 2012. p. 144–54. <CEUR-WS.org>. ISSN 1613-0073.

[65] Cohen T, Schvaneveldt R, Rindflesch T. Predication-based semantic indexing: permutations as a means to encode predications in semantic space. AMIA Annu Symp Proc 2009:114–8.

[66] <http://www.nlm.nih.gov/mesh/mbrowser.html>.

[67] Bath PA, William H. Information retrieval: a health and biomedical perspective. New York, NY: Springer; 2003. p. 517. ISBN: 0387955224 89.95

[68] <http://www.nlm.nih.gov/mesh/>.

[69] Aronson A, Mork J, Gay C, Humphrey S, Rogers W, et al. The NLM indexing initiative's medical text indexer. Medinfo 2004;11(Pt 1):268–72.

[70] Huang M, Lu Z. Learning to annotate scientific publications. In: Proceedings of the 23rd international conference on computational linguistics: posters; 2010. p. 463–71.

[71] Cortes C, Vapnik V. Support-vector networks. Mach Learn 1995;20(3):273–97.

[72] Vapnik V. The nature of statistical learning theory. Springer; November 1999.

[73] Joachims T. In: Learning to classify text using support vector machines: methods, theory and algorithms, vol. 186. MA, USA: Kluwer Academic Publishers Norwell; 2002.

[74] Boser BE, Guyon IM, Vapnik VN. A training algorithm for optimal margin classifiers. In: Proceedings of the fifth annual workshop on computational learning theory; 1992. p. 144–52.

[75] Uzuner Ö, Goldstein I, Luo Y, Kohane I. Identifying patient smoking status from medical discharge records. J Am Med Inform Assoc 2008;15(1):14–24.

[76] Clark C, Good K, Jezierny L, Macpherson M, Wilson B, Chajewska U. Identifying smokers with a medical extraction system. J Am Med Inform Assoc 2008;15(1):36–9.

[77] Sahlgren M, Coster R. Using Bag-of-Concepts to improve the performance of support vector machines in text categorization. In: Proceedings of the 20th international conference on computational linguistics, COLING; 2004. p. 2004.

[78] Ding CHQ, Dubchak I. Multi-class protein fold recognition using support vector machines and neural networks. Bioinformatics 2001;17(4):349–58.

[79] Leslie C, Eskin E, Noble WS. The spectrum kernel: a string kernel for SVM protein classification. In: Pacific symposium on biocomputing; 2002. p. 564–75.

[80] Vert J-P. A tree kernel to analyse phylogenetic profiles. Bioinformatics 2002;18(Suppl. 1):S276–84.

[81] Noble WS. In: Bernhard Schölkopf J-PV, Tsuda Koji, editors. Support vector machine applications in computational biologyin Kernel methods in computational biology. MITPress; 2004.

[82] Hartigan JA, Wong MA. Algorithm AS136: A k-means clustering algorithm. J Roy Statist Soc Ser C (Appl Statist) 1979;28(1):100–8.

[83] Schütze H. Automatic word sense discrimination. Comput Linguist 1998;24(1):97–124. [online]. <citeseer.nj.nec.com/schutze98automatic.html>

[84] Newton G, Callahan A, Dumontier M. Semantic journal mapping for search visualization in a large scale article digital library. In: Second workshop on very large digital libraries at the European conference on digital libraries (ECDL); 2009.

[85] Salton G, Fox EA, Wu H. Extended boolean information retrieval. Commun ACM 1983;26(11):1022–36.

[86] Widdows D. Orthogonal negation in vector spaces for modelling word-meanings and document retrieval. In: Proceedings of the 41st annual meeting of the association for computational linguistics (ACL), Sapporo, Japan. Japan: Sapporo; 2003.

[87] Birkhoff G, von Neumann J. The logic of quantum mechanics. Ann Math 1936;37:823–43.

[88] Widdows D, Peters S. In: Word vectors and quantum logic. In: Proceedings of the eighth mathematics of language conference, Bloomington, Indiana

[89] Gärdenfors P. In: Conceptual spaces: the geometry of thought. Bradford Books MIT Press; 2000.

[90] Bruza PD, Widdows D, Woods J. A quantum logic of down below. Elsevier; 2009. p. 625–60.

[91] Kanerva P. Hyperdimensional computing: an introduction to computing in distributed representation with high-dimensional random vectors. Cognit Comput 2009;1(2):139–59.

[92] Cohen T, Widdows D, Schvaneveldt R, Rindflesch T. Finding schizophrenia's prozac: emergent relational similarity in predication space. In: Proceedings of the fifth international symposium on quantum interaction; 2011.

[93] Gayler RW, Slezak Peter. Vector symbolic architectures answer jackendoff's challenges for cognitive neuroscience. In: ICCS/ASCS international conference on cognitive science. Sydney, Australia: University of New South Wales; 2004. p. 133–8.

[94] Jones MN, Mewhort DJK. Representing word meaning and order information in a composite holographic lexicon. Psychol Rev 2007;114:1–37.

[95] Fishbein JM. Integrating structure and meaning: using holographic reduced representations to improve automatic text classification; 2009.

[96] Kanerva P. Binary spatter-coding of ordered k-tuples. Artif Neural Netw—ICANN 1996;96:869–73.

[97] Plate TA. In: Holographic reduced representation: distributed representation for cognitive structures. Stanfpord, CA: Springer; 2003.

[98] Rindflesch TC, Fiszman M. The interaction of domain knowledge and linguistic structure in natural language processing: interpreting hypernymic propositions in biomedical text. J Biomed Inform 2003;36:462–77.

[99] Kilicoglu H, Shin D, Fiszman M, Rosemblat G, Rindflesch TC. SemMedDB: a PubMed-Scale repository of biomedical semantic predications. Bioinformatics 2012.

[100] Cohen Trevor, Widdows Dominic, Schvaneveldt Roger, Rindflesch Thomas. Finding schizophrenia's prozac: Emergent relational similarity in predication space. In: QI'11. Proceedings of the 5th international symposium on quantum interactions. Aberdeen, Scotland. Springer-Verlag, Berlin, Heidelberg; 2011.

[100] Cohen Trevor, Widdows Dominic, Schvaneveldt Roger, Rindflesch Thomas. Finding schizophrenia's prozac: emergent relational similarity in predication space. In: QI'11, Proceedings of the fifth international symposium on quantum interactions, Aberdeen, Scotland. Berlin, Heidelberg: Springer-Verlag; 2004. p. 133–8.

[101] Widdows D, Ferraro K. Semantic vectors: a scalable open source package and online technology management application. In: Sixth international conference on language resources and evaluation (LREC2008); 2008.

[102] Widdows D, Cohen T. The semantic vectors package: New algorithms and public tools for distributional semantics. In: IEEE Fourth International Conference on Semantic Computing (ICSC); 2010. p. 9–15.

[103] Widdows D, Cohen T. Real, complex, and binary semantic vectors. In: Quantum Interaction: 6th International Symposium, QI 2012, Paris, France, June 27–29. LNCS. vol. 7620. Springer-Verlag. Berlin, Heidelberg. p 24–35.

[104] <http://code.google.com/p/semanticvectors/>.

Biomedical Natural Language Processing and Text Mining

Kevin Bretonnel Cohen

*Computational Bioscience Program, University of Colorado School of Medicine,
Department of Linguistics, University of Colorado at Boulder, USA*

6.1 NATURAL LANGUAGE PROCESSING AND TEXT MINING DEFINED

Natural language processing is the study of computer programs that take natural, or human, language as input. Natural language processing applications may approach tasks ranging from low-level processing, such as assigning parts of speech to words, to high-level tasks, such as answering questions. *Text mining* is the use of natural language processing for practical tasks, often related to finding information in prose of various kinds. In practice, natural language processing and text mining exist on a continuum, and there is no hard and fast line between the two.

6.2 NATURAL LANGUAGE

Natural language is human language, as opposed to computer languages. The difference between them lies in the presence of ambiguity. No well-designed computer language is ambiguous. In contrast, all known natural languages exhibit the property of ambiguity. *Ambiguity* occurs when an input can have more than one interpretation. Ambiguity exists at all levels of human language. (For illustrative purposes, we will focus on written language, since that is the domain of most biomedical natural language processing, with the exception of speech recognition applications.) Consider, for example, the word *discharge*. This word is ambiguous in that it may be a noun or a verb. In this example, we see both cases:

> *With a decreased LOS, inpatient rehabilitation services will have to improve FIM efficiency or discharge patients with lower discharge FIM scores. (PMID 12917856)*

In the case of *discharge patients*, it is a verb. In the case of *discharge FIM scores,* it is a noun. Suppose that an application (called a part of speech tagger) has determined that it is a noun. It remains ambiguous as to its meaning. In these examples, we see two common meanings in biomedical text:

> *Patient was prescribed codeine upon discharge*
> *The discharge was yellow and purulent*

In the first case, *discharge* has the meaning "release from the hospital," while in the second case, it refers to a body fluid. Once an application has determined which is the correct meaning, it remains ambiguous as to its relationship to the words with which it appears—i.e., there is syntactic ambiguity. Should *discharge FIM scores* be interpreted as *discharge* modifying *FIM scores*, or as *discharge FIM* modifying *scores*? The correct analyses—noun versus verb, release from hospital versus body fluid, and *discharge [FIM scores]* versus *[discharge FIM] scores*—are so obvious to the human reader that we are typically not even consciously aware of the ambiguities. However, ambiguity is so pervasive in natural language that it is difficult to produce a sentence that is not ambiguous in some way, and the ambiguity that humans resolve so easily is one of the central problems that natural language processing must deal with.

The statistical properties of language would be much different if the same ideas were always presented the same way. However, one of the predominant features of human language is that it allows for an enormous amount of variability. Just as we saw that ambiguity is a fact at all levels of language, variability occurs at all levels of language as well.

On the most basic level, corresponding to the sounds of spoken language, we have variability in spelling. This is most noticeable when comparing British and American medical English, where we see frequent variants like *haematoma* in British English versus *hematoma* in American English.

At the level of morphemes, or word parts, we see ambiguity in how words should be analyzed. Given a word such as *unlockable* (PMID 23003012), should we interpret it as [un[lockable]] (not capable of being locked), or as [[unlock]able] (capable of being unlocked)?

At the level of words, the phenomenon of synonymy allows for using different, but (roughly) equivalent, words. For example, we might see *cardiac surgery* referred to as *heart surgery*. One common type of synonymy comes from using abbreviations or acronyms, such as *CAT* for *computed axial tomography*. Of course, synonymy multiplies the chances for ambiguity—it is commonly the case that biomedical synonyms can have multiple definitions.

Variability exists at the syntactic level, as well. Consider, for example, how many syntactic constructions can express a simple assertion about binding between a protein and DNA:

- *Met28 binds to DNA*
- *…binding of Met28 to DNA…*
- *Met28 and DNA bind…*
- *…binding between Met28 and DNA…*

Of course, additional modifying material can make any one of these variants take many more forms:

- *…binding of Met28 to DNA…*
- *…binding under unspecified conditions of Met28 to DNA…*
- *…binding of Met28 to upstream regions of DNA…*

Ambiguity and variability together are the primary challenges that natural language processing applications face.

6.3 APPROACHES TO NATURAL LANGUAGE PROCESSING AND TEXT MINING

Two approaches to natural language processing and text mining dominate the field. They are known as *rule-based* or *knowledge-based* on the one hand, and *statistical* or *machine learning based* on the other. Although there are theoretical issues that may drive the individual researcher toward a preference for one or the other, we will focus on the practical aspects of choosing an approach.

Knowledge-based approaches to natural language processing make use of one or more sources of knowledge about the domain. Two kinds of knowledge may be brought to bear on a natural language processing problem. One is knowledge about language and about how facts are typically stated in biomedical documents. Systems that make use of this kind of knowledge are known as *rule-based* systems. Rules may consist of linguistic patterns, for instance. The other kind of knowledge that may be used is real-world knowledge about the domain. For example, a natural language processing application may benefit from knowing that *cancer* is something that receives treatment, while *phenobarbital* is something that is used to perform treatment. Natural language processing applications may make use of one or both of these types of knowledge.

Statistical or *machine learning*-based systems are based on providing a computer application with a set of labeled training examples and letting it learn how to classify unseen examples into one or more classes. The classes will vary depending on the exact problem that we are trying to solve. For example, a machine learning application might be presented with fifty examples of *discharge* meaning "release from hospital" and fifty examples of *discharge* meaning "body fluid." Based on features of the context in which the 100 examples appear, the application will learn how to classify a new, previously unseen example of *discharge* as having one meaning or the other.

From a practical perspective, most natural language processing systems are a hybrid of rule-based and machine learning-based approaches—to paraphrase Oscar Wilde, natural language processing is never pure and rarely simple. The two approaches may be combined loosely or as tightly integrated components of the system. A typical example of loose combination is the use of machine learning to handle common examples with a rule-based post-processing step to fix errors on more difficult cases. An example of tight combination would be to use rules as an integral part of the learning system. For example, a popular approach to parsing (i.e., syntactic analysis) is based on statistical properties of the head of the noun phrase (roughly, the main noun of a group of words that is centered on a noun, such as *scores* in *discharge FIM scores*). However, to determine which word in the noun phrase is the head noun, a set of simple heuristic rules is applied—e.g., removing any prepositional phrase that follows the noun.

Knowledge-based and machine learning-based approaches each have their advantages and disadvantages. Knowledge-based approaches can work because the linguistic rules and domain knowledge that they use are psychologically, formally, and empirically real in some sense. They also have the advantage that they can be developed on the basis of intuition—we do not need a large set of training data to know that if *discharge* is preceded by a color, it is probably a noun and probably does not have the meaning "release from the hospital." Knowledge-based approaches have the disadvantage that they can require considerable manual effort to build the rules and the necessary knowledge bases. For example, it is likely that since the 1960s a majority of linguists in the world have been working on the problem of English syntax, but we still do not have a comprehensive formal grammar of the English language on which there is wide consensus. Machine learning-based approaches have the advantage that no domain-specific knowledge is required to build them (at least in the case where features are kept simple). They can work well because some of the phenomena that we are interested in occur frequently enough to be statistically tractable. They have the disadvantage that it requires considerable effort to build the large bodies of training data that they require. They also have the disadvantage that the available data is often very sparse—some phenomena occur frequently, but it is the nature of natural language that an enormous number of phenomena occur very rarely. (Zipf's law [54] describes this phenomenon.) This is especially an issue in biomedicine, where we care deeply about rare events—most people who present to the emergency department with chest pain are not having a myocardial infarction, but we never want to miss the one who is. Often the choice between the two boils down to a financial one—will it be cheaper to invest time in building more rules, or will it be cheaper to invest time in labeling sufficient training examples? Again, the most common solution is to combine the two approaches. There is no evidence that one works better than the other in any objective sense.

6.4 SOME SPECIAL CONSIDERATIONS OF NATURAL LANGUAGE PROCESSING IN THE BIOMEDICAL DOMAIN

To date, most research in natural language processing has focused on "newswire text," primarily because of its wide availability and the fact that various collections of newswire text with a variety of types of labels that we have already seen to be important (part of speech, word senses, syntactic structure, etc.) have been made available free of copyright considerations. Such work is generally considered to be "general domain" natural language processing. "Specialized domains," such as the biomedical domain, present both special problems and special opportunities for natural language processing.

Biomedical natural language processing generally deals with two genres of input texts: (1) scientific journal articles and (2) clinical documents. Scientific journal articles have a number of characteristics that make them difficult for natural language processing. One of these is the heavy use of parenthesized text. In general, parenthesized text poses problems for the syntactic analysis of sentences. It also causes problems for finding the scope of "hedging" statements, which express uncertainty about a statement. Parenthesized material may be useful to scientists, but confusing to lay people. For these reasons, some systems delete parenthesized text. However, parenthesized text can also have a number of uses. Parenthesized text can be used for determining (and disambiguating) abbreviation meanings, gene names and symbols, establishing rhetorical relationships between papers, and various bibliometric applications. For this reason, it has been found useful to be able to classify the contents of parentheses into a variety of classes, including citations, data values, P-values, figures or table pointers, and parenthetical statements. Scientific papers also often contain crucial information in tables and figures, which are in general difficult for natural language processing applications to handle.

Clinical documents present a range of difficulties of their own. One prominent example is the predominance of sentence fragments in many types of clinical documents. For example, *No fever or chills.* is a typical example of a "sentence" in a clinical document. It is sentence-like in that it is an independent unit and has sentence-final punctuation, but is unlike a sentence in that it contains no verb, subject, or object.

A useful way to begin thinking about the special aspects of biomedical text in general and clinical text in particular is to approach them from the viewpoint of the sublanguage. A *sublanguage* is a genre of language that has special characteristics as compared to the language from which it is derived (e.g., general English in the case of English-language medical documents). Various researchers have focused on different aspects of sublanguages and how they differ from the related language. One commonly accepted characteristic is that in a sublanguage, there is a restricted semantic range of entities that are discussed and that can be the arguments of verbs or other predicators (an *argument* is a participant in the action of a verb or nominalization). Another characteristic of sublanguages is that they typically make use of a restricted set of lexical items and syntactic structures, as compared to the base language. Some disagreement exists over whether sublanguages are subsets of the base language or whether they also allow constructions that would not be considered grammatical (i.e., do not follow syntactic rules) in the base language.

The notion that there is a restricted semantic range of entities that are discussed in a sublanguage and that verbs have restrictions on the semantic classes of their arguments is important in natural language processing because it allows the use of inference in interpreting inputs [27,46]. For example, given an input like *X-ray shows perihilar opacities and peribronchial thickening*, we can make a number of inferences. One is that the *X-ray* refers to an *X-ray* of the lungs; another is that it is the patient's lungs that have been examined by the X-ray. Another is that given a sentence like *No fever or chills.* we can infer that there was an event of measurement, and that the subject of the measurement was the patient.

The notion that sublanguages use a restricted set of the possible constructions in the language suggests that it might be more tractable to process language that fits the sublanguage model, even if those constructions do not fit the normal syntactic rules of the language, simply because there are fewer constructions in total. So, although *No fever or chills.* might present problems for a syntactic parser that was developed to process general English, we can write rules for parsing such constructions and hope for broad coverage because this is such a common construction in the clinical sublanguage.

In general, clinical sublanguage has a clear bearing on the theoretical question of whether sublanguages are simply subsets of the general language or whether they contain additional elements, since clinical language is full of constructions like *No fever or chills.* that clearly do not exist in general English.

One genre-specific problem that is receiving growing attention is the challenge of dealing with full-text scientific journal articles. The early history of applying biomedical natural language processing to scientific publications focused almost entirely on the abstracts of journal articles. These were considered to present sublanguage-like difficulties of their own. For example, early abstracts were typically restricted to a 500-word length, and authors were thought to utilize convoluted sentence structures to keep their abstracts within these limits. However, as the full text of journal articles began to become widely available, it quickly became apparent that they presented additional challenges that had not been confronted when language processing focused on abstracts. For example, scientific articles typically contain a *Materials and Methods* section. These sections turn out to be the cause of rampant false positives for some types of language processing applications [7,50], such as gene mention systems (see below). For that reason, much early research tried to apply techniques to find such sections and exclude them from processing. A number of differences have been noted between abstracts and the full text of journal articles, a number of which have implications for natural language processing [18]. As noted earlier, one example is the use of parenthesized text [15]. Parenthesized text is uncommon in abstracts. However, it is very common in the full text of journal articles. Parenthesized text poses problems for a number of both lower-level and higher-level processing tasks, such as syntactic parsing and finding the scope of indicators of uncertainty. Some researchers have attempted to deal with this by deleting parenthesized text entirely. However, parenthesized text sometimes contains content that is actually quite useful to interpreting the input. For example, parenthesized references to figures or tables are often good indicators that a sentence contains highly reliable information or that it would be useful to include in a summary of the document. Parentheses may contain statistical values that could allow a system to assign weights to the certainty of an assertion in a sentence. They may contain data on the number of subjects in an experiment that is important for use in constructing systematic reviews. They may contain important primary data, such as coordinate values for fMRI studies. Therefore, it is important to be able to classify the contents of parentheses before making a decision about whether to ignore it or, on the contrary, to try to extract it. Comparisons of the performance of language processing tools on abstracts versus full text have found degradations in performance on full text. For example, gene mention systems typically perform worse, and sometimes much worse, on the full text of journal articles than on abstracts. Part-of-speech taggers also perform better on abstracts than on full text. Despite the presence of these and other complicating factors, it is clear that processing full text is important for a number of applications, and in fact can improve performance on information retrieval, so it is likely and important that research continue into the challenges of handling full text.

6.5 BUILDING BLOCKS OF NATURAL LANGUAGE PROCESSING APPLICATIONS

Text mining applications are often built as pipelines of components that perform specific, often low-level, processing tasks. Again, at each level, ambiguity and variability are issues.

6.5.1 **Document Segmentation**

Frequently, a necessary first step is segmenting an input document into sections. In the case of scientific publications, we often see some version of an introduction, materials and methods section, results section, discussion, and bibliography. In practice, the actual section structure can vary from journal to journal and from article type to article type within a journal. For example, systematic reviews will have a very different structure from research articles. One recent competition on natural language processing involving answering questions given a large body of journal articles—the 2006 Text Retrieval Conference genomics track—required writing 17 different document structure parsers for just the products of a single publisher. Within sections, further processing may be necessary—for example, it is very useful to be able to identify figure and table captions. Different sections of a scientific journal article present different advantages and challenges. Materials and methods sections are a prime example. They are frequent sources of false positives for many kinds of natural language processing applications, including gene name finders and programs that look for evidence of Gene Ontology functions. For this reason, many early biomedical natural language processing applications tried to identify materials and methods sections and ignore their contents. However, as work in the field has progressed toward doing a better job of establishing the context of assertions made in journal articles, it has been recognized that extracting methods from journal articles is an important task in and of itself, and researchers may now find themselves in the position of needing to find materials and methods sections and focus on them.

Clinical documents present a wide range of section-related issues. First of all, there are many distinct types of clinical documents. X-ray reports, pathology reports, ICU progress notes, cross-coverage notes, and discharge summaries are just a small sample of classes of clinical documents. Any hospital will produce a wide range of clinical documents. The structure of these documents will vary from hospital to hospital. Furthermore, the structure of these documents is likely to vary from department to department, and even from physician to physician within a department. This makes the diversity of document structure parsers that need to be written for scientific journal articles seem simple. However, it is crucial to be aware of document structure when working with clinical documents. For example, finding a medication listed in the history section of a discharge summary carries very different connotations from finding it in the treatment plan section of a discharge summary.

6.5.2 **Sentence Segmentation**

The standard unit of analysis in most natural language processing applications (and in linguistics in general) is generally the sentence. Following the determination of the structure of a document, the next step is often to split it into sentences. Even scientific journal articles present problems here. The conventions of general scientific writing sometimes violate general rules of sentence formation. For example, an abstract may contain text like the following:

> *INTRODUCTION: The development of acute coagulopathy of trauma (ACoT) is associated with a significant increase in mortality. (PMID 23272297)*

A colon (:) would not normally be treated as sentence-final text. However, in this case, it clearly functions as a sentence-like boundary between *INTRODUCTION* and a sentence that begins *The development of acute coagulopathy...* A standard sentence segmenter will fail here, and a knowledge-based system that is aware of the specifics of this specialized domain is probably necessary. Sentences in scientific journal articles also do not necessarily start with upper-case letters. For example, when a sentence begins with a gene name or symbol and a mutant form of the gene is being discussed, the sentence may begin with a lower-case letter, as in *p21(ras), a guanine nucleotide binding factor, mediates T-cell signal transduction through PKC-dependent and PKC-independent pathways.* (PMID 8887687) This violates a basic expectation of any standard sentence segmentation algorithm.

6.5.3 **Tokenization**

After segmenting the input into sentences, a common step is to segment those sentences. A *token* is any individual separable unit of the input. This will obviously include words, but also includes punctuation. For example, *pathways.* at the end of the previous example consists of two tokens, *pathways* and the sentence-final period.

Biomedical text shares some tokenization issues in common with general-domain text. For example, the best treatment for negative contractions is an open question. *Don't* can reasonably be separated into *do* and *n't*, but how should *won't* be handled? Biomedical text also presents many tokenization issues that are specific to the domain. For example, in medical text, $+fever$ indicates the presence of fever, and the $+$ and *fever* must be separated into distinct tokens to obtain the correct semantic interpretation (e.g., in contrast to $-fever$, which indicates the absence of fever), while H^+ should be kept as a single token identifying a particular ion.

6.5.4 **Part of Speech Tagging**

Having identified the tokens, the next step is often to assign them a part of speech. This is essential if steps such as syntactic analysis will be attempted later. Natural language processing applications may recognize as many as eighty parts of speech. We get from the eight parts of speech of our traditional education to the eighty parts of speech of natural language processing in part by subdividing the well-known parts of speech into finer subdivisions. For example, the class of verbs may be subdivided into the separate parts of speech of bare verb, third person present tense singular verb, past tense verb, past participle verb, and present participle verb. (See [31] for a typical set of part-of-speech tags for natural language processing; the British National Corpus uses over a hundred tags.)

Part of speech tagging is much more domain-specific than might be expected. General-domain part of speech taggers do not work well on scientific journal articles, and part of speech taggers for just such textual genres have been developed. Part of speech tagging in clinical documents is even more fraught; it has been found that a part of speech tagger that works well for documents from one hospital may not work well for documents from another hospital.

6.5.5 **Parsing**

A final processing step may be *parsing,* or syntactic analysis. Various approaches to parsing exist. One of the fundamental differences is between shallow parsing and full parsing. *Shallow parsing* attempts to find groups of words that go together, typically focusing on a "head" word of a specific part of speech, such as a noun or verb, without attempting to determine the complete syntactic structure of a sentence. For example, given the sentence *The development of acute coagulopathy of trauma (ACoT) is associated with a significant increase in mortality.* (PMID 23272297), a shallow parser might try to produce the following output:

The development

of

acute coagulopathy

of

trauma (ACoT)

is associated

with

a significant increase

in

mortality

.

In contrast, *full parsing* attempts to determine the complete structure of a sentence, identifying the phrases that a shallow parser would identify, but also showing the relationships between them.

Full parsers include constituency parsers and dependency parsers. *Constituency parsers* are focused on phrasal relationships and dominance and precedence. In contrast, *dependency parsers* detect relationships between individual words, and classify the types of those relationships. Because those relationships include labels like *subject*, dependency parses are sometimes thought to be more direct reflections of the semantics of the sentence. Constituency parsing is much further developed than dependency parsing, and constituency parser output can be converted to a dependency parse representation.

6.6 ADDITIONAL COMPONENTS OF NATURAL LANGUAGE PROCESSING APPLICATIONS

The preceding building blocks are the basic components that are likely to be found in any text mining application. Other components, including word sense disambiguation, negation detection, temporal link detection, context determination, and hedging can be important parts of a system, as well.

6.6.1 Word Sense Disambiguation

Word sense disambiguation is the task of determining which of multiple "senses," or meanings, a given token of a word has. An example is the noun *discharge*, discussed earlier. The word sense disambiguation task is sometimes divided into two classes—all-words word sense disambiguation and targeted word sense disambiguation. In all-words word sense disambiguation, the goal of the system is to disambiguate every word in the text. In targeted word sense disambiguation, the system focuses only on specific words of interest.

A classic knowledge-based approach to word sense disambiguation is the Leskian paradigm [35]. The Leskian paradigm requires a dictionary. The intuition behind the Leskian paradigm is that given a sentence containing an ambiguous word and multiple definitions for that word, we calculate the similarity between the sentence and between the definitions. The most similar definition will belong to the correct sense of the word.

6.6.2 Negation Detection

Detection of negation is important both in scientific publications and in clinical documents. Failure to detect negation is a classic source of false positives in co-occurrence-based approaches to text mining, in which the occurrence of two concepts within some window of analysis (e.g., a sentence or a journal article abstract) is assumed to indicate a relationship between those concepts. Many early studies on information extraction simply ignored negation and removed negated sentences from their evaluation data. However, negation detection is now a prominent focus of research in natural language processing. In clinical documents, negation detection is critical; one study found that about half of all clinical concepts in some classes of clinical documents are negated [10]. Depending on the report type, one or another type of negation might predominate. *Constituent negation* is the negation of a phrase, typically a noun phrase, e.g., *No fever or chills.* *Proposition negation* is the negation of an entire assertion—e.g., *Patient has not had any previous surgery.* Much domain-specific phraseology is used to indicate negation in clinical documents, such as the use of the verb *deny*, as in *He denies any chest discomfort at this time.* Interestingly, regular expressions have been found sufficient to identify negated clinical concepts in clinical documents [11]; this is in contrast to many linguistic phenomena, which require greater computational power than regular expressions.

6.6.3 **Temporality**

Detection of temporal relations is an important part of interpreting both scientific publications and clinical documents. In scientific publications, it may be important to know when some event occurs relevant to some particular frame of reference, such as the cell cycle. In clinical documents, relative times between events is important as well. For example, if we are looking for adverse drug events, it might be important to know whether symptoms of a rash preceded or followed the administration of a medication.

Besides the granular level of relations between individual events, there is also a larger frame of reference for temporality, in which we try to differentiate facts that are current, that are part of the patient's history, or that are part of the family history. We discuss those separately under the topic of context.

6.6.4 **Context Determination**

The notion of "context" can refer to widely varying concepts in scientific publications and in clinical documents [12]. In scientific publications, it refers primarily to biological or experimental context. For example, a finding reported in a paper may be true only at a specific pH, or in a specific growth medium, or in a specific cell line. Failure to extract context may decrease the willingness of biologists to trust the output of text mining applications. However, this aspect of context remains largely unexplored and is a very open area for research.

In clinical documents, context is more related to temporality. The most prominent aspects of context are the relationships between clinical concepts mentioned in a document and the patient's current situation. For instance, a clinical concept may be true of the patient's current condition, it may be true of the patient's history with or without being true of the patient's condition, or it may be an aspect of the patient's family history.

6.6.5 Hedging

Hedging occurs when speakers qualify their statements in a way that allows them to not fully commit to their veracity [40]. This is a common phenomenon in clinical text, where we are often considering multiple diagnoses, possible findings, etc.

- *treated for a presumptive sinusitis*
- *It was felt that the patient probably had a cerebrovascular accident involving the left side of the brain. Other differentials entertained were perhaps seizure and the patient being post-ictal when he was found, although this consideration is less likely*
- *R/O pneumonia*

The phenomenon of hedging is a good illustration of the fact that we cannot assume that mention of a concept in a document implies the presence of that concept in the world. Not surprisingly, hedging cues can be ambiguous— even *or* can be a device for hedging [40]:

- *Findings compatible with reactive airway disease or viral lower respiratory tract infection*
- *Nucleotide sequence and PCR analyses demonstrated the presence of novel duplications or deletions involving the NF-kappa B motif*

Once a hedge has been detected, determining the scope of the hedging cue is a challenge. Hedges may even be multiply embedded, as in *These results suggest that expression of c-jun, jun B, and jun D gene might be involved in terminal granulocyte differentiation or in regulating granulocyte functionality.*

…which is analyzed in the BioScope corpus [51], which annotates negation, speculation, and their scopes, as:

These results <xcope id="X7.5.3"><cue type= "speculation" ref="X7.5.3"> suggest </cue> that <xcope id= "X7.5.2">expression of c-jun, jun B, and jun D genes <cue type= "speculation" ref= "X7.5.2"> might </cue> be involved <xcope id="X7.5.1">in terminal granulocyte differentiation <cue type= "speculation" ref="X7.5.1" >or</cue> in regulating granulocyte functionality </xcope></xcope></xcope>.

6.7 **EVALUATION IN NATURAL LANGUAGE PROCESSING**

Evaluation techniques in natural language processing fall into three general categories: (1) evaluation against a gold standard, (2) post hoc judging, and (3) testing with a structured test suite.

Evaluation against a gold standard is the most common approach. Gold standard preparation is typically manual and labor-intensive. To evaluate the quality of a gold standard, one often has some or all of the gold standard marked by multiple annotators and then determines the extent to which the annotators agree with each other. If this *inter-annotator agreement* is high, it is generally taken as evidence that the task was well-defined, the guidelines are clear, and the task is actually tractable. Inter-annotator agreement is sometimes taken as an estimate of the best possible performance for a natural language processing system. If inter-annotator agreement is low, we suspect that whether due to poor task definition, poor guidelines, or the inherent difficulty of the task, the gold standard itself is of poor quality.

Post hoc judging is often applied when a dataset is too large for every element of it to be classified. For example, if given a set of over 100,000 clinical documents and asked to retrieve all documents related to patients that fit particular criteria for cohort definition, the outputs of a system might be manually judged for correctness, rather than trying to classify all 100,000 documents in advance.

Various metrics are used in the evaluation of natural language processing applications, depending on the task type. The most common ones are precision, recall, and *F*-measure.

Precision is the positive predictive value. It reflects how many of a system's outputs are correct. It is defined as

$$P = \frac{TP}{TP + FP},$$

where *TP* is true positive outputs and *FP* is false positive outputs.

Recall is the sensitivity. It reflects how often a system found something if it was present in the input. It is defined as

$$R = \frac{TP}{TP + FN},$$

where *FN* is false negatives.

F-measure is the harmonic mean of precision and recall. It is usually defined as

$$F = 2 * \frac{P * R}{P + R}.$$

The metrics of precision, recall, and *F*-measure have been applied to many types of natural language processing tasks. Many other metrics exist as well, some of them building on these basic measures. For example, an information retrieval application might be evaluated with the P@10 metric, or precision for the top ten results returned by the system.

Structured test suites are used not to characterize overall performance, but to test software for bugs and to perform fine-grained evaluation of performance on particular classes of inputs. Structured test suites are discussed further in this chapter within the section on software engineering in natural language processing.

Evaluation in clinical natural language processing has been plagued since the inception of the field by the lack of availability of publicly shareable data. Individual research institutions built their own gold standards that they were not allowed to share (usually due to protection of human subjects concerns), making it difficult to evaluate the quality of the evaluation and impossible to replicate work. One of the most important changes taking place in clinical natural language processing at this time is the changing of this situation, while still appropriately accommodating the necessary human subjects protections. Multiple initiatives to prepare shareable clinical gold standard data are in progress and stand to change the face of research into clinical natural language processing radically.

Evaluation of text mining as applied to scientific journal articles has profited from the availability of copyright-free texts and various community efforts to build gold standards. A number of these have been used in shared tasks that have had a large influence on the direction and progress of research in biomedical text mining. In a *shared task*, a group of participants agrees on a task definition, a gold standard for judging performance, and a set of metrics for quantifying performance. Then training materials are made publicly available, the public is invited to work on the task, and all systems are judged on the same test data. Tasks are typically repeated for multiple years, allowing for improvement in performance.

6.8 PRACTICAL APPLICATIONS: TEXT MINING TASKS

6.8.1 Information Retrieval

One of the earliest text mining tasks was information retrieval. It remains one of the most commonly performed. *Information retrieval* is the task of finding documents relevant to some information need. In the global context, the best-known version of information retrieval is finding web pages with a search engine. In the biomedical domain, the analog is finding scientific journal articles. In a clinical context, it might consist of finding documents that establish that a patient can be ruled in or out of some cohort.

Early information retrieval required the assistance of a trained medical librarian who was familiar with indexing systems based on a fixed set of categories [25]. The availability of publications in electronic form made possible the first approach to automatic information retrieval—keyword search of the contents of a publication. The most basic approach to information retrieval is simple Boolean search. In this technique, the user enters one or more keywords. If a document contains the keyword(s), the system returns it. Ordering of results is likely to be by some aspect of the metadata about the document, such as publication date. For example, the PubMed search engine returns the newest documents at the top of the list.

More sophisticated approaches to information retrieval (such as geometric approaches that were described in Chapter 5) try to determine not just whether or not a document is relevant to the user's information need, but how relevant it is, relative to other documents. The classic approach makes use of the concepts of term frequency and inverse document frequency. The intuition behind term frequency is that the more often a keyword occurs in a document, the more relevant that document is to the user. The intuition behind inverse document frequency is that the more documents a keyword occurs in, the less useful it is in determining relevance and therefore the less it should be weighted in calculating relevance. To give an extreme example, the word *the* probably occurs in every document in PubMed, so if it occurs in a query, we should give it no weight in deciding whether or not a document is relevant to the user. (In practice, words like *the* are called *stopwords* and are generally removed from consideration in queries altogether.)

One heavily studied aspect of information retrieval in the general domain and in the biomedical domain has been the issue of synonymy. Many approaches to biomedical information retrieval have struggled to find large-scale, publicly available knowledge resources that could be used for *query expansion*—automatically adding synonyms to a query in an attempt to increase recall. The verb *struggle* is used here deliberately, because in general the approach has been difficult to implement. As in the general domain, there is the phenomenon that every new word added to the query adds to the potential for polysemy (multiple meanings of words—a source of ambiguity). In the biomedical domain there is the additional problem that many of the publicly available resources for query expansion contain a considerable amount of cruft and can only be used with very careful attention to which synonyms and what kinds of synonyms are utilized.

6.8.2 **Named Entity Recognition**

Named entity recognition is the task of finding all mentions of some semantic class in text. The original semantic classes were people, places, and organizations, leading to the "named entity" categorization. In more recent years within the biomedical domain, the type of semantic class has broadened very widely, to include things like biological processes or molecular functions that are not clearly either named or entities. Nonetheless, the terminology has remained.

In the domain of scientific journal articles, the classic named entity recognition task has been finding mentions of genes and proteins. The first system to attempt this was rule-based [23], but machine learning approaches long ago came to dominate the field. One of the early surprising findings of this research was that having a dictionary of gene names as a resource was of no help unless one's system had terrible performance without the dictionary [53]. Systems for named entity recognition of genes and proteins use features that are common to named entity recognition systems in general. However, they also typically incorporate many features related to typography and orthography, to reflect the varied forms that gene names can take, such as including Arabic numerals, Roman numerals, hyphens, parentheses, Greek letters, etc.

The highest-performing systems have generally been differentiated from the average system by their ability to get gene name boundaries correct. Most systems can find at least part of a gene name; the best systems then employ a variety of tricks to extend the boundary of the candidate gene name to the left or right until the actual boundaries are found.

As the field has matured, the number of semantic classes that named entity recognition systems have attempted to recognize has increased considerably. Table 6.1 lists a variety of these semantic classes.

In the clinical domain, it has been difficult to separate the problem of named entity recognition from the problem of named entity normalization. We turn to this topic in the next section.

6.8.3 **Named Entity Normalization**

Given some semantic class of a named entity, it may not be sufficient simply to recognize when one is mentioned in text (the named entity recognition task). Rather, it is often desirable or necessary to map that named entity to some entity in a database, or to some concept in a controlled vocabulary.

Table 6.1 Semantic classes of named entities in biomedicine. Adapted from Jurafsky and Martin.

Semantic Class	Examples	Citations
Cell lines	*T98G, HeLa cell, Chinese hamster ovary cells, CHO cells*	[47]
Cell types	*Primary T lymphocytes, natural killer cells, NK cells*	[30,47]
Chemicals	*Citric acid, 2-diiodopentane, C*	[19]
Drugs	*Cyclosporin A, CDDP*	[43]
Genes/proteins	*White, HSP60, protein kinase C, L23A*	[48,53]
Malignancies	*Carcinoma, breast neoplasms*	[29]
Medical/clinical concepts	*Amyotrophic lateral sclerosis*	[1,2]
Mouse strains	*LAFT, AKR*	[8]
Mutations	*C10T, Ala64 → Gly*	[9]
Populations	*Judo group*	[52]

In the clinical domain, a wide variety of controlled vocabularies have developed over the years. These have a wide range of sometimes very specialized uses, ranging from billing, classifying diagnoses for epidemiological purposes, and dictating pathology reports, to indexing scientific literature. We can consider all members of any one vocabulary as constituting named entities for the purpose of named entity recognition. However, for a text mining system to be useful, it is crucial that systems not just recognize mentions of these named entities, but determine *which* entity it is.

For many years, the standard tool for doing this with clinical text has been MetaMap [1,2]. MetaMap takes as its input a set of biomedical vocabularies (typically the entire Unified Medical Language System Metathesaurus, although it can be used with other vocabularies, and can also be configured to output only concepts from a specific vocabulary) and some text. In that text, MetaMap finds all mentions of concepts from the biomedical vocabularies, outputting the identifier of that concept (i.e., normalizing it) and giving a measure of confidence in the recognition and normalization. It also includes options of performing word sense disambiguation, negation detection, and other advanced features.

MetaMap begins by performing a shallow parse of the input. For each phrase, many variant forms are calculated, manipulating such things as inflectional morphology, derivational morphology, acronym generation, and spelling variants, as well as identifying parts of phrases that can commonly be ignored. MetaMap then tries to match the various forms to terms from the various biomedical vocabularies. Potential candidates are scored on four characteristics:

- Whether or not the head noun matches.
- The edit distance between the phrase and the potential candidate.
- How much of the phrase and of the potential candidate match each other, ignoring gaps.
- How much of the phrase and of the potential candidate match each other, not ignoring gaps.

Although MetaMap was originally developed for clinical texts, it has been found to be applicable to scientific journal articles, as well. Furthermore, although it has been claimed that MetaMap is appropriate only for offline processing due to its execution speed, it is also available as a Java API that has been successfully deployed for relevance ranking. MetaMap has also been proposed as an appropriate baseline for cohort retrieval studies [16]; although most groups that have worked in this area have found the Lucene API to be a difficult baseline to beat, MetaMap can do so. (Lucene is a publicly available application programming interface for building search applications. It includes classes for representing documents and queries, methods for building and searching indexes, etc.)

In the biological domain, the predominant target for normalization has been genes and proteins. This has become known as the *gene normalization* task. The earliest work in this area applied techniques from descriptive linguistics to determine what parts of gene names and symbols are most meaningful and what parts can be ignored in normalization, by examining large numbers of gene names and symbols from the Entrez Gene database (LocusLink at the time) [17]. The general approach was to account for how often particular linguistic, typographic, positional, and orthographic features were associated with contrast and how often they were associated with variability. *Contrast* occurs when a feature is used to mark the difference between two different genes. For example, two different numbers at the right edge of a gene name or symbol most likely indicate that two different genes are being referred to, and should not be ignored in the normalization process. *Variability* occurs when a feature does not indicate a difference between two different genes in the database. For example, whether a Roman numeral or an Arabic numeral is used typically does not mark a difference between two different genes, but rather may typically be used freely to indicate the name of the same gene. Such differences can be ignored in the normalization process.

This early work was based entirely on the contents of the database. Subsequent work moved to the next step, mapping from mentions in text to entities in a database. The field moved gradually from easier to more difficult formulations of the problem, but even the easier formulations of the problem were instructive. In early work, the task was, given a database of genes for some species and a set of documents, to produce the database identifiers for all genes mentioned in the document. Note that mention-level accuracy is irrelevant here—scoring is on the basis of the document. For example, given a document that mentions X, Y, and Z, the system must realize that Y and Z refer to the same entity in the database and that only two gene identifiers should be returned. These early studies artificially inflated performance, since the species was a given. (Many genes with the same name exist in different species—at least 22 species in EntrezGene have the BRCA1 gene.) However, the results were illustrative. The first work focused on the species yeast, fly, and mouse [26]. Most systems were able to perform quite well on yeast, with F-measures in the 0.90s frequently achieved. In contrast, performance on mouse was significantly lower, and performance on fly was both lower and all over the map. These early findings led to the hypothesis that length was a contributor to the difficulty of gene normalization. Subsequent work on human genes showed similar results to the early work on the mouse [41]; the two species have similar gene names, supporting the initial analysis.

After going through the period where species were known a priori, research in gene normalization progressed to the next step—normalization of genes in documents containing mentions of arbitrary species [38]. This required the development of systems capable of recognizing species first; then the task is to relate a mention of a gene to the species. This is often complicated by the fact that a single paper may mention any number of species.

6.8.4 **Information Extraction**

Information extraction, also known as relation extraction, is the task of finding relationships between things that are mentioned in text. For example, we might want to find proteins that interact with other proteins, or genes that are related to specific diseases. Information extraction requires the ability to perform named entity recognition or named entity normalization, but adds the ability to characterize relationships between named entities.

In the biological domain, the earliest work in information extraction was on finding protein-protein interactions. From the very beginning, researchers took both rule-based and machine learning-based approaches. The first machine learning approach [20] assumed that protein names could be identified by dictionary look-up, found sentences that contained two protein names, and used a simple bag-of-words representation and a Bayesian classifier to classify sentences as asserting or not asserting a relationship between the two proteins. The first rule-based approach [5] also assumed that proteins could be identified by dictionary look-up, and used simple regular expressions to recognize assertions about protein-protein interactions. Both rule-based and machine learning-based systems continue to be used to this day. The rule-based OpenDMAP system [28] has outperformed other systems in the BioCreative shared task on two occasions, once using manually constructed rules [3] and once using automatically learned rules [24]. Most systems now employ support vector machines and a much more elaborate set of features than the earliest machine learning-based systems, typically employing a dependency parse. This approach has been dominant in the BioNLP-ST shared tasks [32,33].

Methods for evaluating information extraction systems have varied in different research programs. The first machine learning-based system for detecting protein-protein interactions was evaluated based on a "lightly annotated" gold standard, constructed not manually but by automatic extraction from databases. The first rule-based system was evaluated based on its ability to reconstruct two known protein interaction pathways in Drosophila. Recent work has seen evaluations in which protein-protein interaction databases withhold manually curated data, releasing only the publications that they used to find these interactions; then systems are tested on the held-out data, which is subsequently released to the public.

Information extraction has been attempted for a variety of types of relationships. It is difficult to compare performance in these cases, since it is likely that some types of relationships are simply more difficult to extract than others. Table 6.2 gives examples of some of the types of relationships that have been attempted.

Table 6.2   A sample of information extraction tasks.

Protein and cellular component	[20]
Protein binding	[34]
Drugs, genes, and diseases	[43]
Disease and treatment	[44]
Inhibition relations	[42]
Protein transport	[37]
Cell types and gene expression	[28]
Genes and keywords	[13]

Early work in information extraction, primarily carried out as part of the Message Understanding Conferences, dealt with filling multi-part templates with many information components. However, when information extraction work began in the biological domain, it tended to deal with simple binary relations—one single relation type between two entities, whether of the same or different semantic classes. These were typically genes or proteins, and the most common relation type was undifferentiated interaction.

Later advances in the field included work in which an attempt was made to extract multiple types of binary relationships [44]. The participants were always diseases and treatments, and the relationships between them were always binary, but the system attempted not just to recognize relationships, but also to identify what the type of relationship between them was:

■ Treatment CURES disease.
■ Treatment PREVENTS disease.
■ Disease is a SIDE EFFECT of treatment.
■ Treatment DOES NOT CURE disease.

In later work, this approach was extended to the protein-protein interaction domain; they differentiated between ten different relationship types [45].

A further advance in the field was to go beyond binary relationships to relationships with multiple participants. An example of this was work on protein transport [4,28], in which the goal was to extract four participants in a given relation:

■ A transported protein.
■ The transporting protein.
■ The origin of the transported protein.
■ The destination of the transported protein.

The most recent work on information extraction in the biological domain has evolved toward an event recognition model [32,33]. This representation models assertions about relationships as events, with participants that are in some relationship to each other. The model has been extended to single-participant events (e.g., gene expression), two-participant events (e.g., protein binding), and events that can have other events as participants—e.g., as causes of some event. Performance declines as one proceeds along this continuum.

In the clinical domain, MedLEE [22] is an example of an information extraction system that has been specialized for a number of applications, including extraction of elements of radiology reports, adverse event discovery, breast cancer risk, and associations between diseases and drugs.

MedLEE is a rule-based system that makes use of a semantic grammar and a limited amount of syntactic structure. Semantic grammars can mix terminals and non-terminals and can have semantically typed non-terminals. Semantic types in the MedLEE grammar that is applied to radiology reports include bodily location, radiology finding, device, disease, position, procedure, and technique. MedLEE also makes use of a limited syntactic grammar to handle difficult linguistic constructions such as coordination and relative clauses. An example of a very abstract semantic pattern is *DEGREE + CHANGE + FINDING*—e.g., *mild increase in congestion*. The developers make the theoretically controversial assumption that the nature of the sublanguage and the restricted set of semantic relations that it can express limits normal ambiguity, so that, for example, in the *DEGREE + CHANGE + FINDING* pattern, we can always imply the interpretation that the degree modifies the change (*mild increase*) and these in turn modify the finding. After applying the semantic parser, MedLEE normalizes recognized concepts to a controlled vocabulary. The exact vocabulary depends on the application.

The following shows an example of MedLEE output. Some things to notice about this output are:

- The sentences have been through shallow parsing (see above).
- The system finds the concept *codeine* and recognizes that it is a change to the patient's situation, specifically a prescription.
- In the same sentence, *discharge* is analyzed as an expression of temporality and is correctly identified as the time for provision of codeine.
- In the second sentence, *discharge* is correctly identified as a problem.
- In the same sentence, *purulent* and *yellow* are correctly identified as modifiers of *discharge*.

```
<tt><sent id =  "s1">Patient <phr id = "p4">was</phr>
  <phr id
= "p6">prescribed</phr> <phr id = "p8">codeine</phr>
  <phr id
= "p10">upon</phr> <phr id =
"p12">discharge</phr>.</sent><sent id = "s2">

The <phr id = "p18">discharge</phr> <phr id =
"p20">was</phr> <phr id = "p22">yellow</phr> and
  <phr id =
"p26">purulent</phr>.</sent></tt>

med:codeine
        certainty>> high
```

```
                    idref>> 4
            change>> prescription
                    idref>> 6
            idref>> 8
            parsemode>> model
            sectname>> report unknown section item
            sid>> 1
            timeper>> discharge
                    idref>> 12
                    reltime>> on
                            idref>> 10

problem:discharge
            certainty>> high
                    idref>> 20
            descriptor>> purulent
                    idref>> 26
            descriptor>> yellow
                    idref>> 22
            idref>> 18
            parsemode>> model
            sectname>> report unknown section item
            sid>> 2
```

6.8.5 **Summarization**

Summarization is the task of taking one or more input texts and producing an output text that is shorter than the input(s) and preserves the important information in it [39]. A number of questions immediately present themselves, such as how short is useful and what counts as important. Summarization is useful both in the biological domain, where over 65,000 publications mention the single gene p53, and in the clinical domain, where a single patient's health record might run to volumes in length.

Two approaches to summarization exist. *Extractive summarization* selects text from the input and uses it as output. *Abstractive summarization* does not output original input text, but rather extracts some aspect of the meaning of the input and outputs it in altered form. Extractive summarization is the most common.

One interesting biological application that combines information extraction and summarization is Chilibot [13]. Chilibot was originally designed for analyzing gene lists produced by high-throughput assays such as microarray experiments. Given a list of gene names and optionally keywords, Chilibot produces a graph showing which genes interact with each other. A number on each link shows the number of publications in which evidence was found for the interaction. For each interaction, the application has a separate window that characterizes the specific type of the interaction and then displays the best sentence providing evidence for the interaction.

6.8.6 Cohort Retrieval and Phenotype Definition

One natural application of text mining is in ruling patients in or out of cohorts for clinical trials and in refining phenotypes for translational research. As an example of the latter, one study in genetic associations of pulmonary fibrosis found no genes associated with the disease. Narrowing of the phenotype was attempted. A diagnosis of pulmonary fibrosis in the medical record was not sufficient; other attributes were considered, which in 7% of cases required manual review of the health record. With this narrowing of the phenotype, 191 genes associated with the disease were uncovered [6,49]. If that step of manual review were automated, many more patients could be screened for inclusion in such studies.

The TREC Electronic Medical Record track [52] sponsored an evaluation of technologies for finding patients who could be ruled into or out of cohorts for clinical effectiveness studies. Participants were given a set of over 100,000 clinical documents and a set of 35 queries specifying particular types of patients. These queries presented a number of challenges for natural language processing that were simultaneously opportunities to showcase the power of natural language processing, since these challenges also make retrieval based on fielded data surprisingly difficult.

- Patients with hearing loss.
- Patients with complicated GERD who receive endoscopy.
- Hospitalized patients treated for methicillin-resistant *Staphylococcus aureus* (MRSA) endocarditis.
- Patients diagnosed with localized prostate cancer and treated with robotic surgery.
- Patients with dementia.
- Patients who had positron emission tomography (PET), magnetic resonance imaging (MRI), or computed tomography (CT) for staging or monitoring of cancer.
- Patients with ductal carcinoma *in situ* (DCIS).
- Patients treated for vascular claudication surgically.
- Women with osteopenia.
- Patients being discharged from the hospital on hemodialysis.

- Patients with chronic back pain who receive an intraspinal pain-medicine pump.
- Female patients with breast cancer with mastectomies during admission.
- Adult patients who received colonoscopies during admission which revealed adenocarcinoma.
- Adult patients discharged home with palliative care / home hospice.
- Adult patients who are admitted with an asthma exacerbation.
- Patients who received methotrexate for cancer treatment while in the hospital.
- Patients with Post-traumatic Stress Disorder.
- Adults who received a coronary stent during an admission.
- Adult patients who presented to the emergency room with anion gap acidosis secondary to insulin dependent diabetes.
- Patients admitted for treatment of CHF exacerbation.
- Patients with CAD who presented to the Emergency Department with Acute Coronary Syndrome and were given Plavix.
- Patients who received total parenteral nutrition while in the hospital.
- Diabetic patients who received diabetic education in the hospital.
- Patients who present to the hospital with episodes of acute loss of vision secondary to glaucoma.
- Patients co-infected with Hepatitis C and HIV.
- Patients admitted with a diagnosis of multiple sclerosis.
- Patients admitted with morbid obesity and secondary diseases of diabetes and or hypertension.
- Patients admitted for hip or knee surgery who were treated with anticoagulant medications post-op.
- Patients admitted with chest pain and assessed with CT angiography.
- Children admitted with cerebral palsy who received physical therapy.
- Patients who underwent minimally invasive abdominal surgery.
- Patients admitted for surgery of the cervical spine for fusion or discectomy.
- Patients admitted for care who take herbal products for osteoarthritis.
- Patients admitted with chronic seizure disorder to control seizure activity.
- Cancer patients with liver metastasis treated in the hospital who underwent a procedure.

Challenges include specifications of temporal relationships, such as *in the hospital* representing a time span; abbreviations, whether with or without definitions in the body of the query; and the requirement for inference, as in the case of specifying *adults*.

Many participants found it difficult to beat the baseline of an out-of-the-box application of the Lucene information retrieval API. The highest-performing system [21] illustrated some of the points that have been discussed elsewhere in this chapter. It modeled queries as questions, mapping their components to the evidence-based medicine clinical question frame of patient/problem, intervention, comparison, and outcome. A robust document structure parser was built, and specific elements of the clinical question frame were searched for in specific document sections. Concept recognition was done with MetaMap, and queries were then carefully expanded. It is also probably important that the system-builders increased the amount of "training data" considerably by working with a clinician to generate more queries than were provided by the task organizers. In any case, the resulting system achieved a P@10 of 0.73, while a baseline Lucene system managed only 0.44.

6.9 SOFTWARE ENGINEERING IN NATURAL LANGUAGE PROCESSING

Years of research into both biological and clinical natural language processing have advanced our knowledge of the practical and theoretical issues to the point where practical, useful applications can now be built. However, a number of issues must be dealt with in turning a research project into a deployed application. These include issues of architecture, scaling, and software testing and quality assurance.

6.9.1 Architectures

The typical text mining application is built as a pipeline of linearly ordered natural language processing components. The order of components discussed earlier in this chapter would constitute a typical pipeline. This may seem obvious, but architectures have been proposed in which no commitment is made to earlier stages of analysis until later stages of analysis have been considered. For instance, given an input like *Discharge patient to skilled nursing care*, such a system might not assign a part of speech to *discharge* until it has reached a decision about whether or not the sentence is an imperative. However, such systems remain largely in the research stage. (Hidden Markov Models make optimal sets of decisions, rather than isolated decisions, but this is a different matter from systems that defer decisions until later expectations are met, or not.) A typical early system might store the output of each processing step in a file and use a scripting language to launch successive applications.

More recent work has seen the emergence of architectures that streamline passage of data from one processing component to another. One example of such an architecture is the Unstructured Information Management Architecture (UIMA). Although it has its weaknesses, it illustrates the power of a very simple design system for assembling pipelines. UIMA components never alter the original input data file. Rather, all of their output is generated with respect to character offsets in that original file. This is the central principle of UIMA. This very simple "contract" between processing components—to communicate all results from one "Analysis Engine" (AE) to another by means of character offsets into the original data file—is sufficient to allow the assemblage of applications as complex and powerful as IBM's Watson. UIMA accretes output from successive analysis engines in a data structure called a Common Analysis Structure (CAS). A CAS is created for each input document, and the CAS is passed along the pipeline from analysis engine to analysis engine, accumulating outputs as it goes. Finally it is passed to a component known as a "CAS consumer," which turns the final output into the desired product. It should be noted that although UIMA is a Java-based architecture, Analysis Engines can call applications written in any programming language.

Competitors to UIMA exist, such as GATE and the BioCreative project on software communicability. They differ in details such as how information is passed from processing component to processing component, with the BioCreative initiative favoring a file-based approach. However, increasingly the momentum in architecture design is toward non-destructive processes that pass along information in terms of character offsets.

One of the major design issues in text mining is whether an application is meant to run in batch mode or whether it can produce real-time results. The vast majority of applications process documents offline in batch mode. This is sufficient for many applications, such as aiding in the interpretation of high-throughput data analysis. However, if text mining is to find a role in the clinic, faster applications capable of real-time processing will have to be built.

Another major architectural issue in text mining, particularly in the clinical domain, is the integration of natural language processing applications into larger software contexts. The current trend toward electronic health records is both an opportunity and an obstacle to the implementation of natural language processing in clinical contexts. The multiplicity of electronic health record systems in the past posed a largely intractable problem for deploying text mining systems that integrated with the health record. However, as the industry has come to be dominated by a much smaller number of players, new opportunities arise to focus on a much smaller number of targets, making deployment of text mining systems that interface with the electronic health record increasingly plausible.

6.9.2 **Scaling**

Part of the effort to extend work in the field beyond research prototypes has involved dealing with issues of scale. This is most obviously an issue in the case of systems that aim to do information extraction or other higher-level tasks from all of MEDLINE. However, it is often not the higher-level tasks that present the biggest bottlenecks, but the lower-level processing tasks. For example, running a typical syntactic parser over a MEDLINE abstract might take a minute and a half. Multiplied by all of MEDLINE, this would take close to 21,000 days.

Various approaches to such scaling issues exist. One is to reduce the number of inputs. For example, an experiment on extracting assertions about gene expression might run all MEDLINE abstracts through a gene mention system first—gene mention systems typically run on the order of 15 seconds per abstract—and then only parse those abstracts that contain a mention of a gene name. Search-based filters can be even more efficient—for example, if we know that we are only interested in lung disease, we can begin with an information retrieval step that retrieves only documents that mention some word related to the lungs. Often this will not be possible, however—for example, unlike words related to "lung," gene names cannot be enumerated.

Where inputs cannot be filtered or otherwise reduced, software engineering approaches are required. These typically involve parallel and distributed programming. These can be difficult skills to master, and a number of solutions have been developed to simplify the task of running an application in such a fashion. As one example, the UIMA Asynchronous Scaleout (UIMA-AS) architecture allows a UIMA processing task to be deployed across multiple machines or across multiple processes within a single machine. The typical UIMA pipeline works on a single document collection as input and aggregates outputs via a single CAS Consumer. When UIMA Asynchronous Scaleout is used, the capability of using a single document collection as input is maintained. Separate instances of the various Analysis Engines can be started as separate processes, with multiple CASes being passed between them. At the end of processing, the multiple CASes are handled by a single CAS consumer, enabling the production of unified output for the single input document collection. UIMA Asynchronous Scaleout allows specifying options for error recovery.

A more generalized solution is exemplified by the MapReduce approach. The intuition behind MapReduce is to abstract apart the problems of running the application (in this case, but not necessarily, a language processing application) and aggregating the results [36]. A similarity to the goals of UIMA Asynchronous Scaleout will be apparent. The mapping function shepherds an input through various processing steps via the simple data structure of the key/value pair. The reduce function performs the final step of aggregating outputs from intermediate processing steps that share the same key. Hadoop is a popular Java implementation of the MapReduce functionality. Like UIMA, although it is written in Java, Hadoop allows calling applications written in any language.

6.9.3 Quality Assurance and Testing

Evaluation of natural language processing software in terms of global performance metrics like precision, recall, and F-measure is relatively well-understood. Such evaluation is the standard for publication and is useful for broad comparisons between systems. However, an enormous amount of detail about the specifics of what a system is good at and what it is bad at can be lost in these global performance metrics. Granular evaluation of natural language processing applications requires approaches that have more in common with software testing than with tweaking a system to maximize the value of some figure of merit.

In addition, natural language processing software is software like any other, and as such requires testing. This is true both for deployable systems and for research prototypes. In the case of deployable systems, although natural language processing software is not considered a medical device and is not subject to the legal provisions of Section 201(h) of the Federal Food, Drug, and Cosmetic Act, Title 21 of the Code of Federal Regulations Part 820, or 61 Federal Register 52602, there is an ethical requirement to ensure that any software that affects patients or health decision-making or research is of the highest possible quality. In the case of research prototypes, software testing is still of paramount performance. Buggy software is not behaving as intended, and as such it does not test the hypothesis that the researcher thinks it is testing. As Rob Knight has put it, "For scientific work, bugs don't just mean unhappy users who you'll never actually meet: they mean retracted publications and ended careers. It is critical that your code be fully tested before you draw conclusions from results it produces" (personal communication).

Taking a testing approach to natural language processing software serves the dual purposes of granular evaluation of performance that is more revealing than global performance metrics, and of finding bugs. However, testing and quality assurance for natural language processing applications presents challenges that differ from the normal software testing situation.

Software testers often say that "software is different," by which they mean that testing it presents different engineering challenges than the ones presented in a typical product testing situation. In most quality assurance, the relationship between cause and effect is clear. We can relate the percentage of broken light bulbs dropped from various heights to the resulting impact quite clearly. However, software is characterized by often unclear relationships between components, and it is often a mystery why perturbing a parameter in one part of the system should affect the function of some seemingly independent part of the system. Language is similar to software in this respect—it is characterized by interactions between different components of the grammar that are often obscure, difficult to detect, and more difficult to understand.

The solution is to approach a natural language processing application as if it were an unknown language. A body of techniques for doing this exists in the field of descriptive linguistics. The process of eliciting data that will provide insight into an unknown language turns out to have an enormous amount in common with constructing a test suite using the techniques of software testing. Application developers will find it helpful to obtain the assistance of a linguist in assembling test data for text mining systems.

Software test suites and instruments for investigating unknown languages are constructed by the same set of principles. One attempts to delineate the components of the system and the ways that they can interact. In the case of language, this constitutes the parts of the language and the contexts in which they can occur. For example, in testing a named entity recognition system for genes, one might enumerate the features of gene names and the contexts in which they can appear in sentences.

In testing an application, we want to explore the parameter space of the possible inputs as fully as time and resources allow. An important part of constructing a test suite is to be sure to include both expected and unexpected inputs. As an example of an unexpected input, for a function that takes two numbers as its inputs we might pass in letters instead of numbers, or null values.

As suggested above, time and resources for testing (and software development in general) are finite. However, the number of possible test inputs for any non-trivial software program is demonstrably infinite. The art and science of software testing therefore consists in part of determining the set of test inputs that is most likely to actually uncover bugs (or elucidate performance in a more fine-grained fashion than traditional metrics), with the maximum of efficiency. One approach to doing this is to determine how to partition inputs into equivalence classes. An *equivalence class* is a set of inputs that are all likely to uncover the same bug. We then pick a small number of inputs from the (probably large number of) members of the equivalence class.

One approach to guiding software testing is to attempt to execute all of the code that has been written. This is more complex than it sounds. *Code coverage* is a measure of what percentage of the code is executed by a test suite. There are various measures of code coverage, including *line coverage* (the percentage of lines of code that are executed), *branch coverage* (the percentage of paths through the logical flow of the program that have been executed), and others. Line coverage is actually a relatively weak indicator of code coverage; branch coverage is a better indicator.

The intuition behind code coverage is that if code is not executed, then we will not discover any bugs that it might hold. One might assume that the way to maximize code coverage in natural language processing applications is to run the largest possible amounts of data available through the system. This turns out not to be the case. One study compared the code coverage achieved by running a very large corpus through a natural language processing application with the code coverage achieved by running a moderately sized test suite written according to principles of linguistics and software testing through the application [14]. The results showed that *much* higher coverage was achieved with the test suite than with the very large corpus. Furthermore, running the corpus through the application took several hours, while running the test suite took only 11 seconds. This made it possible to run the tests multiple times throughout a day's work, quickly catching any bugs introduced by additions or modifications to the code.

6.10 CONCLUSION

Natural language processing or text mining is the processing of human language by computers. It is made difficult by the ambiguity and variability that characterize human language. Biomedical language, whether in scientific journal articles or in clinical documents, has special characteristics that add to the challenge of biomedical natural language processing. Biomedical text mining software must be tested to industry standards, whether it is a research prototype or a deployed application.

ACKNOWLEDGMENTS

Thanks to Leonard D'Avolio, Wendy Chapman, Dina Demner-Fushman, and John Pestian for examples. Carol Friedman provided assistance with MedLEE. Christophe Roeder provided assistance with the section on scaling. Dina Demner-Fushman has had an enormous influence on my thinking about how to communicate the concepts of natural language processing to informaticians.

REFERENCES

[1] Aronson A, Lang F. An overview of MetaMap: historical perspective and recent advances. J Am Med Inform Assoc 2010;17(3):229–36.

[2] Aronson AR. Effective mapping of biomedical text to the UMLS Metathesaurus: the MetaMap program. Proc AMIA; 2001:17–21.

[3] Baumgartner Jr WA, Lu Z, Johnson HL, Caporaso JG, Paquette J, Lindemann A, et al. Concept recognition for extracting protein interaction relations from biomedical text. Genome Biol 2008;9(Suppl. 2).

[4] Bethard S, Lu Z, Martin JH, Hunter L. Semantic role labeling for protein transport predicates. BMC Bioinform 2008;9(277).

[5] Blaschke C, Andrade MA, Ouzounis C, Valencia A. Automatic extraction of biological information from scientific text: protein-protein interactions. Intell Syst Mol Biol 1999:60–7.

[6] Boon K, Bailey NW, Yang J, Steel MP, Groshong S, Kervitsky D, et al. Molecular phenotypes distinguish patients with relatively stable from progressive idiopathic pulmonary fibrosis (IPF). PLoS ONE 2009;4.

[7] Camon EB, Barrell DG, Dimmer EC, Lee V, Magrane M, Maslen J, et al. An evaluation of GO annotation retrieval for BioCreAtIvE and GOA. BMC Bioinform 2005;6(Suppl. 1).

[8] Caporaso GJ, Baumgartner Jr WA, Cohen KB, Johnson HL, Paquette J, Hunter L. Concept recognition and the TREC Genomics tasks. In: The 14th text REtrieval conference (TREC 2005) proceedings; 2005.

[9] Caporaso JG, Baumgartner Jr WA, Randolph DA, Cohen KB, Hunter L. MutationFinder: a high-performance system for extracting point mutation mentions from text. Bioinformatics 2007;23:1862–5.

[10] Chapman WW, Bridewell W, Hanbury P, Cooper GF, Buchanan B. Evaluation of negation phrases in narrative clinical reports. Proc AMIA Symp 2001; 105–9.

[11] Chapman WW, Bridewell W, Hanbury P, Cooper GF, Buchanan BG. A simple algorithm for identifying negated findings and diseases in discharge summaries. J Biomed Inform 2001;34:301–10.

[12] Chapman WW, Chu D, Dowling JN. ConText: an algorithm for identifying contextual features from clinical text. In: BioNLP 2007: Biological, Translational, and Clinical Language Processing. Association for Computational Linguistics; 2007.

[13] Chen H, Sharp BM. Content-rich biological network constructed by mining PubMed abstracts. BMC Bioinform 2004;5.

[14] Cohen KB, Baumgartner Jr WA, Hunter L. Software testing and the naturally occurring data assumption in natural language processing. In: Software engineering, testing, and quality assurance for natural language processing. Association for Computational Linguistics; 2008. p. 23–30.

[15] Cohen KB, Christiansen T, Hunter L. Parenthetically speaking: classifying the contents of parentheses for text mining. Am Med Inform Assoc Fall Symp; 2011.

[16] Cohen KB, Christiansen T, Hunter LE. MetaMap is a superior baseline to a standard document retrieval engine for the task of finding patient cohorts in clinical free text. In: Proceedings 20th Text Retrieval Conference; 2011.

[17] Cohen KB, Dolbey A, Acquaah-Mensah G, Hunter L. Contrast and variability in gene names. In: Natural Language Processing in the Biomedical Domain. Association for Computational Linguistics; 2002. p. 14–20.

[18] Cohen KB, Lanfranchi A, Corvey W, Baumgartner Jr WA, Roeder C, Ogren PV, et al. Annotation of all coreference in biomedical text: guideline selection and adaptation. In: Proceedings BioTxtM: second workshop on building and evaluating resources for biomedical text mining; 2010.

[19] Corbett P, Batchelor C, Teufel S. Annotation of chemical named entities. In: Biological, translational, and clinical language processing. Association for Computational Linguistics; 2007. p. 57–64.

[20] Craven M, Kumlien J. Constructing biological knowledge bases by extracting information from text sources. In: Seventh international conference on intelligent systems for molecular biology, ISMB-99. AAAI Press; 1999.

[21] Demner-Fushman D, Abhyankar S, Jimeno-Yepes A, Loane R, Rance B, Lang F, et al. A knowledge-based approach to medical records retrieval. In: 20th Text retrieval conference. National Institute of Standards and Technology; 2011. p. 163–72.

[22] Friedman C, Alderson PO, Austin JH, Cimino JJ, Johnson SB. A general natural-language text processor for clinical radiology. J Am Med Inform Assoc 1994;1(2):161–74.

[23] Fukuda K, Tsunoda T, et al. Toward information extraction: identifying protein names from biological papers. Pac Symp Biocomput 1998.

[24] Hakenberg J, Leaman R, Vo NH, Jonnalagadda S, Sullivan R, Miller C, et al. Efficient extraction of protein-protein interactions from full-text articles. IEEE/ACM Trans Comput Biol Bioinform 2010;7(3):481–94.

[25] Hersh W. Information retrieval: a health and biomedical perspective. 3rd ed. Springer; 2010.

[26] Hirschman L, Colosimo M, Morgan A, Yeh A. Overview of BioCreative Task 1B: normalized gene lists. BMC Bioinform 2005;6(Suppl. 1).

[27] Hirschman L, Sager N. Automatic information formatting of a medical sublanguage. In: Sublanguage: studies of language in restricted semantic domains. Walter de Gruyter; 1982. p. 27–80.

[28] Hunter L, Lu Z, Firby J, Baumgartner Jr WA, Johnson HL, Ogren PV, et al. OpenDMAP: an open-source, ontology-driven concept analysis engine, with applications to capturing knowledge regarding protein transport, protein interactions and cell-specific gene expression. BMC Bioinform 2008;9(78).

[29] Jin Y, McDonald RT, Lerman K, Mandel MA, Carroll S, Liberman MY, et al. Automated recognition of malignancy mentions in biomedical literature. BMC Bioinform 2006;7.

[30] Johnson HL, Cohen KB, Baumgartner Jr WA, Lu Z, Bada M, Kester T, et al. Evaluation of lexical methods for detecting relationships between concepts from multiple ontologies. Pac Symp Biocomput 2006:28–39.

[31] Jurafsky D, Martin JH. Speech and language processing: an introduction to natural language processing, computational linguistics, and speech recognition. Pearson Prentice Hall; 2008.

[32] Kim J-D, Ohta T, Pyysalo S, Kano Y, Tsujii J. Overview of BioNLP'09 shared task on event extraction. In: Proceedings of natural language processing in biomedicine (BioNLP) NAACL 2009 workshop: shared task; 2009.

[33] Kim J-D, Pyysalo S, Ohta T, Bossy R, Tsujii J. Overview of the BioNLP shared task 2011. In: BioNLP Shared Task 2011 Workshop; 2011.

[34] Krallinger M, Leitner F, Rodriguez-Penagos C, Valencia A. Overview of the protein-protein interaction annotation extraction task of BioCreative II. Genome Biol 2008;9(Suppl. 2).

[35] Lesk M. Automatic sense disambiguation using machine readable dictionaries: how to tell a pine cone from an ice cream cone. In: SIGDOC '86: Proceedings of the fifth annual international conference on systems documentation. ACM Press; 1986. p. 24–6.

[36] Lin J. Exploring large-data issues in the classroom: a case study with MapReduce. In: Third workshop on issues in teaching computational linguistics. Association for Computational Linguistics; 2008. p. 54–61.

[37] Lu Z. Text mining on GeneRIFs. University of Colorado School of Medicine; 2007.

[38] Lu Z, Kao H-Y, Wei C-H, Huang M, Liu J, Kuo C-J, et al. The gene normalization task in BioCreative III. BMC Bioinform; 2012.

[39] Mani I. Automatic summarization. John Benjamins Publishing Company; 2001.

[40] Morante R, Daelemans W. Learning the scope of hedge cues in biomedical texts. In: BioNLP 2009. Association for Computational Linguistics; 2009. p. 28–36.

[41] Morgan A, Lu Z, Wang X, Cohen A, Fluck J, Ruch P, et al. Overview of BioCreative II gene normalization. Genome Biol 2008;9(Suppl. 2).

[42] Pustejovsky J, Castaño J, Zhang J, Kotecki M, Cochran B. Robust relational parsing over biomedical literature: extracting inhibit relations. Pac Symp Biocomput 2002:362–73.

[43] Rindflesch TC, Tanabe L, Weinstein JN, Hunter L. EDGAR: extraction of drugs, genes and relations from the biomedical literature. Pac Symp Biocomput 2000:515–24.

[44] Rosario B, Hearst MA. Classifying semantic relations in bioscience texts. In: Proceedings of ACL; 2004. p. 430–7.

[45] Rosario B, Hearst MA. Multi-way relation classification: application to protein-protein interactions. In: Proceedings of the HLT-NAACL 5. 2005.

[46] Sager N. Syntactic formatting of scientific information. In: AFIPS conference proceedings 41. Walter de Gruyter; 1972. p. 791–800.

[47] Settles B. ABNER: an open source tool for automatically tagging genes, proteins and other entity names in text. Bioinformatics 2005;21(14):3191–2.

[48] Smith L, Tanabe L, Johnson nee Ando R, Kuo C-J, Chung I-F, Hsu C-N, et al. Overview of BioCreative II gene mention recognition. Genome Biol 2008.

[49] Steele MP, Speer MC, Loyd JE, Brown KK, Herron A, Slifer SH, et al. Clinical and pathologic features of familial interstitial pneumonia. Am J Respir Crit Care Med 2005.

[50] Tanabe L, Wilbur JW. Tagging gene and protein names in full text articles. In: Proceedings of the workshop on natural language processing in the biomedical domain. Association for Computational Linguistics; 2002.

[51] Vincze V, Szarvas G, Farkas R, Mora G, Csirik J. The BioScope corpus: biomedical texts annotated for uncertainty, negation and their scopes. BMC Bioinform 2008;9(Suppl. 11).

[52] Voorhees EM, Tong RM. Draft overview of the TREC 2011 medical records track. In: Text Retrieval Conference 2011. National Institute of Standards and Technology; 2011. p. 94–8.

[53] Yeh A, Morgan A, Colosimo M, Hirschman L. BioCreative task 1A: gene mention finding evaluation. BMC Bioinform 2005;6(Suppl. 1).

[54] Zipf GK. Human behavior and the principle of least effort: an introduction to human ecology. 1949.

References 177

Knowledge Discovery in Biomedical Data: Theory and Methods

John H. Holmes

University of Pennsylvania, Philadelphia, PA, USA

7.1 INTRODUCTION

7.1.1 Characteristics of Biomedical Data

Biomedical data often overwhelm due to the depth and complexity of the knowledge contained therein. We have traditionally sought out that knowledge through the use of various statistical tools, including frequency distributions, descriptive statistics, and more advanced, multivariable methods such as logistic and other regression techniques. However, the application of statistical methods typically presupposes a hypothesis, or at least a suggestion of one, even if one is searching through the data to generate hypotheses. Furthermore, these data are often of such high dimensionality that traditional statistical analytic approaches are untenable. For example, one could spend days scanning through a seemingly endless list of contingency tables to find a two-variable interaction that should be accounted for in a regression. And, if one comes to such data with a pre-formed hypothesis, it is entirely possible that another, more compelling hypothesis might be ignored, if only because it wasn't thought of in the first place. As a result, biomedical data is very fertile ground for the exploration and discovery of new knowledge, a process we call *knowledge discovery in databases*, or simply, *KDD*.

So what is knowledge? It would be good to consider the *Information Hierarchy*, proposed by several writers, but perhaps best articulated by Ackoff [4]. According to Ackoff, there are five ordered categories in the hierarchy: (1) Data, (2) Information, (3) Knowledge, (4) Understanding, and (5) Wisdom. The first three of these concern us directly in our quest to discovering knowledge in data, but Understanding is an important, and usually overlooked component of this endeavor.

Data are characterized as a set of symbols, wherein there are certain syntactical conventions that govern how and when these symbols are used. In the hierarchy, data, in and of themselves, have no particular meaning or significance. However, data provide the grist of all that comes afterward in the hierarchy; data are the *sine qua non* of information, which is data that has taken on some informative meaning to a receiver, human, or otherwise. Data become *information* when they take on meaning through some form of semantic or relational convention. When information becomes useful and usable in a given context, it becomes *knowledge*, considered here to be a set of one or more concepts that describes a concept. However, it is important to recognize that knowledge can be reducible to something that can be memorized. The typical knowledge-based ("expert") system contains a knowledge base of if-then rules that are triggered or fired in response to a given stimulus or condition from the environment. As such, knowledge can be naïve, although it is utterly important to what decisions are made and when and how they are made in a medical context. For this reason, we often equate data mining and knowledge discovery, although one could successfully argue that they are part of a process: we mine data to discover knowledge. And this is where the fourth level, *understanding*, often ignored in the knowledge hierarchy of many information scientists, comes into importance. Understanding involves making higher-order, or "meta" knowledge-based decisions, such as we see in learning (rather than memorizing). The reason that understanding is so important to KDD is that it drives our capacity to winnow out trivial from significant findings that are generated when applying the tools of data mining to databases.

There are a number of characteristics of biomedical data that differentiate them from many other types of data. First, biomedical data are typically collected with a single goal in mind. Data from electronic health records (EHRs), diagnostic instruments, or microarrays are collected with one specific purpose. In the case of EHRs and diagnostic instruments, the data they contain were collected for the delivery of clinical care; microarray data are typically collected for a specific analysis. While there are numerous examples of data from other domains such as banking that also collect data for a single purpose, they are relatively rarely used for secondary purposes (the Michael Milken story being a counter-example). We often use biomedical data for secondary purposes that have nothing to do with the original purpose for which they were collected. For example, we use EHR data for retrospective studies such as post-marketing drug surveillance.

Second, biomedical data are often large, in the sense that they may contain many observations, many variables, or a combination of both. Furthermore, biomedical data often contain repeated measurements, for example vital signs that are collected many times over the course of a patient's hospital stay. Interactions between variables also contribute to the largeness of biomedical data. These may be simple, where a database may include height and weight, but also body-mass index, which is calculated from the former two. Such an interaction can cause considerable confusion when analyzing these data. Complex interactions, those that are subtler, and are manifest only with deeper analysis, can lead to confounding and ultimately biased inferences drawn from the data. Ultimately, the largeness of biomedical data impacts on our ability to analyze these data efficiently.

With the advent of distributed research networks, there is an increasing appreciation of the value of data from multiple sites. This is especially the case in the domain of comparative effectiveness research, where a single site's data may be insufficient for a particular research question. These distributed data resources not only contribute to the largeness of biomedical data, but also raise a number of issues with regard to governance, data harmonization, and especially analysis technique (as highlighted in Chapter 2).

Biomedical data frequently contain missing values, even to the extent that a particular data element may not be analyzable. There are several reasons why missing data occur. The most common is when the data are simply not collected, for whatever reason. For example, missing data may occur from instances where a question might not be asked, or if a part of a physical examination was not recorded. On the other hand, data might be corrupted due to deficiencies in transmission over a network or malfunctioning mass storage equipment. Of particular importance is the type of "missingness" that occurs when data for a particular element are missing because they depend on the value of another data element. Whatever the cause, missing data can result in inaccurate analyses and subsequently, the inferences made from them.

7.1.2 Traditional Methods for Analyzing Biomedical Data

We often analyze biomedical data for associations between some set of exposures and a given outcome or set of outcomes. In these types of analyses, outcomes are considered to be, in machine learning parlance, classes. And to the extent that many types of biomedical data represent the real world, these classes are often unbalanced. For example, breast cancer, defined as an outcome or class variable with the values "absent" or "present," is actually rare in the general population: there are many more women without cancer than afflicted with it. We would say that the class is unbalanced as a result, and this has serious ramifications for any analysis we would perform using these data. Study design strategies have been developed to account for this; the case-control study is a good example, where one selects the number of controls based on the number of cases available. However, in case-control studies where multiple controls are selected relative to the number of cases, one is still faced with the unbalanced class problem. There are statistical methods for dealing with this, but some of the data mining methods we will examine here do not cope as well, and require some type of data preparation or sampling routine.

Many times, the data we analyze do not have specific class variables, or at least weren't collected for so specific a purpose that a class variable is needed. The many survey databases available through the National Center for Health Statistics (http://www.cdc.gov/nchs) are ample examples of these kinds of data. Analyses of these survey data are often highly descriptive, without considering a particular exposure-outcome relationship. However, this does not preclude a more sophisticated analysis that would address such a relationship. Here, the analyst would specify, from the list of all available variables, one or a set of variables that could be considered an "outcome." An example of this would be a study that examined the relationship between various demographic factors and having had a prostate-specific antigen test, as recorded on the Behavioral Risk Factor Surveillance System (http://www.cdc.gov/brfss/).

7.1.3 A First Look at Knowledge Discovery in Databases: Mining Data

Knowledge discovery in databases (KDD) takes place in a continuum of activities, some automated, and others not. One automated activity is *data mining*, which produces a variety of different outputs, such as decision trees and variants thereof, rules of various types, clusters, and visualizations. But before we discuss each of these in turn, we need to define more precisely what we mean by a *class*. A class is what separates a dataset into two or more partitions. While a class is defined within a class variable, that variable serves as a *hyperplane*, where records in the data are divided by the hyperplane that runs through the data. The relationship of a hyperplane to data is illustrated in Figure 7.1.

If one conceptualizes each value of the class variable (in this case, the variable is dichotomous, so only two values) as dispersed throughout a space of all instances, or records, in the data, one can see that the hyperplane divides

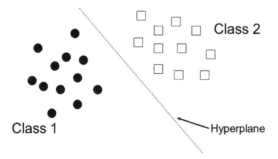

■ **FIGURE 7.1** The classification problem. The two classes in this example are separated by a hyperplane, a boundary that is typically determined through the application of a statistical or machine learning algorithm.

the data instances into two segments, one for each value of the dichotomous class variable. Each instance has a specific membership—it is in one or the other segment, as defined by the hyperplane. The goal of much of KDD is to find that hyperplane which best separates between the classes. This is the fundamental characteristic of classification.

We use classification in our daily lives, all the time. Classification provides us with the means whereby we are able to deal with a highly complex world, and KDD is really not much different. If one could stretch a point, our environment and all that it contains—people, things, places—represents a huge search space consisting of data. In order for us to navigate that space effectively, perhaps avoiding dangerous situations like crossing the street against a red light, we classify these objects in our environment, and draw upon our experience to make inferences based on that classification. Even if we have never seen a red light at a pedestrian crossing before, but we have seen one while driving, we would probably infer that it is best to wait until that light turns green before walking into the intersection, just as we would do if we were behind the wheel of a car.

As in our daily experience, classification and inference are at the heart of KDD. But in order to apply these effectively, we need the capacity to learn. Expert systems, in their purest form, use deductive logic to arrive at conclusions that are often classification problems, and they do not have this learning capacity.

7.2 KNOWLEDGE DISCOVERY AS A PROCESS: DATA MINING IN PERSPECTIVE

One of the best, and long-used, definitions of knowledge discovery in databases, or KDD, is: "…the data-driven identification of valid, novel, potentially useful, and ultimately meaningful patterns in databases" [1]. This definition is packed with important terms. First, KDD is data-driven; that is, data, not pre-formed hypotheses, drive the analysis, which is itself characterized as the identification of patterns in the data. These patterns may take many different forms, as we shall see shortly, but for now, they could be if-then rules, trees, clusters, or other structures. Second, these patterns must be valid—that is, valid in the context of a particular knowledge domain. A pattern that suggests that thinner people are less likely to develop hypertension than those who are obese seems, at least initially, a pattern that is not valid in the face of current knowledge about the causes of hypertension. A pattern should be novel, in the sense that it suggests something new, not previously seen. Part of novelty is the ability of such a pattern to suggest a new hypothesis; it is directly a result of novelty and its attendant surprise, that a pattern can generate a new hypothesis. Finally, such patterns must be meaningful, or not trite. KDD is not about pointing out the obvious, which is part of the reason why a pattern should be novel, but a pattern that indicates an already-known relationship is not only not novel, it is not particularly meaningful. The other side of meaningfulness is that a discovered pattern has some degree of utility; that is, it can be used to formulate hypotheses and subsequent analyses that may have an impact on future analyses and ultimately to the benefit of patients.

It is important to recognize that KDD is not necessarily coterminous with data mining, although the two terms have been used interchangeably for quite some time. It is useful to think of data mining as the application of specialized software and cognitive tools in the process of KDD. Such software tools will be described shortly, but it is important to remember that the discovery of knowledge, and certainly an understanding of that knowledge, is fundamentally a cognitive process that requires substantial intellectual investment by those using these software tools, but most critically experts in the domain of the data being mined. It literally takes a village to engage in the KDD process, and requires people to bring their specific expertise to the table during that process.

7.3 A BRIEF OVERVIEW OF MACHINE LEARNING

Much of data mining focuses on the application of machine learning-based algorithms to the discovery of knowledge in data. It is worthwhile to introduce the basic principles of machine learning before considering the process of KDD (Chapters 8 and 9 describe in more detail advanced machine learning techniques). Machine learning is the discipline that seeks to create computer systems that learn concepts from data. It focuses on inductive processes, that is, learning from examples and generalizing that learning to other, similar problems. Machine learning is the opposite of deductive reasoning, such as that embodied in expert systems, where predefined rules populate a knowledge base that provides a pool of possible answers to questions or problems posed to the system. In machine learning, that knowledge base is developed over time, as the system learns from its environment. In many cases, the goal of KDD is classification, which is the discovery of a surface to which a particular set of data might belong.

In some cases, that environment is a physical one, such as an obstacle course or a maze that has to be learned by a robotic system. These types of systems often use a type of machine learning that involves examples, but those examples are not "labeled" in the sense that the classification of a particular decision is not evaluated against a known classification at the time the

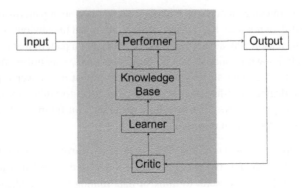

■ **FIGURE 7.2**   A simple machine learning system. Inputs and outputs come from an environment, which in KDD is usually a database. The system, demarcated in gray, communicates with the environment through the Performer, and during learning, with the Critic. The Knowledge Base contains the examples, learned over time during training, and the Learner is responsible for improving the accuracy of the Knowledge Base using the evaluation provided by the Critic.

decision is made. Rather, such a system learns over time from a sequence of decisions, and is rewarded for correct decisions (and punished for incorrect ones) toward or at the end of the maze. The system is not aware of the classification of a training case, and must build its own classification model. This is an example of *unsupervised learning*, which is most commonly used in KDD in clustering methods. *Supervised learning* involves the use of "labeled" data, such that each decision is evaluated against the known label for a given case, or instance. This type of learning has been referred to as "stimulus-response" learning, because the decision-reward cycle is so tightly coupled. Supervised learning is the type most commonly used in KDD, being implemented in decision tree induction, certain types of evolutionary computation, some neural networks, classification and association rule induction, and prediction.

Figure 7.2 demonstrates a generic machine learning system during learning. The gray outer square represents the environment, which in KDD is usually a database. The light purple[1] square represents the machine learning system proper, with four components shown in blue. These components, Performer, Knowledge Base, Learner, and Critic function in sequence during learning to learn the environment problem, which in much of KDD is classification. However, before classification can occur a concept, or set of concepts, must be learned.

---

[1] For interpretation of color in Figure 7.2, the reader is referred to the web version of this book.

7.3.1 **Concept Learning**

A concept is related to a category, or a generalization of a phenomenon or relationship that can be applied to similar situations as they are encountered. As such, a concept is learned, rather than memorized. There are numerous theories of and approaches to concept learning that are beyond the scope of this chapter. However, one approach that is particularly germane to data mining is induction, which is found in many machine learning algorithms. Induction involves learning concepts from examples that are drawn from an environment, such as a set of data. These concepts can be represented in the learner in a variety of ways, such as rules or trees, but in any case, successful or accurate learning depends on the construction of concepts that can be generalized to similar, but as-yet unseen situations. Such learning takes place during a period of training, and the generalizability of the concepts formed during training is evaluated during testing.

7.3.2 **Training and Testing Regimes**

Data mining, by definition, relies on data in order to construct the concepts needed for accurate classification and knowledge discovery. These data may come from such sources as electronic health records, insurance claims, or disease registries. In order to mine these data they need to be prepared as *datasets*, in such a way that the software can use them. Methods such as *n*-fold cross-validation and other bootstrapping approaches, as well as split-sample validation may be used. In cross-validation, one decides into how many segments a dataset should be divided; a common number is 10, where each of the 10 segments contains an equal number of randomly selected records. During the training phase, one segment is held out for testing, while the remaining nine segments are used for training. Each training case is presented to the system for concept learning, and each of the 10 segments is tested in an iterative fashion, such that each record is used for training or testing once. The results of the testing cycles are then averaged or otherwise voted upon to create a final concept set (see Figure 7.3).

Another common method for training is split-sample validation, in which some proportion (often 50% or 67%) records are randomly selected from the main dataset to form a training set. The remaining records are held out for testing after training is complete. Each training case is presented to the system for learning at least once, but usually many times over a training period. Since training usually takes place over such a length of time that in order for the target accuracy to be attained, it is required that each case is sampled more than once, it is usual to sample the cases with replacement, such that each case is presented to the system multiple times (see Figure 7.4).

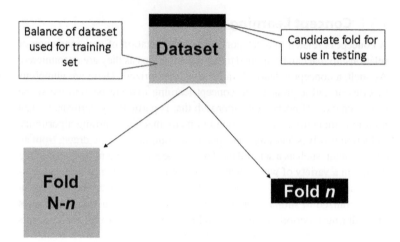

■ **FIGURE 7.3** An example of *n*-fold cross-validation. The dataset is partitioned into *n* folds, or groups of records, usually of equal size. Folds are iteratively selected for testing, and the remaining folds are used for training, until all folds have been tested. It is good practice to ensure that the class distribution is maintained in each fold, such that the testing data resembles the training data with respect to the number of records in each class.

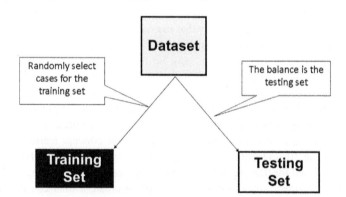

■ **FIGURE 7.4** An example of a split-sample validation regime. A pre-determined proportion, typically between 50 and 75%, of the records in a dataset are randomly selected for training. The balance of the dataset, sometimes referred to as a "hold out," is used for testing. It is good practice to ensure that the class distribution is maintained in both training and testing sets, such that the testing data resembles the training data with respect to the number of records in each class.

During the training period, the system makes educated guesses as to the correct course of action, such as a classification of a given training case. This period can be viewed as a time during which hypotheses are proposed and evaluated using some form of feedback from the environment. Ideally, the system

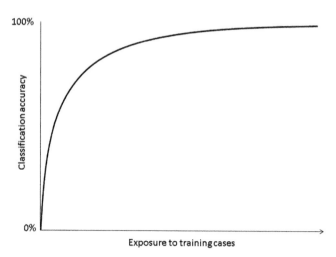

■ **FIGURE 7.5** A learning curve. As the learner is exposed to an increasing number of training cases, it should attain an increasing degree of classification accuracy.

will make fewer errors over time, asymptotically reaching a target accuracy, which can be measured using one of a variety of metrics; these are described in Section 7.4.3.7 of this chapter. For our purposes now, simple accuracy, or the proportion of correct decisions made divided by the total number of decisions. Figure 7.5 illustrates a training period in terms of accuracy over time; accuracy increases as training cases are presented to the system.

A third family of training-testing regimes is the ensemble. In an ensemble method, multiple data mining algorithms are applied to the data to improve classification or prediction performance. Several popular approaches to ensemble classification are bagging, boosting, and Bayesian model averaging and combination. In bagging (bootstrap aggregation), each model gets an equal vote during the training period and their results are averaged to provide the classification for a given case. Boosting redoubles exposure to a training case that has been misclassified so that it is oversampled from the training set in order to improve classification performance. This procedure can increase classification accuracy, but at the expense of overfitting, such that a problematic training case is memorized, rather than generalized, leading to poor classification performance on the testing set. Bayesian model averaging selects a model in each ensemble, weighting it by its prior probability and log likelihood, and then averaging across all models. Bayesian model combination is similar to the averaging method, but it samples from all possible models in the ensemble. As a result, it addresses the overfitting that can occur with the averaging method, which focuses on only one model.

7.3.3 **Supervised Learning**

There are two types of learning in the machine learning paradigm. The first of these is supervised learning, where each training case is labeled; that is, its classification is ultimately made known to the system. This classification serves as a gold standard against which the classification proposed by the system is evaluated. In Figure 7.2, the *Critic* serves this function, passing on information about the comparison to the Learner. For example, if the proposed classification is "Diseased" and the actual classification of the training case is also "Diseased," then the *Learner* is informed that the system made a correct decision, and the *Learner* updates the *Knowledge Base* in such a way that the overall accuracy of the system is improved. However, if the system made an incorrect decision, where the proposed classification differs from the gold standard classification, the overall accuracy of the system will be diminished. How system accuracy is actually calculated, and by what value that accuracy is changed is discussed in Section 7.4.3.7, where evaluation metrics are described.

7.3.4 **Unsupervised Learning**

Unsupervised learning differs from supervised in that the gold standard classification is not known to the system each time a training case is presented. Instead, in unsupervised learning the system is led over time to a solution of the problem posed by the environment, based on a pattern of deferred reinforcement. For this reason, reinforcement learning algorithms are often used rather than the stimulus-response algorithms that are used in supervised learning. Maze environments, in which the learner has to learn a path to a correct decision and is rewarded only upon successful reaching a target at the end, are excellent environments for unsupervised learners. In data mining, clustering algorithms are well-known examples of unsupervised learning, where a class is not known to the system at all. Rather, the purpose of the system is to learn during training what cases aggregate into one cluster or another. These clusters are not automatically labeled by the system; rather, this is the responsibility of the analyst, who, upon examining the features and their values within each cluster, determines how each cluster should be labeled.

7.4 **A KNOWLEDGE DISCOVERY LIFE CYCLE**

We can think of the process of KDD in a life cycle framework, as shown in Figure 7.6, adapted from Fayyad et al. [1]. Defined as such, the KDD process consists of four discrete phases: (1) data preparation, (2) data reduction, (3) data mining, and (4) evaluation. Like most systems development life cycle models, the process is highly iterative. It is common that one must

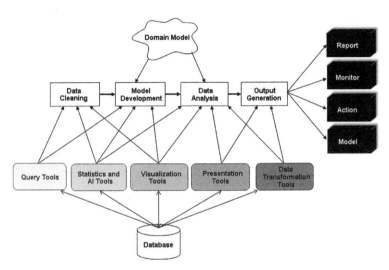

■ **FIGURE 7.6** A schematic of the knowledge discovery process as it includes sources of data, tasks and tools for accomplishing KDD, and the all-important domain model, which drives the process.

revisit some aspect of data preparation after applying a data mining routine that was found to be sensitive to the way the data were prepared, but this was not discovered until after running the routine.

7.4.1 **Data Preparation**

There are myriad things to think about when preparing data for any analysis, and data mining is no exception. In fact, many of the same issues we need to address in statistical analysis are the same when preparing data for mining. The first problem to confront in preparing data is its "cleanliness." As noted earlier, biomedical data are notoriously dirty, in that they are rife with missing data, illogical relationships between two or more variables, and of range data, just to name three. Just as we encounter similar data cleaning issues in data mining as we do in statistical analyses, we have similar tools to address these issues.

7.4.1.1 *Variable/Value Standardization*

Variables and their value labels are often represented in different ways, especially in multi-site studies. For example, one site might call a variable Sex, while another would call it Gender. In addition, each might be coded numerically in a different way, where for the first site Females are represented with a value of 1 and at the second site with a 2. This problem is not limited to multi-site studies. When merging historical with current data, or merging data from two different sources at the same site, these kinds of labeling discrepancies are often found. It is extremely important to resolve these discrepancies through a process called harmonization, where an authority list is developed that translates these labels and values to the same system. Without this list, and enforcing it in the creation of a final dataset for analysis, one runs the risk of having an unanalyzable dataset. As a result, this is the very first step in preparing data for mining. The easiest method for harmonizing the data is to create a table in a database or spreadsheet, listing each variable on a row, followed by all of its names across all data sources. The first column should be the name of the variable to which the disparate variable names will be harmonized. On the same row, the process should be repeated for each of the variable values.

7.4.1.2 *Out-of-Range Values*

Every variable in a dataset has a value, whether it is discrete or continuous, numeric, or text. In addition, most variables have a legal range of values, beyond which a value would be deemed unacceptable, and potentially not analyzable. When the value of a variable does not fall into the acceptable range of values for that variable, we say that the value is out of range, and we call such values "outliers." Such values need to be identified and corrected before analysis or mining, because they can cause one to make incorrect inferences from the data. Identifying outliers is straightforward. The simplest method is the frequency distribution, where each value that is present in the dataset for a given variable is listed, along with its frequency (the number of times that value appears). A visual scan of a frequency distribution will quickly identify any outliers, and these can be investigated through queries of the data to identify the record(s) that contain those outliers. Once identified, one would edit the data, preferably using data from the original source, if possible. If an outlier cannot be resolved, it should be replaced with a missing or imputed value (see Section 7.4.1.6). It is always best to obtain and closely examine the frequency distribution for each variable in a dataset prior to proceeding with any of the next steps in data cleaning.

7.4.1.3 *Logical Inconsistencies*

When the observed relationship between the values of one variable compared with the values of another is discordant, there is an inconsistency in the logical nature of the relationship. This anomaly occurs not because the inconsistency is possible, but because of some error, such as might occur during data entry. One example of a logical inconsistency is the case of the "pregnant male." In this case, there are two variables: Gender, which takes on the values Male and Female, and Pregnant, which takes on the values Yes, No, Don't Know, and Not Applicable. If one finds a combination such as Male/Yes, or Male/Don't Know for Gender and Pregnant, respectively, then we have a logical inconsistency between these two variables. In fact,

		Sex	
		Female	Male
Pregnancy status	Pregnant	30	2
	Not pregnant	67	5
	Not applicable	3	98

■ **FIGURE 7.7** A 2×2 contingency table. Often referred to as a "confusion matrix," this table provides a simple method for identifying discordant pairs in classification. Two such pairs are illustrated here in the shaded cells. They are discordant because males cannot become pregnant, nor can they be classified as "not pregnant" when a "not applicable" category is available. Females can become pregnant, and they can be not pregnant; in addition, the "not applicable" category can apply to females who have not reached menarche or are past menopause, or have had some condition or surgery that renders them unable to become pregnant.

the only legal combination for males would be Male/Not Applicable. For females, any combination is possible, even Female/Not Applicable, if that were used to indicate women who were beyond childbearing years or who had a hysterectomy. The logical inconsistency can be found by creating a cross-tabulation of the two variables in question, as shown in Figure 7.7.

After identifying the discordant variable-value pairs (indicated in Figure 7.7 as the shaded cells), one can query the data to find the records with this discordance. As with the out-of-range value, the problematic records should be edited after resolving the discordance using original source data. The variables of discordant pairs that cannot be resolved in this way should be set to a missing value or possibly imputted (see Section 7.4.1.6).

7.4.1.4 *Variable Transformation*

In some cases, most often due to the requirements of analytic software routines, one may need to transform the variable to another scale. One example is in certain types of cluster analyses, where in order for an accurate distance metric to be enforced, the data must be prepared in such a way as to minimize the effect of variable-value distributions. For example, body temperatures might be normalized to a scale over the range -1 to $+1$ in order to remove the effect of the distribution, which could be heavily concentrated around 37 °C, but with significant numbers of values above a normal temperature. Most statistical and data mining software packages support automatic normalization procedures, so that the data are normalized within the analytic routine, although it is possible that analysts will need to run a standalone normalization procedure on the data prior to running the clustering algorithm.

7.4.1.5 *Discretization*

It is occasionally required by a data mining routine that variables be discretized. This involves creating "cutpoints" across a variable's distribution, such that the values for the variable are now placed in discrete categories. For example, body temperature, which is commonly expressed as a continuous variable, might be discretized into two categories: Febrile and Afebrile, with a cutpoint of 37.5°C. In this case, anyone with a body temperature of less than or equal to 37.5 would be labeled Afebrile, and those with a higher temperature would be labeled as Febrile. Discretization is performed in a variety of ways. The simplest is to inspect the frequency distribution and create cutpoints based on that distribution. Related to this method is to look at the output from a simple descriptive statistics routine, which usually includes a quantiles distribution, most often as quartiles. The values used to create the quantiles function as cutpoints. Other methods, such as entropy-based discretization, are often used for variable discretization, and this will be discussed later in this chapter.

7.4.1.6 *Missing Data*

As discussed previously, biomedical data are plagued with variables for which there are no values. Such missing data might result from someone forgetting or refusing to fill in an item on a form, or possible corruption of the data. In some cases, such missing data are ignorable, meaning that they can be left as-is in the data, perhaps represented with a special code to indicate that they are missing, and should not be included in an analysis. Such data, the missingness of which is not dependent on the value of that variable or any other variable in the dataset, would be considered to be missing completely at random. In other cases, the value of a variable might be missing because it is dependent on the value of another variable, but not on the variable with the missing data. An example would be that men are less likely to report their smoking history, regardless of whether or not they smoke; this is missing at random, and may be ignorable. Other missing data might not be ignorable, however. If men were not reporting their smoking history if they were smokers, this would be not missing at random.

The choice of how to handle any of these types of missing data is largely left up to the analyst, but she is constrained by the requirements of the data mining software. Some routines, such as neural networks, are highly sensitive to missing data, while decision trees are less sensitive. But first, one must decide how to handle missing values. There are several strategies for this, the simplest being to represent missing values with some form of code that is recognized by the data mining software as "missing." Usually this is a question mark (?) or a number than can be used in an instruction to the software to convert that to an internal missing value code. In statistical software, this code is usually an astronomically high number that the software is programmed to recognize as missing.

A more complicated approach to handling missing data is *imputation*, or more simply, filling in the missing data with some value. There are several types of imputation, the simplest of which is replacing the missing value with a number randomly selected from within the range of accepted values for the variable. Another is the so-called "hot deck imputation," in which the missing value is replaced with a value that is conditioned on the value of some other variable. For example, missing systolic blood pressure in a male might be replaced with the mean (or mode) systolic blood pressure over all males who have a non-missing value for this variable. Finally, a more complicated approach, but one that has gained some acceptance, is *multiple imputation*. In this procedure, one uses a Monte Carlo method or creates a series of regression models using the variables of interest to generate point estimates and confidence intervals for the missing values. In this way, missing values are replaced on a probabilistic basis, not the deterministic or naïve basis of the previous methods. Regardless of which method is used to handle missing data, it should be documented carefully and completely in order to understand the ramifications of the data mining analysis results, once obtained. These results can be influenced considerably by the specific method of handling missing data.

7.4.2 **Data Reduction**

The goal of data reduction is to make the data mining process, that is, applying and interpreting the results obtained from data mining methods, tractable. This means better mining efficiencies in order to adhere to the constraints of the data mining software, while reducing the amount of output in order to make the results of data mining more easily interpretable. Biomedical data are often of extraordinarily high dimensionality, as described in the Introduction of this chapter. Large numbers of variables and records contribute to the dimensionality biomedical data, but so too does the temporality of such data, where multiple hospitalizations, clinic visits, measurements, and the like are recorded over time on the same individual. Microarray and other genomic data are particularly complex, containing hundreds or thousands of variables. This embarrassment of data riches has overwhelmed even the most sophisticated data mining algorithms to the extent that much effort often needs to be expended in reducing the dimensionality of a dataset prior to running some data mining routines. Fortunately, there has been a substantial amount of work on developing algorithms that effectively reduce data for mining without compromising the accuracy of these routines. These techniques include variable selection, numerosity reduction, and sampling.

7.4.2.1 *Feature Selection*

Also called variable selection, this process involves finding the best suite of variables that contribute the most to knowledge discovery. Those familiar with stepwise procedures in regression will be comfortable with these techniques as they are used in data mining and dimensionality reduction. Forward selection, illustrated in Figure 7.8, is one such technique, where one starts with an empty list of variables, or feature set. Each candidate variable is evaluated one by one by some criterion to determine if it adds substantively to explaining a target function, such as classification. Variables are added to the feature set until no more variables meet the criterion. Backward selection (Figure 7.9) is the reverse of forward, in that the procedure starts with a complete feature set—that is all candidate variables are in the feature set. Each variable is evaluated in turn by a criterion and removed from the feature set if it does not meet the criterion. The process continues until no

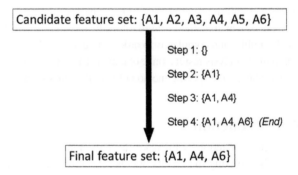

■ **FIGURE 7.8**　An illustration of forward feature selection. In this regime, the feature set is empty at start of selection, and features are *added* iteratively until the final feature set is complete.

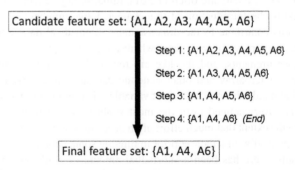

■ **FIGURE 7.9**　An illustration of backward feature selection. In this regime, the feature set consists of all features in the dataset at start of selection. Features are then *removed* iteratively until the final feature set is complete.

more variables can be removed from the feature set without compromising the accuracy of the set in explaining the target function.

A second method of feature selection is correlation-based feature selection [55]. It is based on the premise that candidate variables can be tested for their correlation with a classification task, but not be related to each other. A third method of feature selection uses decision tree induction to discover not only the variables that contribute to the specific value of a class, but also the relationships between these variables. Decision trees will be discussed in more detail in Section 7.4.3.3. Finally, feature selection can be accomplished through the use of traditional statistical methods. In the case of categorical variables, one can use contingency table analysis with the chi-square statistic as a criterion for selection. In this approach, one would cross-tabulate the class variable with each variable in the dataset individually in order to obtain a chi-square point estimate. The cutoff of the point estimate at which variables should be retained can be determined through consulting a critical values table of the chi-square distribution in any statistics text, but one could also consider the significance level (p-value) or confidence interval around the point estimate as the criterion. For continuous variables, an unpaired t-test would serve the same function as the chi-square does for categorical variables.

7.4.2.2 *Numerosity Reduction*

A second method of data reduction involves reducing the complexity of the data by representing groups of variables with models; thus, the group of variables becomes a single variable. Such models could be obtained through a variety of techniques, most notably multivariable methods such as regression, log-linear modeling, and principal component analysis, as well as cluster analysis. This numerosity reduction is appropriate when it would be difficult to interpret the output from a data mining routine due to the number of variables included in that output.

7.4.2.3 *Sampling*

So far, the discussion about data reduction has focused on variables. A third method of data reduction focuses instead on records; it involves sampling these from the dataset using one or more of several sampling approaches. Each of these assumes that the resulting sampled data subsets will be analyzed either individually, or as a suite of subsets to be analyzed separately. In the first case, one would sample from the dataset, and apply the desired data mining routines to it, and the analysis would stop there. In the second case, the routines would be applied to a series of subsets sampled from the dataset; this approach requires some way to coalesce the separate analytic results into a single result. There are two primary sampling regimes: with replacement and without replacement. When records are sampled with replacement, each record has some probability of being selected many times; thus a record could appear more than once in a resulting subset of the data. More common is sampling without replacement; in which records, once sampled, are not eligible for selection again. Thus, each record is represented once and only once in a resulting subset of the data.

Within these two regimes, there are several methods for sampling data. The first is systematic sampling, in which one would select every *n*th record until the desired sample size is created. This method is rarely used in data mining because of its propensity for bias and resulting lack of representativeness in the sample. More common is simple random sampling, where records are selected based on digits drawn from a random number table or applying a randomization program as part of a database query. Under this method, each record has an equal probability of being sampled. The third method is stratified sampling, where the data are divided into pre-determined strata based on some categorizing variable such as sex or race. Simple random sampling may be applied then to each stratum separately, or one may employ blocking to ensure that the strata are evenly balanced and that a stratum is not over-represented in the resulting data subset. In any case, one should ensure that the number of selected records in each stratum approximates the proportion of records in each stratum in the dataset. That is, if females comprise 70% of the main data, the selected female records should comprise 70% of the total records selected. Other methods such as cluster sampling are not used as frequently in data mining.

7.4.3 **Data Mining Methods**

There are two major families of methods for data mining: statistical or probabilistic, and machine learning. As KDD grows to include other types of data, such as text and images, additional methods such as those from the natural language processing and feature recognition domains, respectively, are added to the data mining armamentarium. We focus here on data mining, however, and will concentrate our discussion on first the statistical and probabilistic methods and then the machine learning methods for mining numeric data.

7.4.3.1 *Statistical Classification*

It is important to remember that KDD is a process that utilizes a variety of methods in its primary goal, which is the discovery of knowledge. One isn't limited in this process to only the most sophisticated software tools, and there are many valid reasons to recommend the use of frequentist, or statistical methods to mine data. Univariate methods, such as frequency distributions and descriptive statistics, have already been mentioned as ways to identify the characteristics of a dataset, among them outliers and logical inconsistencies. This application is in itself a type of KDD; through the application of univariate statistical methods one discovers much about the data at hand.

7.4.3.1.1 **Univariable Methods**

Univariate methods, such as frequency distributions and descriptive statistics, have already been mentioned as ways to identify the characteristics of a dataset, among them outliers and logical inconsistencies. This application is in itself a type of KDD; through the application of univariate statistical methods one discovers much about the data at hand.

7.4.3.1.2 **Multivariable Methods**

Multivariable methods, such as various forms of regression (such as least squares, logistic, Poisson, etc.), factor analysis, principal components analysis, and can also be used in KDD. In fact, exploratory statistical analyses, where the focus is on hypothesis generation or exploration rather than testing, are a type of KDD. These methods presuppose a class variable that serves as the dependent variable. The *vector* of independent variables is then examined in stepwise fashion, or sometimes as "fixed," where all variables are evaluated together at once. The resulting models are then examined for variables that have an association with the dependent variable, but now adjusted for the other independent variables in the model. As a result, the multivariable methods provide more information about the complexity of the relationship between the independent variables and the class variable.

7.4.3.1.3 **Clustering**

Most multivariable methods are developed using a process that is analogous to supervised learning. That is, records are drawn from a training set, run through the model algorithm, and their importance in explaining the variance of the model is evaluated. However, a special type of multivariable method, *cluster analysis*, often uses a method that is analogous to unsupervised learning. In cluster analysis, the goal is to identify those cases from the dataset that cluster within a certain distance from a centroid, or the center of a cluster, in other words, to find the cases that are most similar to each other and to exploit those similarities (and dissimilarities) in defining the characteristics of those cases. In cluster analysis, an analyst will specify the number of clusters (always greater than one), and a distance metric, often a Euclidean or Manhattan distance that provides a maximum for the clustering algorithm to evaluate a case. The clusterer will iteratively evaluate each case drawn from the dataset in serial fashion against the other cases it has already drawn, using the distance metric as the criterion for membership in the cluster. Cases that are farther from the centroid are less likely to be placed in that cluster, while cases that are closer will be defined as members of that cluster.

There are several clustering families used in data mining, including partitioning clustering, hierarchical, density, grid, and model-based clustering. A well-known partitioning method is the k-means algorithm. In k-means, k is specified by the analyst as the number of clusters to create, and these are assembled by grouping cases closest to the mean of some variable within that cluster. As a result, these clusters tend to be spatially similar. Another well-known clustering method is the expectation-maximization (EM) algorithm. Instead of assignment to a cluster based on means, EM uses mixtures of normal distributions, resulting in clusters that are spatially diverse. Other clustering methods used in data mining include COBWEB, which is a type of hierarchical clustering. In hierarchical clustering, clusters are nested within others in a subordinate-superordinate relationship, and can be represented as a tree structure. Hierarchical clustering can be agglomerative, where each case in the data is a cluster and clusters are recursively aggregated to create larger clusters; the process stops when the pre-specified number of clusters has been constructed. In divisive hierarchical clustering, the process begins with one large cluster that is recursively decomposed until the pre-specified number of clusters has been constructed.

The major advantage of using a clusterer to mine biomedical data is the lack of need for a class variable. Clustering methods are very robust, and especially valuable in descriptive analyses where the research question might focus on what makes one case different from another, or more largely, a group of cases from another group. The primary disadvantage with clustering is the need for a suitable distance metric for a given database. Selecting the metric is often a heuristic process, starting with an approximation of what would be suitable, but then parameterizing the metric with a range of values is often required to ensure that the clusters represent a good characterization of the data.

Clustering algorithms have been used in data mining where class membership is not explicitly defined. These methods might be particularly useful in analyzing survey data, where an outcome variable is not obvious, but they have gained wide acceptance in analyzing microarray data [5,7,19,30,71,74,122], adverse event detection [57], document clustering [85,135], image classification [135], complex patient identification [51,66,101], telemedicine [123], cognitive status assessment [125], survival analysis [125,137], and disease screening [141].

7.4.3.1.4 **Kernel Methods**

Each record in a dataset can be represented as a feature vector in a high dimensional feature space. One can think of these vectors as Euclidean coordinates where the relationships between them need to be characterized as the purpose of the data mining exercise. However, evaluating each coordinate can become rapidly intractable, computationally. It is more efficient to employ a kernel function, which uses the dot product (or inner product, given that it operates in Euclidean space) to compute the coordinate relationships between all ordered pairs of features. In essence, a kernel is a similarity function that maps a nonlinear problem to a linear classifier.

One of the best known examples of a kernel method that is used extensively in data mining is the support vector machine (SVM) [16]. The SVM operates on two principles. First, a decision boundary that separates two or more classes can be constructed and there are instances from each class that approach that boundary; these instances are called support vectors. Second, a linear discriminant function is used to optimally separate the support vectors. It is important to note that decision boundaries are not required to be linear; they can be quadratic, cubic, or polynomial, and thus curvilinear. For now, let us consider the linear SVM. In this case, the boundary is linear, as shown in Figure 7.10.

We can consider this boundary to be a classifier, in that it separates the two classes. It serves as the hyperplane discussed earlier in this chapter.

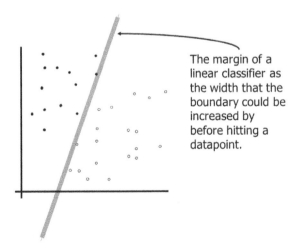

The margin of a linear classifier as the width that the boundary could be increased by before hitting a datapoint.

■ **FIGURE 7.10** A linear classifier and its margin. The margin indicates a boundary around the hyperplane. The margin is defined as the maximum width that boundary can be attained without intersecting an individual observations in a database. The margin is most usefully understood as a maximum margin linear classifier, as illustrated in Figure 7.11.

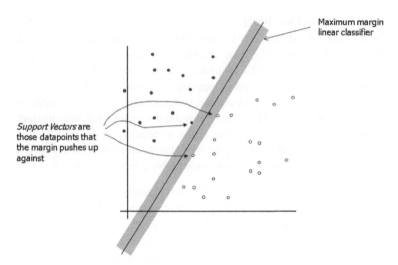

■ **FIGURE 7.11** An illustration of support vectors, which are observations or datapoints that the maximum margin linear classifier touches.

Note that the boundary in Figure 7.10 has a margin; that is, it is not simply a single line separating the two classes, but has a border that can be extended until it just touches upon an instance in each class. The function that extends that margin is called a *maximum margin classifier*, otherwise known as the linear classifier with the largest possible margin. The maximum margin classifier is the simplest form of SVM, and is shown in Figure 7.11. Figure 7.12 illustrates the boundaries of each of the two classes, as defined by convex hulls.

There are several advantages associated with the support vector machine in data mining. First, the boundary between classes need not be linear. This is very important when the data are noisy, with contradictions that make it difficult to classify a case because it does not neatly fit in one class or another. Second, SVMs generalize very well from training data. Third, SVMs tend to produce simple, single solutions to classification. There are two disadvantages, however, most importantly the lack of an easily understood and immediately available knowledge model. While SVMs are very accurate and fast classifiers, they offer no information about how the classification was actually made. Additional software is required to visualize the margin. A second important disadvantage is the need to understand the complex parameters that are required to fine-tune the SVM. These parameters are data sensitive, and as with the neural network and some evolutionary computation methods, require some trial and error in finding the right combination of parameter values.

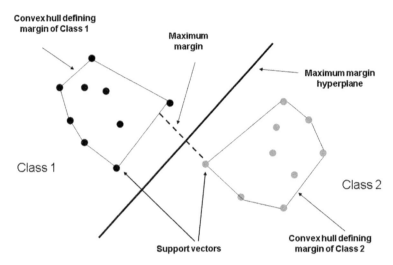

■ FIGURE 7.12 An illustration of how classes are differentiated by a support vector machine. Each class can be thought of as enclosed by a boundary (the convex hull shown here), and separated by the maximum margin linear classifier. The center of the classifier is the maximum margin hyperplane, and the support vectors are those datapoints closest to the hyperplane.

Kernel-based methods have been used widely in mining biomedical data. For example, support vector machines have been applied in genomics [15,104,110,111,140], proteomics [26,35,42,82], disease classification and prediction [6,82,110], and text mining [17,20,54,75,115]. Variations of kernel methods have also been developed and applied, which extend or otherwise modify the SVM paradigm [36,39,70,77,79,83,103,128,133,138,149,154].

7.4.3.1.5 **Probabilistic Methods**

There are several probabilistic approaches to data mining that extend beyond the statistical classification methods described above. These include latent variable models, maximum likelihood estimation, and Bayesian approaches. Of these, the Bayesian methods are arguably the most common, especially naïve Bayes classifier which is based on Bayes' Theorem expressed here as a joint probability function:

$$P(C|V_1..V_n) = P(C) * P(V_1 \cdots V_n|C), \tag{7.1}$$

where C is a class, such as Diseased/Not Diseased, and $V_1 \cdot V_n$ is a vector of predictor variables. Bayes' Theorem estimates the posterior probability $(P(C|V_1 \cdots V_n))$, given the prior probability $(P(C))$ times the likelihood $(P(V_1 \cdots V_n|C))$. While Bayes' Theorem assumes strong independence between the features, naïve Bayes ignores this independence assumption, based on the reality that such independence rarely occurs empirically. However, naïve

Bayes is an accurate classifier, especially in two-class problems, and it can handle large datasets with a high degree of efficiency.

Another Bayesian approach uses a directed acyclic graph representation, where nodes represent the variables in a dataset, with a distinct probability function, and the links between them represent the probabilistic relationships between the nodes. The probabilities are learned as priors empirically from the data. Once learning is complete the probabilities in the network are static and can be used for classification. Because of this representation, it is possible that once constructed from training data, the network could be used to determine the classification of a new case with a probability of class membership. It is also possible to update the node and link probabilities with new training cases over time. In examining the structure of the network, one can get a sense of the complex relationships between the variables in a set of data. As a result, the Bayesian network is a useful data mining technique as well as a tool for classification or prediction.

The advantages of Bayesian approaches are several. They are very simple to implement and apply to even complex databases. The theory behind these approaches is also relatively easy to understand and explain to domain experts who might not be familiar with other data mining approaches; this is especially the case with Bayesian networks. Finally, they are remarkably accurate for classification, even when exposed to a relatively small number of training cases, compared to the number required by other methods. The primary disadvantage of naïve Bayes is the independence assumption, which might not hold true in certain databases that could contain many interactions between the predictor (independent) variables. Bayesian networks suffer from the requirement that priors be specified for each node, and these may be difficult to obtain when there are effects from variables that haven't been included in the data. This is analogous to the "unmeasured confounding" problem that affects many statistical analyses of biomedical data.

The naïve Bayes classifier has been applied to a variety of data mining analyses in a large number of domains. These include signal detection and classification [12], diagnosis [2], prediction [72] and clinical decision making [157]. Bayesian networks have been applied in anatomic mapping of magnetic resonance images [27], disease risk factor identification [10], and genetic epidemiology [116,117]. There have been numerous extensions to Bayesian methods, or incorporation of these in other data mining approaches and these are well represented in feature selection [109], microarray analysis [28], rule learning [53], identifying gene-gene interactions [143], and particularly pharmacovigilance using adverse event reporting data [8,46,47,84,121,127,134]. Additional details on Bayesian approaches are given in Chapter 8.

7.4.3.2 *Instance-Based Methods*

In instance-based learning, testing cases are presented one at a time to the system and compared with training cases that are represented with their correct classification. The training case closest to the testing case is used to output a predicted class for the testing case. Instance-based learning thus requires the specification of a distance metric. One such metric is Euclidean, which compares the differences between sums of squares for each attribute-value pair for the testing case and training case. Another is the Manhattan distance, which compares differences between each attribute-value pair, without squaring.

One well-known instance-based algorithm is k-nearest neighbors (k-NN). The parameter k is an integer, defined in advance of the training regime, which indicates how many neighbors in the vicinity of a training case should be considered in evaluating a testing case. When k is greater than 1, the classification of the testing case is determined by a vote of k training cases that fall within the vicinity of the testing case. Thus, if $k = 5$, and three of the five training cases that are nearest to the testing case classify the testing case as "disease positive," the classification proposed by the system will be "disease positive." The advantage of the k-NN method is that it is very simple to understand and implement. It also performs well for mining many databases. However, one must specify a distance metric that is uniformly applied to all cases, and this assumes that the metric cannot change over time as the system is exposed to additional cases that may influence the appropriateness of that metric. In addition, k-NN speed and accuracy can be hampered by large, complex databases.

k-NN methods have been applied to mining biomedical data to identify drug interaction networks [25], for image classification and retrieval [96,112,153,155], for text mining [156], and various applications in bioinformatics [67,94,100,144].

7.4.3.3 *Tree-Based Methods*

Tree-based methods follow a general paradigm of the directed acyclic graph. Like the Bayesian network described above, nodes represent variables and links represent the relationships between them in terms of the values the variables can take on. Pathways from the root, or starting, node to the leaf, or class node, are expressed as conjunctions that can be translated to IF-THEN rules. An example of a decision tree that could be used to

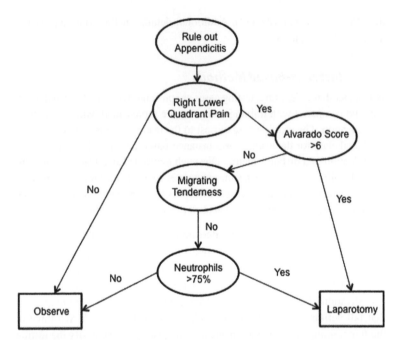

■ **FIGURE 7.13** A simple decision tree for determining treatment of possible appendicitis. Like most such trees, each node represents a single decision point, the direction of the path from the node being determined by the value of the variable or feature represented by the node.

determine if surgery is warranted for clinical signs and symptoms related to appendicitis is illustrated below in Figure 7.13.

Decision trees are induced from data using recursive partitioning, wherein the data are split by evaluating the contribution a variable and its respective values make to some criterion, such as an entropy metric, at a given time step. The process is repeated for each variable in the dataset until a tree that provides the optimal value for the metric is obtained. The earliest implementations of knowledge discovery using decision tress include ID3 and C4.5. Decision tree induction using variants of C4.5, such as C5.0 and CART (Classification and Regression Trees), is very popular in the biomedical domain, and is available in many statistical packages and most data mining suites.

Decision trees are created, or induced from data by means of such measures as Gini index or an entropy-based metric, information gain. These are used to select recursively the attribute that best separates the data into separate classes at a given node. This procedure is repeated recursively for each subtree until the data have been exhaustively partitioned. A decision tree for a two-class problem is based on the relative frequency of each class.

For example, given a dataset with disease-positive and disease-negative classes, the tree will be constructed so as to determine what variables and values should discriminate between these. The following equation defines the expected information needed to make this discrimination:

$$I(p,n) = -\frac{p}{p+n} \log_2 \frac{p}{p+n} - \frac{n}{p+n} \log_2 \frac{n}{p+n},$$

where p is the frequency of positives, n of the negatives, and $I(p,n)$ is the information gain across the dataset including both classes.

As the tree is constructed at each time step, a variable as a node in the tree. This variable is selected based on the expected information if variable A were selected as a node:

$$E(A) = \sum_{i=1}^{v} \frac{p_i + n}{p + n},$$

where $E(A)$ is the expected information for a given variable. The variable with the highest $E(A)$ is selected as the node at a given iteration.

Finally, the information gained by branching on node A is:

$$\text{gain}(A) = I(p,n) - E(A).$$

The goal is to choose the variable for branching that yields the most gain.

A simple example, based on a rabies treatment scenario, is provided here to illustrate how decision tree induction works. In this example, a small dataset contains five candidate predictors and one class variable:

	Variable Name	Description
Candidate predictors	BITTEN	Was patient bitten by an animal?
	PRESENT	Was rabies present in the area?
	CAPTURED	Was biting animal captured?
	VACCINATED	Was biting animal vaccinated for rabies?
	NORMAL_BRAIN	Did animal have normal brain on necropsy?
Class	TREAT	Should patient be treated for rabies?

Each candidate predictor is coded dichotomously (Yes/No) and the class variable is coded Treat/NoTreat. There are 32 records, identified with a record number which is included for reference. The data are shown below:

RECORD	BITTEN	PRESENT	CAPTURED	VACCINATED	NORMAL_BRAIN	TREAT
1	No	No	No	No	No	NoTreat
2	No	Yes	No	No	No	NoTreat
3	No	No	Yes	No	No	NoTreat
4	No	No	No	Yes	No	NoTreat
5	No	No	No	No	Yes	NoTreat
6	No	Yes	Yes	No	No	NoTreat
7	No	Yes	No	Yes	No	NoTreat
8	No	Yes	No	No	Yes	NoTreat
9	No	No	Yes	Yes	No	NoTreat
10	No	No	Yes	No	Yes	NoTreat
11	No	No	No	Yes	Yes	NoTreat
12	No	Yes	Yes	Yes	No	NoTreat
13	No	Yes	Yes	No	Yes	NoTreat
14	No	Yes	No	Yes	Yes	NoTreat
15	No	No	Yes	Yes	Yes	NoTreat
16	No	Yes	Yes	Yes	Yes	NoTreat
17	Yes	No	No	No	No	NoTreat
18	Yes	No	Yes	No	No	NoTreat
19	Yes	No	No	Yes	No	NoTreat
20	Yes	No	No	No	Yes	NoTreat
21	Yes	No	Yes	Yes	No	NoTreat
22	Yes	No	Yes	No	Yes	NoTreat
23	Yes	No	No	Yes	Yes	NoTreat
24	Yes	No	Yes	Yes	Yes	NoTreat
25	Yes	Yes	No	No	No	Treat
26	Yes	Yes	No	Yes	No	Treat
27	Yes	Yes	No	No	Yes	Treat
28	Yes	Yes	No	Yes	Yes	Treat
29	Yes	Yes	Yes	Yes	No	NoTreat
30	Yes	Yes	Yes	Yes	Yes	NoTreat
31	Yes	Yes	Yes	No	No	Treat
32	Yes	Yes	Yes	No	Yes	NoTreat

The goal of this exercise is to induce a decision rule that identifies those individuals in need of treatment, based on patterns of the exposure attributes (predictors):

Step 1: The first thing to do is calculate the overall information (I) in the data as a whole:

$$I(Rabies) = -\frac{5}{32}\log_2\left(\frac{5}{32}\right) - \frac{27}{32}\log_2\left(\frac{27}{32}\right) = 0.625.$$

Step 2: Now that we know how much information the *entire* dataset contributes, we need to partition the data so that we can determine the *relative* information contributed by each of the exposure attributes. To do this, we calculate a measure of *expected information (E)*:

$$E(P) = \sum_{i=1}^{n} \frac{C_i}{C} I(C_i),$$

where C is a set of training instances and C_i is a subset of C, partitioned on the n values of attribute P.

We need to calculate this for each exposure attribute, starting with the first one in the dataset, BITTEN. The calculation for BITTEN is as follows:

General characteristics:

Total not bitten: 16.

Total bitten: 16.

C_1 (not bitten): 16/16, all in the no-treat class.

C_2 (bitten): 11/16 in the no-treat class, 5/16 in the treat class.

Step 2a: To calculate $E(Bitten)$:

$$E(Bitten) = \frac{16}{32} I(C_1) + \frac{16}{32} I(C_2).$$

Step 2b: To calculate $I(C_1)$:

$$I(C_1) = -\frac{16}{16} \log_2 \frac{16}{16} = 0.$$

Step 2c: To calculate $I(C_2)$:

Thus:

$$I(C_2) = -\frac{11}{16} \log_2 \frac{11}{16} - \frac{5}{16} \log_2 \frac{5}{16} = 0.896.$$

$$E(Bitten) = \frac{16}{32} * 0 + \frac{16}{32} * 0.896 = 0.448.$$

Step 2d: We do this series of calculations (Steps 2a–c) for each of the remaining exposure attributes, and obtain the following results:

BITTEN	0.448
PRESENT	0.448
CAPTURED	0.574
VACCINATED	0.621
NORMAL_BRAIN	0.621

Step 3: We next compare each of these expected information measures with the overall information in the dataset. We do this via the gain:

$$\text{gain}(P) = I(C) - E(P),$$

where $I(C)$ is the total information content in the entire dataset and $E(P)$ is the expected information from attribute P. Thus, knowing that $I(C) = 0.625$:

Predictor	E(P)	Gain(P)
BITTEN	0.448	0.177
PRESENT	0.448	0.177
CAPTURED	0.574	0.051
VACCINATED	0.621	0.004
NORMAL_BRAIN	0.621	0.004

The attribute with the highest gain is selected as the first node to be expanded. We can see that BITTEN and PRESENT are tied the top contenders in the competition for the root node (because this is the first pass). As it happens, because BITTEN comes first in the data, it will be selected as the root node at this iteration and PRESENT will be evaluated on the next iteration to determine where it appears in the decision tree.

The next step is to determine the split for BITTEN, for which we return to a count of instances in each value of BITTEN, conditioned on the class (see Figure 7.14):

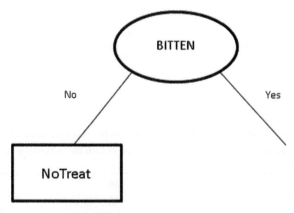

■ **FIGURE 7.14** Step 1 in the creation of a simple decision tree to determine treatment for possible rabies in the case of an animal bite. "Bitten" was selected first, because it provided the most information relevant to treating someone for rabies.

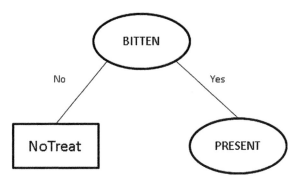

FIGURE 7.15 Step 2 in creating the decision tree includes the next most informative feature, "Present."

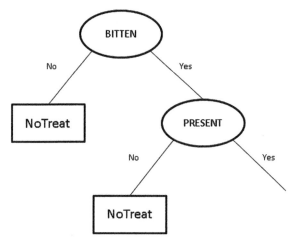

FIGURE 7.16 Step 3 evaluates the values of "Present" to determine the subsequent paths from this node.

C_1 (not bitten): 16/16, all in the no-treat class.

C_2 (bitten): 11/16 in the no-treat class, 5/16 in the treat class.

Thus, BITTEN will be split with NoTreat as the leaf, or terminal node, and PRESENT (because it tied with BITTEN) is now added to the tree (see Figure 7.15).

Based on the results of Step 3, the next node to be expanded is PRESENT (see Figure 7.16).

CAPTURED had the next highest gain from Step 3, so it is selected as the next node (see Figure 7.17).

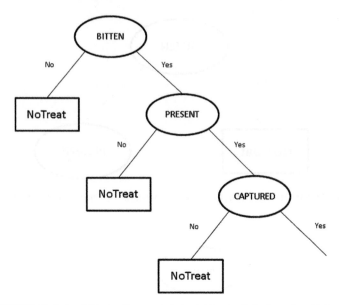

■ **FIGURE 7.17** In step 4, "Captured" was evaluated and determined to be the next most informative feature. The values of the feature were evaluated to determine the next path.

And finally, VACCINATED and NORMAL_BRAIN tied on gain in Step 3 and would have the same expansion based on their value so the first of these variables is selected as the terminal node in the tree (see Figure 7.18).

The final tree shown below Figure 7.18 was induced from the data, and could be used in the treatment of a patient presenting to the emergency department with an animal bite.

Decision trees are a commonly used approach in data mining. They are very fast, they can handle missing data, and they are easily transferred to IF-THEN rule representations. However, they can become very large in terms of width and depth, depending on the complexity of the data. "Bushy" trees can be pruned, and there are numerous algorithms for accomplishing this, but there is often a trade-off between pruning and tree size that can impact on the accuracy of the tree when applied to classification tasks and especially when using decision tree induction for hypothesis generation or feature selection.

There are times when a single decision tree may not afford optimal classification accuracy or even computing tractability. This is often the case where a dataset is huge, with many variables or records, or both; an example would be microarray data. An approach to these data using a decision tree paradigm is to use a number of decision trees, each of which randomly selects a

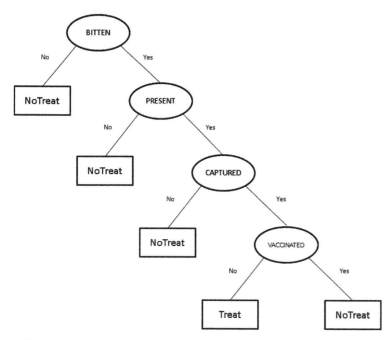

■ **FIGURE 7.18** The final decision tree for determining rabies treatment for a patient presenting with an animal bite.

variable from the dataset on which to construct each node the decision tree. This approach, *random forests*, is an example of a "metaclassifier" in that it is an ensemble of classifiers. The process of selecting the random sample of features is analogous to bootstrapping, wherein a variable is selected as each node is constructed. At the end of learning, there are N trees in the "forest" which can be used for classification of test cases. Each testing case is run through each tree, the classifications assigned to the testing case tallied, and the most frequent class value is used as the classification for the testing case.

There are several advantages to tree-based methods that make them especially attractive for use in mining biomedical data. First, they do not require any pre-specified domain knowledge. A decision tree inducer can be applied to any set of data without setting any parameters, except perhaps for pruning. Second, they can process categorical and continuous data. In fact, decision trees are often used to determine the cutpoints for categorizing complex, continuous data. Third, they automatically prune out variables that do not add any information to the overall tree, and are thus useful for feature selection. Finally, the tree representation is very accessible, and is easily translated to IF-THEN rules.

Decision trees feature prominently in the biomedical data mining literature, with a variety of applications. These include clinical outcome prediction [23,29,41,65,81,99,124], diagnosis [48,78,132,147], screening [68], clinical decision making [139], risk assessment [69], feature selection [3,105], signal detection [80,129], adverse event detection [24], and genomics [90,91,107]. An excellent review of the use of decision trees in drug discovery is found in [56]. Random forests are gaining wide acceptance in biomedical data mining as well. In the bioinformatics domain, they have been used in genome-wide association studies [21,111], identification of gene-gene interactions [40], proteomics [73], and microarray analysis [91]. They have also been used for classification in clinical applications [52,63,93] and feature selection [11].

7.4.3.4 *Rule-Based Methods*

In machine learning, a rule is an expression that contains an antecedent (condition) and a consequent (action):

$$\{V_1 \cdots V_n\} \rightarrow C,$$

where $\{V_1 \cdots V_n\}$ is a vector of variables each of which is associated with a value, and represents the "IF," or condition of the rule. The arrow translates to "THEN" and C is a class variable. Logically, the condition is a conjunction, with each variable in the condition a conjunct that may be joined with a Boolean operator (AND, OR, NOT). Populated in plain English, a possible rule would be:

IF (right-lower-quadrant-pain = Yes AND Alvarado-Score > 6)

THEN Perform-Laparatomy.

Rules are a particularly common form of knowledge representation in data mining, and this is seen in the number of rule discovery algorithms that are available, a few of which will be discussed here. In general, the process of rule-based knowledge discovery seeks to identify conjunctions of variables that indicate possible associations between sets or variable, or to identify the variables and associated values that classify or predict class membership.

7.4.3.4.1 Association Rule Discovery

Association rule mining focuses on discovering the relationship between any variables or sets of variables in a dataset. Thus, the consequent of an association rule does not have to be the class variable. The method comes from market basket analysis, where the products purchased together in a single basket or cart are analyzed for how often they co-occur across all purchases. Thus, if a record in a database were considered a "purchase," and each variable a "product" that is defined as present or absent, a model of how often such variables occurred together from record to record could indicate possible associations between them. Another name for this approach is frequent itemset discovery, where an item set is a basket of products.

The best known approach to association rule mining is the *a priori* algorithm. In *a priori*, itemsets are constructed starting with one candidate variable (item) at a time and evaluating it for frequency as a proportion of all instances (records) in the database. The evaluation requires a two-step calculation that involves assessing two metrics: support and confidence. Support is simply the proportion of records in the database that contain a specific itemset over all records in the database; thus, support indicates the strength of a given itemset, represented in [2] as X:

$$Support(X) = \frac{Records\ in\ database\ containing\ X}{Total\ number\ of\ records\ in\ database}.$$

Confidence indicates the strength of a rule derived from the itemset based on its support:

$$Confidence(X \rightarrow Y) = \frac{Support(X \cup Y)}{Support(X)}.$$

Association rule discovery is best understood by working through an example. The Pima Indians Diabetes Database [50] contains 768 records of women, 268 of whom have diabetes. There are a total of nine variables, eight predictors, and one class variable (diabetes yes/no). For the example below, the database has been reduced to two predictors, diastolic blood pressure (DIASTOLIC, coded as HiBP and NormBP) and skinfold thickness (SKINFOLD, coded as Obese and NotObese). The class variable is Diabetes (DM, coded as DM and NoDM):

Step 1: Create the candidate 1-itemsets. The purpose of this and the subsequent itemset creation steps is to determine, based on support, which variables will go into the final *n*-itemset. Since there are three variables, the maximum itemset size is 3. The support for each variable will be calculated; those variables with a support less than the threshold of 0.20 will be dropped from the 1-itemset (see Figure 7.19).

Step 2: Create the candidate 2-itemsets. The algorithm proceeds to evaluate variable pairs in this step. Note that only the itemsets (variables in this step) from the final 1-itemset are included as candidates at this step. The support for each variable pair will be calculated, and based on the threshold of 0.20, evaluated for membership in the 2-itemset (see Figure 7.20).

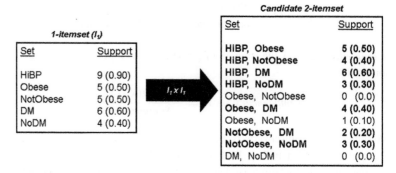

Dataset
HiBP, Obese, DM
HiBP, Obese, NoDM
HiBP, Obese, DM
HiBP, NotObese, NoDM
NormBP, NotObese, NoDM
HiBP, NotObese, DM
HiBP, NotObese, DM
HiBP, NotObese, NoDM
HiBP, Obese, DM
HiBP, Obese, DM

Candidate 1-itemset

Set	Support
HiBP	9 (0.90)
NormBP 1	1 (0.10)
Obese	5 (0.50)
NotObese	5 (0.50)
DM	6 (0.60)
NoDM	4 (0.40)

■ **FIGURE 7.19** The creation of a candidate 1-itemset, using the A Priori algorithm for association rule discovery. Each single feature is evaluated for support; those features meeting the threshold support value will be included in the final 1-itemset shown in Figure 7.20.

1-itemset (I₁)

Set	Support
HiBP	9 (0.90)
Obese	5 (0.50)
NotObese	5 (0.50)
DM	6 (0.60)
NoDM	4 (0.40)

$I_1 \times I_1$

Candidate 2-itemset

Set	Support
HiBP, Obese	5 (0.50)
HiBP, NotObese	4 (0.40)
HiBP, DM	6 (0.60)
HiBP, NoDM	3 (0.30)
Obese, NotObese	0 (0.0)
Obese, DM	4 (0.40)
Obese, NoDM	1 (0.10)
NotObese, DM	2 (0.20)
NotObese, NoDM	3 (0.30)
DM, NoDM	0 (0.0)

■ **FIGURE 7.20** The candidate 2-itemset is created by performing a Cartesian join on each feature in the 1-itemset. Support is calculated for each pair in the candidate 2-itemset and used to determine which pair will be included in the final 2-itemset, as shown here in bold and in Figure 7.21.

Step 3: Create the candidate 3-itemsets. In this step, variable triplets are evaluated for inclusion in the 3-itemset. Only the itemsets included from Step 3 that pass the support threshold are included (see Figure 7.21).

Step 4: Create the rules for each of the three 3-itemsets derived from Step 3. The rules will be constructed from all possible combinations of the variables in each of the 3-itemsets. Note that the class variable may appear anywhere in the rule (see Figure 7.22).

Step 5: Determine which rules created in Step 4 are added to the final association rule set (see Figure 7.23).

It is important to note that many association rules represent trivial concepts, and at times can even be counterintuitive or nonsensical. The does not mean

2-Itemset (I_2)

Set	Support
HiBP, Obese	5 (0.50)
HiBP, NotObese	4 (0.40)
HiBP, DM	6 (0.60)
HiBP, NoDM	3 (0.30)
Obese, DM	4 (0.40)
NotObese, DM	2 (0.20)
NotObese, NoDM	3 (0.30)

$I_2 \times I_2$

Candidate 3-itemset

Set	Support
HiBP, Obese, DM	**4 (0.40)**
HiBP, Obese, NoDM	1 (0.10)
HiBP, NotObese, DM	**2 (0.20)**
HiBP, NotObese, NoDM	**2 (0.20)**
HiBP, DM, NoDM	0 (0.0)
HiBP, Obese, NotObese	0 (0.0)
Obese, NotObese, DM	0 (0.0)
Obese, NotObese, NoDM	0 (0.0)
Obese, DM, NoDM	0 (0.0)
NotObese, DM, NoDM	0 (0.0)

■ **FIGURE 7.21** Similarly to the creation of the 2-itemset, the candidate 3-itemset is created by performing a join of all pairs from the final 2-itemset.

Itemset 1: **HiBP, Obese, DM**	Itemset 2: **HiBP, NotObese, DM**	Itemset 3: **HiBP, NotObese, NoDM**
HiBP $\Rightarrow$ Obese and DM	HiBP $\Rightarrow$ NotObese and DM	HiBP $\Rightarrow$ NotObese and NoDM
HiBP and Obese $\Rightarrow$ DM	HiBP and NotObese $\Rightarrow$ DM	HiBP and NotObese $\Rightarrow$ NoDM
HiBP and DM $\Rightarrow$ Obese	HiBP and DM $\Rightarrow$ NotObese	HiBP and NoDM $\Rightarrow$ NotObese
Obese $\Rightarrow$ HiBP and DM	NotObese $\Rightarrow$ HiBP and DM	NotObese $\Rightarrow$ HiBP and NoDM
Obese and DM $\Rightarrow$ HiBP	NotObese and DM $\Rightarrow$ HiBP	NotObese and NoDM $\Rightarrow$ HiBP
DM $\Rightarrow$ HiBP and Obese	DM $\Rightarrow$ HiBP and NotObese	NoDM $\Rightarrow$ HiBP and NotObese

■ **FIGURE 7.22** Candidate association rules are created from each triplet in the final 3-itemset.

they should be ignored, because such rules can lead the analyst toward an association that ultimately does make sense.

7.4.3.4.2 Classification Rules

Classification rules are a form of knowledge representation that differ from association rules in that the consequent always includes the class label [34]. Thus, a classification rule states the condition (in the antecedent) that defines class membership (represented as the consequent). Classification rules can be learned *directly* from data using such methods as RIPPER (described below), or *indirectly* from decision trees, some evolutionary computation algorithms such as learning classifier systems, or neural networks. Classification rule algorithms typically create a set of rules, although one algorithm, 1R, generates one rule only [62]. 1R is a direct rule learner that determines which features should be included in the rule based on error

Rule	Confidence
HiBP $\Rightarrow$ Obese and DM	4/9 (0.44)
HiBP and Obese $\Rightarrow$ DM	4/5 (0.90)
HiBP and DM $\Rightarrow$ Obese	4/4 (1.00)
Obese $\Rightarrow$ HiBP and DM	4/5 (0.90)
Obese and DM $\Rightarrow$ HiBP	4/4 (1.00)
DM $\Rightarrow$ HiBP and Obese	4/6 (0.67)

R1: If HiBP and Obese then DM
R2: If HiBP and DM then Obese
R3: If Obese then HiBP and DM
R4: If Obese and DM then HiBP

■ **FIGURE 7.23** The candidate rules will be evaluated; those rules meeting the predetermined threshold for confidence will be included in the final association rule set.

rate. In this regard, it is one of the simplest knowledge discovery algorithms available, as seen in the following pseudocode:

```
Initialize empty rule R
For each attribute Ai
    For each value j of Ai
        Count frequency of each class
        Determine prevalent class
        Assign class to Aij in R
    Calculate classification error e of R
Select R with lowest e
```

Another well-known direct rule discovery algorithm is RIPPER (Repeated Incremental Pruning to Produce Error Reduction) [32]. RIPPER is a propositional rule learner that grows rules in supervised environments by greedily adding one antecedent at a time until the rule is correct, based on training data. Candidate antecedents are evaluated for information gain and those with the highest gain are added first. Information gain here is calculated according to the same metric in an algorithm for concept learning, FOIL (First Order Inductive Learner) [113]. This process is repeated until a set of rules is created that has at least 50% accuracy overall. After the rule set is constructed, each rule is pruned based on its classification accuracy, and the final rule set is then evaluated for accuracy.

Initialize empty rule R
    While information gain improves and R covers negative examples
        Add antecedent a to R
        Prune R ($v = (p - n)/(p + n)$, where $p =$ positive examples
                              covered by rule
                      $n =$ negative examples
                              covered by rule
        Remove antecedents that maximize v

Other direct rule learners include such as PRISM [22], CN2 [31], and the numerous descendants of AQ [97].

7.4.3.4.3 Prediction Rules

Prediction rules are classification rules that are used to predict class membership of an object whose class is unknown. Predictions may be expressed as membership in one class or another, or as a probability of being in a specific class. In applying a prediction rule, a case with an unknown class is presented to the system and a prediction of that class, typically as a probability, is returned. There are several statistical methods for prediction, such as least-squares regression, the discriminant function, and logistic regression. All of these use a vector of independent variables (predictors) that have been weighted in some way, depending on the algorithm. The dependent variable is the class that is predicted by applying the weights or coefficients to the respective predictor variables.

7.4.3.5 *Data Mining Approaches Inspired by Nature*

Nature has inspired the development of a number of interesting algorithms and computational approaches for discovering knowledge in data. These include evolutionary computation, neural networks, artificial immune systems, swarm intelligence, and ant colony optimization.

7.4.3.5.1 Evolutionary Computation

Evolutionary computation has a long history. Even as early as the 1950s, there was interest in using operators from natural genetic variation and natural selection to "evolve" solutions to problems. By the 1960s, an approach called "evolution strategies" was taking hold, maturing into "evolutionary programming," in which genetic operators were applied to finite state machines to identify candidate solutions in a solution space. The rationale for considering evolution as an appropriate metaphor for solving problems is threefold. First, evolution is a process of search for some optimum in time. Second, evolution is an adaptive process; as evolution proceeds, and populations of organisms are allowed to carry over from one generation to the next, the individuals making up the populations are adapting to various pressures exerted upon them by the environment and other factors. Finally, evolution can be seen as effecting a body of metarules that direct, at a very high level, and with a degree of generality, the development of populations over time, from one generation to the next. Ultimately, evolution is a search for solutions to some problem.

Central to the development of evolutionary computation is the genetic algorithm. The goal of the GA is to use the paradigm of natural adaptation as a general problem-solving approach. The GA has been used in function optimization and as a search method, and has been employed in data mining in the learning classifier system and genetic programming. The GA has three essential characteristics. First, it is population based, in that knowledge is represented by "individuals" contained in a population. Individuals may be expressed as a tuple, or record, in a database and the population is the database that contains these records. Each individual in the simplest GA representation is a haploid structure, or a single chromosome, containing a one-dimensional array of genes, each of which takes on a value, and thus acts like an allele in "wet" organisms. The chromosome is analogous to a record in a database, while the genes are similar to database fields, or variables, which are instantiated as alleles. Each individual has a "fitness," or a representation of its ability to solve a problem. For example, an individual that contains a more accurate solution to a problem will have a better fitness than one that is inaccurate. Finally, genetic operators, typically reproduction, crossover, and mutation, are employed to evolve the population over time, expressed as a series of generations.

Reproduction takes place in a simulated mating of two "parents," or individuals selected to be copied into the next generation. Parents can be selected deterministically, where the two individuals with the best fitness are selected for reproduction, or probabilistically, using a weighted roulette wheel. In the latter method, the overall population fitness is calculated, and used as the denominator to calculate the proportion of total population fitness contributed by each individual. The individual with the highest proportional fitness is more likely to be selected as a parent.

Copies of the two parents are created, and with some predetermined probability, crossover is applied at a randomly selected chromosome locus. This exchange of "genetic material" is the way in which the GA explores the hypothesis space and thus forms the core of its search function. Mutation may be applied, typically at very low probability at each gene to rein in the effects of crossover that over time can create wildly inaccurate and low fitness individuals.

A simple GA is represented below:

Initialize a population P of n chromosomes of length l
Evaluate fitness F of each chromosome in the population
Repeat
    Select two chromosomes ("parents") proportional to their fitness
    With probability χ, apply crossover operator to create two new
    chromosomes ("offspring")
With probability μ, mutate each locus on each offspring chromosome
    Insert offspring into P
    Delete two chromosomes from P proportional to fitness
    Evaluate population fitness F_P
Until
    Termination condition is met (defined by target fitness function)
Return final population P_{Final} as the set of best (most "fit")
chromosomes

GAs have been used in a number of data mining applications, most notably in the learning classifier system and in genetic programming [76]. The learning classifier system uses the GA for knowledge discovery through its ability to search a space of hypotheses, although the GA is only one component of the LCS. Like the GA, the LCS uses a population of individuals, but the representation is analogous to a condition-action rule, more precisely, a genotype-phenotype respectively. The other components of the LCS include a performer, which provides interaction between the environment (such as a database) and the population. The performer is responsible for matching the genotype of an input, such as a training case, with the genotypes of the individuals in the population, and then proposing an output based on the phenotype of the population individuals selected to match. A reinforcement component adds or subtracts from the fitness of the individuals in the population that were elected to propose the output. Finally, the genetic algorithm is applied to individuals or the entire population in order to propose new solutions. There have been numerous extensions to the basic learning classifier system first proposed by Holland [59]. These include the Animat [146] and its successors which use a stimulus-response paradigm, such that reward is instantaneous at each time step, and more recently, XCS and their successors, which use reinforcement learning. These are all examples of the Michigan approach to learning classifier systems, and are differentiated from the Pittsburgh approach in that they use a population of individuals, whereas the latter uses populations of rule *sets*, in applying the genetic algorithm. Chapter 9 provides additional details about learning classifier systems.

The advantages of evolutionary computation approaches in data mining are several. First, the knowledge representation is easily understood as individuals with a genotype and a phenotype that is analogous to an IF-THEN rule. In genetic programming, an individual is represented as a program, and each gene can be thought of as a program component, and this representation is similarly accessible. Second, the genetic algorithm is a well-tested method for optimization and subsequently for exploration of the hypothesis space. Third, approaches that use evolutionary computation, such as the learning classifier system, in conjunction with other learning and reinforcement paradigms have gained much credence in the data mining community as tractable, easily implemented, and robust methods for knowledge discovery. Finally, there are numerous evolutionary programs available "off the shelf," typically as add-ins but also standalone software.

There are several disadvantages of using evolutionary computing in mining data. First, there is a limit on the tractability of these systems, particularly when applied to data with a very large number of features. The genotype can be so complex and computationally burdensome that training can take long periods of time, or even fail to converge on an acceptable accuracy standard. Second, even though there are numerous code examples and even compiled software packages that use one evolutionary method or another, they often need to be adapted for a given database. Thus, it is not uncommon that one would need extensive programming knowledge to make such tools useful in mining biomedical data. Third, these methods require very substantial parameterization, often accomplished through trial and error. For example, it is often difficult to anticipate how large a population should be, or how frequently crossover should be performed. Finally, there is so much research in evolutionary computation that it is difficult for a new user to understand which approach to choose. This is especially the case with learning classifier systems, as described in Chapter 9 in this book. In spite of these disadvantages, evolutionary computation of various types has been applied in biomedical data mining. Several examples include detection and classification of EEG signals [126], the application of a learning classifier system to injury surveillance [61], and others [18,60].

7.4.3.5.2 Neural Networks

Neural networks are perhaps the oldest of the naturally inspired computing approaches, being based on theories dating back to the late 19th century, but have only fairly recently been applied to data mining. A neural network is a semantic network, where a set of input/output units ("neurons") are connected to each other, and these connections are weighted relative to the importance or strength of the link between one neuron and the next. These connections are roughly analogous to synapses in biological

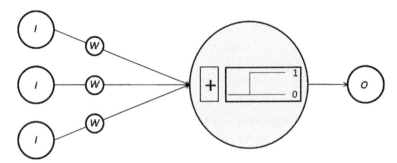

■ **FIGURE 7.24** A simple perceptron. Each input is connected to the neuron, shown in gray. Each connection has a weight, the value of which evolves over time, and is used to modify the input. Weighted inputs are summed, and this sum determines the output of the neuron, which is a classification (in this case, either 0 or 1).

nervous systems. Neural networks learn by adjusting the connection weights during training. Neurons are all-or-none devices that "fire," or transmit a message to the next connected neuron, based on meeting or exceeding some threshold.

An early simulated neuron was the perceptron [118], which incorporates the basis for the neural network. As shown in Figure 7.24, the perceptron takes inputs (I) from the environment, such as a vector of features from a database. Each feature has a specific value such as one would find in the database. Thus, for a vector that includes the three features {Age, Height, Weight}, the values for a given training case could be {32, 61, 120}.

These values are weighted by the connections (shown as "W" in the figure), and these weights evolve over time during training. These weights represent the knowledge model in the perception, and are sent to the perception where they are added and the sum of the weights is evaluated to determine if a threshold is exceeded. The threshold function determines the output of the neuron based on the summed, weighted inputs. Based on the value of the summed weights, the perceptron sends one message such as a decision or classification back to the environment, represented in the figure as either 0 or 1. In the case of supervised learning, the output of the perceptron can be compared to the known class of a training case, and based on the accuracy of the output decision, the weights and the threshold will be adjusted to strengthen or weaken the weights or the threshold, or both. Typically, weight and threshold adjustments are made only when an error occurs in the output. For example, weights can be adjusted at each time step, determined by the exposure of the system to a training case, as follows:

$$w_i(t+1) = w_i(t) + \Delta w_i(t),$$

where w_i = weight of connection i

$$\Delta w_i(t) = (D - O)I_i,$$

where D = known classification and O = classification output by the perceptron.

Numerous extensions have been made to the perceptron model, nearly all of which involve multiple neurons connected in layers, such as an input ("sensory") layer, an output ("effector") layer, and one or more middle ("hidden") layers. The hidden layers build an internal model of the way input patterns are related to the desired output, and as a result, this is where the knowledge representation is implicit in this model—it is the synapses (connectivity) that is the representation proper. In general, the larger the number of hidden layers and the neurons they contain, the less error during training. This type of architecture is used in the *feed-forward, back-propagation neural network*. A schematic of a feed-forward, back-propagation network is shown in Figure 7.25.

This network uses the feed-forward approach of the perceptron, but includes the ability to provide (propagate) feedback about the accuracy of its output to the components. The pseudocode for a feed-forward, back-propagation neural network is shown below:

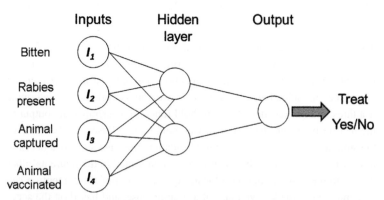

■ **FIGURE 7.25** A feed-forward, back-propagation neural network. In this example, the inputs represent values (yes/no) of four of the features used to determine if a patient who has suffered an animal bite needs to be treated prophylactically for rabies. Each connection is weighted and these weights evolve during training. This simple model is similar to the perceptron in Figure 7.24, except that it includes a hidden layer and that is propagates error back to the input weights during training. The hidden layer provides additional knowledge representation internal to the system, and can provide improvements in classification performance.

```
Initialize weights
For each training case i
        Present input i
        Generate output O_i
        Calculate error (D_i −;O_i)
        Do while output incorrect
                For each layer j
                        Pass error back to each neuron n in layer j
                        Modify weight in each neuron n in layer j
        EndDo
        i = i+1
```

The hidden layer is the workhorse in this type of neural network. Its outputs, whether fed forward or backward through the network, are determined by a variety of different functions, a popular one of which is a logistic function:

$$O_j = \frac{1}{1 + e^{-Nj}},$$

where O_j is the output of hidden layer j and

$$N_j = \sum_i W_{ij} O_i + \theta_j.$$

N_j is the sum of the weighted outputs plus some error term θ.

Neural networks pose several advantages for data mining. They have shown excellent performance in many settings, particularly in prediction, where the trained network can be used to identify the probability of a specific outcome, given the value of an input feature vector for a given patient. In biomedical settings, they are especially useful because of their resistance to noise in the data. However, neural networks pose several challenges to those using them for data mining. Most neural network software requires that the architecture be specified in advance, so that the determination of how many hidden layers (and how many neurons are in those layers) must be made in advance of training. Second, there are many parameters that need to be set in a typical neural network, and some of these are often opaque to a novice user. These include settings that bias the connection weights as the network is trained. Fourth, a neural network can take a long time to train, particularly for some biomedical databases containing many variables, many records, and numerous contradictions in the data. Finally, the knowledge contained in a neural network is not easily translated to something that is readily understandable, such as one would find with a regression model. However, there has been considerable research into extracting the knowledge hidden in neural networks, as noted in [88].

Neural networks have been used in biomedical data mining in such domains as diagnosis [64,92,131], clinical prediction [29,41,102,108], pharmacovigilance [14,134], drug adverse event detection [13,120,136], personalized medicine [119]. Image classification [9,37], and proteomics [26,89,114,142,151]. An excellent introduction to the use of neural networks in mining biomedical data is offered in [150].

7.4.3.5.3 Other Naturally Inspired Methods of Knowledge Discovery

Several other natural-inspired methods of data mining have been developed over the past 10–15 years. One of these is the artificial immune system (AIS), which is based on *in vivo* immune systems [38,49]. The AIS exemplifies learning from the environment, in that once an agent from that environment is encountered, an immune response is set into motion as a cascade of events that attempts to recognize the agent as "friend" or "foe." This recognition is remembered for future encounters, such that friendly agents are ignored and foes result in a reaction that in extreme cases, such as anaphylaxis, result in serious physical harm. The artificial immune system is designed along these same principles, and exhibits similar qualities to the *in vivo* system. These systems have several characteristics that make them particularly useful for data mining. First, they learn from interaction with an environment, and that learning occurs under reinforcement such that learning is rewarded or punished, depending on the response to environmental stimuli. Second, these systems have memory, in that over time they remember environmental inputs from prior experience, so there is an element of recognition. Third, they are adaptive systems, such that response to environmental stimuli can change over time. Finally, they are diverse, in that there are multiple and distributed receptors in the immune pathway. These features translate nearly directly to a computational model of the immune system.

AIS have been used in pattern detection, especially for "intruders," such as computer viruses. In order to determine if an environmental stimulus (antigen) is an invader, however, the pattern must be learned, and this requires data mining. The AIS has this capability through supervised learning that uses an affinity measure that is itself learned over time. The affinity measure is related to a distance metric as used in k-nearest neighbors or clustering, and is used to determine the proximity of an antigen with any matching "antibodies" in the system. Over time, through mutation, cloning, and elimination, the population of antibodies is optimized for recognition of antigens from the environment. Once training has ended, the AIS should be able to detect aberrations from patterns that have been previously encountered. In biomedical domains, AIS have been used in several applications such as clustering of microarray data [87], feature selection [45], and genomics [43].

Another naturally inspired approach is ant colony optimization [44]. Ants are perfect examples of autonomous agents that work independently but in the best interests of a community. An individual ant's behavior may seem random and inherently blind with respect to search. Collectively, however, they exhibit purposive and complex behavior. Examples of this include next building and temperature maintenance, bridge building, and especially food foraging. This latter behavior is a complex of several behaviors including discovery, exploitation, and division of labor. None of these behaviors occurs in a vacuum. Ants communicate stygmergically, in relation to sequential stimuli from their environment and each other. Their seemingly random search for food is a result of a communication between ants that is based on pheromone, which is deposited as they walk, and which creates a guiding path along which ants follow. The strength of the pheromone determines the probability that one path or another will be followed.

Ant colony optimization (ACO) is a machine learning method that is inspired by food foraging behavior in ants. It is a population-based approach that relies on feedback from the environment, In ACO, colonies of software agents work cooperatively to solve problems by following "pheromone" on the links (edges) of a graph that represents the environment. Path choice is determined by pheromone strength. The higher the concentration of pheromone, the more likely a given path on the graph will be explored. The ants do not learn; however, they do have memory. Ant colony optimization has been used in data mining in non-medical domains [86,98], but seems to have attracted little attention for biomedical data mining so far. However, it appears to be a robust method for exploration of large databases, where concepts might be difficult to construct.

7.4.3.6 *Text Mining*

Data mining is not limited to numerical data. Text, such as is found in such documents as medical records and websites, presents a very rich source of data for knowledge discovery. Numerous methods have been developed over the last 10 years for mining text. One of these uses a set of keywords, usually pre-constructed by a content or domain expert, to retrieve concepts from text. In this method, a query is formulated using a vector of keywords, which may be connected with Boolean operators to create a set of concepts. Subsequent queries may return additional concept sets that can in turn be joined by Boolean operators. Anyone who has performed a literature search in PubMed has used keyword retrieval, where the keywords entered by the user are mapped to Medical Subject Headings (MeSH) and used to search for documents indexed by those descriptors. An extension of this method uses similarity retrieval, where search terms that don't map deterministically to terms in a controlled vocabulary are mapped based on a similarity metric.

As described in Chapter 5, another information retrieval-based approach to text mining is latent semantic indexing. This method identifies relationships between words in text based on patterns of their use. This is accomplished through a method from linear algebra, singular value decomposition, which reduces a large matrix to a tractable, and in the case of text mining, meaningful, one. Ultimately, latent semantic indexing works because words that frequently appear together and in similar contexts often have similar meaning. Thus, latent semantic indexing is more likely to return documents or concepts that are similar even if they don't contain the terms expressed in the search query.

A natural language processing method that has been adopted for text mining is information extraction, or IE. This method extracts structured information from unstructured text, such as that seen in progress notes, nursing notes, and consults, but also in web-based documents such as discussion board posts and chat room discussions. There are several components to IE. The first is named entity recognition, where objects ("entities") are searched for in a document using a controlled vocabulary, and once found, the entities are classified by type (person, place, drug, procedure, etc.). These classifications are annotated and stored in a database for further processing. Another step may include determining the semantic relationship between named entities, and then constructing a network of these relationships. This procedure leads to the interpretation of the network to discover the knowledge implicit in the text. Details about the aspects of natural language processing were covered in Chapter 6.

Various approaches to text mining and information extraction have been applied predominantly in genomics and proteomics, where plain-text annotations are used as a primary knowledge representation. The literature is replete with examples of text mining applications in these domains. Recently, there has been a burgeoning interest in applying text mining techniques to components of the electronic medical record, such as progress notes, and this is reflected in a growing literature in this area [20, 33, 58, 95, 106, 130, 145, 148, 152].

7.4.3.7 *Evaluation: Metrics for Classification and Prediction*

Data mining is, by definition, about hypothesis *generating*, not hypothesis *testing*. However, metrics are needed to ascertain the accuracy of classifications and predictions made by data mining programs. Otherwise, the knowledge discovered in databases cannot be put to some useful purpose. Given that so much of data mining is about classification, and often ultimately prediction, the metrics that have been used in medical decision making for the past several decades have found their place in data mining as well. All of these derive from the confusion matrix, a two-dimensional

		Gold standard	
		Disease positive	**Disease Negative**
Rule prediction	**Disease positive**	72 TP	42 FP
	Disease negative	28 FN	58 TN

$$\text{Sensitivity (True Positive Rate)} = \frac{TP}{TP+FN} = \frac{72}{100} = 0.72$$

$$\text{Specificity (True Negative Rate)} = \frac{TN}{TN+FP} = \frac{58}{100} = 0.58$$

$$\text{Positive Predictive Value} = \frac{TP}{TP+FP} = \frac{72}{114} = 0.63$$

$$\text{Negative Predictive Value} = \frac{TN}{TN+FN} = \frac{58}{86} = 0.67$$

■ **FIGURE 7.26** The 2×2 confusion matrix revisited. This table can be used to compare a test against a gold standard for a given classification problem.

table that enables one to compare the results obtained from applying a data mining algorithm with those known to be correct, referred to as the "gold standard." A simple confusion matrix, in this case a 2×2 table that is appropriate for a two-class problem, is illustrated in Figure 7.26.

The gold standard occupies the columns in the table, and the test results (or the results from the data mining classification) appear in the rows. Each cell is occupied with counts of the number of cases (records) classified by the data miner. There are four cells in this table, identified here as TP (true positives, or the number of cases correctly classified as positive), FP (false positives, the number of negative cases incorrectly classified as positive), FN (false negatives, positive cases incorrectly classified as negative), and TN (negative cases correctly classified as negative). These metrics will be used by those developing data mining algorithms, those selecting a data mining algorithm, as well as those who apply them to data in order to fine-tune or parameterize the software.

From this matrix, several useful metrics can be calculated. These include sensitivity, specificity, predictive values, likelihood ratio, and receiver operating characteristic curves. Except for the latter, these metrics reflect a proportion of cases correctly or incorrectly classified by the data miner. The first metric, however, is accuracy, or simply, the proportion correct. It is calculated as $(TP+TN)/(TP+FP+FN+TN)$. While often used in expressing classification accuracy of a given data mining algorithm, it can be misleading, in that if there are a small number of true positives or true negatives in relation to each other (low prevalence, for example), the accuracy metric can be biased toward 100%, and will fail to indicate the error rate. The other metrics are more appropriate for assessing the classification performance of a data mining algorithm.

Sensitivity is proportion of all gold-standard cases classified as positive by the data miner and provides a quantification of the type II error rate. Using the nomenclature of the table in Figure 7.26, sensitivity is calculated as $TP/(TP+FN)$. The sensitivity is often referred to as the true positive rate, although it is not a rate, per se. *Specificity*, or the true negative rate, is the proportion of gold standard-negative cases that are classified as negative (and thus provides a quantification of the type I error rate), and is calculated as $TN/(FP+TN)$. Sensitivity and specificity are often referred to in screening and diagnosis as pretest, or prior probability, and is used to determine if a particular data mining algorithm should be used for classification. An algorithm would be selected to mine a database if its sensitivity and specificity had been shown on similar data to be above some threshold, usually 80% or higher. Sensitivity and specificity indicate how well the data mining algorithm discriminates between the two classes, in advance of applying it to a set of data.

The *positive predictive value* is calculated as $TP/(TP+FP)$, and represents the proportion of cases classified as positive that are truly positive. It is a posterior probability that indicates how good the classification made by the data miner actually classifies positive cases. The *negative predictive value* is the proportion of true negatives that were classified as negative by the data miner: $TN/(TN+FN)$. This metric provides an evaluation of how well the miner classified negative cases.

Another metric that is derived from the confusion matrix and used in evaluating the classification accuracy is the *likelihood ratio*, which is the ratio of two probabilities: the probability of a given classification among those cases that are in that class divided by the probability of that classification among those cases that are not in the class. In a two-class problem, there are two likelihood ratios—one positive, the other negative, and can be considered in terms of sensitivity and specificity:

$$LR_{Positive} = Sensitivity/(1 - Specificity),$$
$$LR_{Negative} = (1 - Sensitivity)/(Specificity).$$

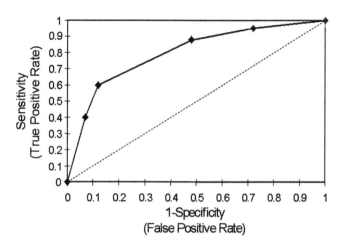

■ FIGURE 7.27 The receiver operating characteristic (ROC) curve. The ROC curve provides a graphical representation of the relationship between sensitivity and specificity for a classifier. The knots, represented as diamonds, indicate specific values of a classifier. For a dichotomous classification, there will be only one knot; in this illustration, there are four knots, as this curve was obtained for a four-class problem. One can see that the tradeoff between sensitivity and specificity is at the second knot from the left, where the true positive rate is 0.6 and the false positive rate is 0.1. The third knot provides much better detection of true positives, but at the expense of specificity.

A useful metric that also incorporates the sensitivity and specificity is the area under the receiver operating characteristic (ROC) curve. If specificity is the true negative rate, then 1-specificity is the false positive rate (FP/(FP + TN) from the table in Figure 7.26). The ROC curve is constructed by plotting the true positive rate against the false positive rate on the X- and Y-axes, respectively, as shown in Figure 7.27.

For a two-class problem, a single point will be plotted and a curve drawn from the origin $(0,0)$ to the destination $(1,1)$. The straight line that runs through the origin and destination represents a classification that is no better than a coin flip, having 50% probability of being correct in terms of positive or negative classifications. One would hope that the curve for a classification algorithm would arc as far as possible away from this line, such that there is minimal probability of a false positive classification and maximal probability of a true positive.

For multi-class problems, a series of sequential 2×2 tables may be constructed for each class. In this situation, one class is selected as the main, and the others comprise the reference. The process is repeated iteratively for each class, and the sensitivity and specificity is calculated at each iteration. In this way, a series of data points are obtained and plotted.

The area under the ROC curve (AUC) can be obtained through integration. As with sensitivity, specificity, and the predictive values, the AUC ranges from 0 to 1, with values closer to 1 indicating a higher degree of classification accuracy. An AUC of 0.5 indicates that the curve is coterminous with the diagonal and thus the classifier operates no better than chance; if it is less than 0.5, this indicates a severely underperforming classifier or that the classes are mislabeled. Two AUCs can be compared using non-parameteric statistics to investigate if there is a significant difference between them. This is useful when comparing the classification performance of two data mining algorithms.

7.5 ETHICAL ISSUES

As with any analysis of biomedical data, the process of data mining as well as the use of the results of that process can pose a number of ethical challenges. First, the source of the data should be considered in terms of several questions. From whom was the data obtained? On whom was the data collected? Is informed consent needed to be obtained from those represented in the data, prior to mining? Will mining the data reveal any information that could be used to identify individuals or business entities? These questions reflect issues of privacy and confidentiality, and these need to be addressed by anyone who plans to mine biomedical data. This is true for all kinds of such data, but especially so for healthcare enterprise data, which may include health records, but also summary data that could reflect the performance of a healthcare institution. Anyone seeking to perform data mining for research purposes is bound by federal law to submit a protocol for approval by his or her institutional review board (IRB). This board has the obligation, again, under federal law, to make the determination about human subjects protections for a given study. However, many pursue data mining in activities outside of the realm of research, per se. Business intelligence and quality improvement studies are examples of these activities, and do not necessarily require IRB approval. These activities still require consideration of the privacy and confidentiality issues described above.

Ideally, data that are intended to be mined should be de-identified, or stripped of any information that could identify an individual or business entity. This would mean deleting the usual primary identifiers, such as name, social security, or medical record numbers, and the like, but also secondary identifiers, such as admission dates. Thus, a "limited dataset," as defined in the Privacy Rule of the Health Insurance Portability and Accountability Act (HIPAA), is not de-identified, and should not be mined except under very stringent conditions that protect privacy and confidentiality and adhere to the HIPAA Privacy and Security Rules. In order to create a fully de-identified database, one will likely need to perform substantial and potentially complex procedures that convert dates and other secondary identifiers to meaningful, yet unidentifiable values. It is important to keep in mind that even with these procedures in place, it still may be possible to re-identify persons or entities.

Another ethical concern is consideration of how the results of mined data will be used. Data mining should be constrained to hypothesis generation, and used in only a limited way in substantive decision making. It would be folly to create a clinical decision rule solely on the basis of the results of a data mining analysis. The basis for a decision rule may be *suggested* by such an analysis, but rigorous biostatistical and epidemiologic methods should be employed to develop and test the rule prior to using it in a clinical setting. The same could be said of enterprise data mining, where it might be used to look for patters suggesting where personnel or financial decisions might be made. Again, these decisions could be informed by a data mining analysis, but should not be made solely on the basis of such an analysis.

Given the increasing ubiquity of data mining across healthcare and biomedical research domains, it is probably reasonable to inform those on whom data are collected—patients, employees, or the general public—that their data may be mined for some purpose. In many cases, it would be appropriate to obtain consent from an individual prior to collecting such data, as is typically done in any research study or in many treatment settings. However, there is some lack of clarity on the requirement for obtaining such consent, especially vis-à-vis HIPAA regulations. At this time, it is arguably best to err on the side of caution with regard to informing and possibly consenting anyone on whom data is collected, since these could be mined at some point in the future.

7.6 SUMMARY

Data mining is part of a larger process of knowledge discovery in databases. Specifically, it is the application of software tools and cognitive processes to the discovery of patterns and other types of phenomena that occur in data that might be missed by traditional analytic means, whether they be statistical methods or in the case of text, simple reading. Most of the methods used in data mining come from the machine learning paradigm, where a learning algorithm is exposed to data and over a period of training develops a model that is generalizable to unseen data from a similar source. This model can be used for classification or prediction, but is first a hypothesis or set of hypotheses generated from the data. These hypotheses require some human expertise to evaluate their plausibility and applicability to a given problem domain. As such, data mining is *automated*, rather than automatic, and the tools of data mining are assistive in the process of knowledge discovery.

While there is much to data mining that is attractive, it is important to remember that in addition to human input in the interpretation of results, consideration of the ethical concerns associated with data mining is needed. These are not inconsequential, and if violated, could cause substantial harm to the entities biomedical data represent.

7.7 ADDITIONAL RESOURCES

There are many resources available to those interesting learning more about data mining as well as to those who are searching for tools to perform it. The most comprehensive resource is kdnuggets (www.kdnuggets.com), which is a one-stop shopping mart of data sources, publications, educational materials and courses, listings of conferences and calls for papers, job openings, and discussion boards. Other resources that will be useful to those exploring data mining are listed below, categorized by type. Note: this list is not comprehensive, as new resources are added frequently.

- Data
    - University of California at Irvine Machine Learning Repository (http://archive.ics.uci.edu/ml/). A repository of over 200 datasets useful for testing data mining algorithms.
    - Amazon Public Data Sets (http://aws.amazon.com/publicdatasets/). Datasets include the 1000 Genomes Project, Google Books *n*-Grams, web crawl corpora, and various website traffic data.
    - Carnegie Mellon University Statlib Archive (http://lib.stat.cmu.edu/datasets/). A comprehensive collection of datasets for use in testing data mining algorithms.
    - National Center for Health Statistics (Centers for Disease Control and Prevention) Surveys and Data Collection Systems (http://www.cdc.gov/nchs/surveys.htm). A collection of health-related survey datasets and instruments.
    - US Department of Energy Comprehensive Epidemiologic Data Resource (https://www3.orau.gov/CEDR/#.UQ2nTGfb6M4). A collection of health data from studies of Department of Energy workers.
- Software

    - CART® (http://www.salford-systems.com/en/). Classification and regression tree software for classification and prediction with graphical models.
    - DBMiner (http://www.dbminer.com/). A Microsoft product designed to work with SQL Server.

- ❑ KNIME (http://www.knime.org/). An open source data mining tool that supports the knowledge discovery life cycle.
- ❑ Orange (http://orange.biolab.si/). Another comprehensive open source data mining suite that uses visual scripting and is available for all computing platforms.
- ❑ SAS® Enterprise Miner™ (http://www.sas.com/technologies/analytics/datamining/miner/). A full-featured data mining suite from SAS Institute.
- ❑ TANAGRA (http://eric.univ-lyon2.fr/~ricco/tanagra/en/tanagra.html) is an open source data mining suite that supports the knowledge discovery life cycle. It is available only for Windows.
- ❑ WEKA (http://www.cs.waikato.ac.nz/ml/weka/). An open source, free data mining suite that supports the entire knowledge discovery life cycle. It runs on all computing platforms and supports visual scripting as well as command line and menu-based mining.
- ❑ Hastie, Trevor; Tibshurani, Robert; Friedman, Jerome: The Elements of Statistical Learning: Data Mining, Inference, and Prediction, Second Edition. New York: Springer Science and business Media, 2009.

REFERENCES

[1] Brachman RJ, Anand T. The process of knowledge discovery in databases: a human-centered approach. In: Fayyad U, Piatetsky-Shapiro G, Smyth P, Uthurusamy R, editors. Advances in knowledge discovery and data mining. Cambridge, MA: MIT Press; 1996.
[2] Abidi SS, Artes PH, Yun S, Yu J. Stud Health Technol Inform 2007;129:2–13.
[3] Acharya UR, Sree SV, Ribeiro R, Krishnamurthi G, Marinho RT, Sanches J, et al. Med Phys 2012;39:4255–64.
[4] Ackoff R. J Appl Syst Anal 1989;16:3–9.
[5] Alabady MS, Youn E, Wilkins TA. BMC Genomics 2008;9:295.
[6] Althouse BM, Ng YY, Cummings DA. PLoS Negl Trop Dis 2011;5:e1258. [electronic resource]
[7] Alves R, Sorribas A. BMC Syst Biol 2007;1:10.
[8] An L, Fung KY, Krewski D. J Biopharm Stat 2010;20:998–1012.
[9] Anderson RW, Stomberg C, Hahm CW, Mani V, Samber DD, Itskovich VV, et al. Biosystems 2007;90:456–66.
[10] Aussem A, de Morais SR, Corbex M. Artif Intell Med 2012;54:53–62.
[11] Baca-Garcia E, Perez-Rodriguez MM, Saiz-Gonzalez D, Basurte-Villamor I, Saiz-Ruiz J, Leiva-Murillo JM, et al. Progr Neuro-Psychopharmacol Biol Psych 2007;31:1312–6.
[12] Bassani T, Nievola JC. Adv Exp Med Biol 2010;657:147–65.
[13] Bate A, Lindquist M, Edwards IR, Olsson S, Orre R, Lansner A, et al. Eur J Clin Pharmacol 1998;54:315–21.

[14] Bate A, Lindquist M, Orre R, Edwards IR, Meyboom RH. Eur J Clin Pharmacol 2002;58:483–90.

[15] Becker K, Pancoska P, Concin N, Vanden Heuvel K, Slade N, Fischer M, et al. Int J Oncol 2006;29:889–902.

[16] Ben-Hur A, Weston J. Methods Mol Biol 2010;609:223–39.

[17] Berchialla P, Scarinzi C, Snidero S, Rahim Y, Gregori D. J Med Syst 2012;36:475–81.

[18] Bernado-Mansilla E, Garrell-Guiu JM. Evol Comput 2003;11:209–38.

[19] Bolshakova N, Azuaje F. Methods Inf Med 2006;45:153–7.

[20] Botsis T, Nguyen MD, Woo EJ, Markatou M, Ball R. J Am Med Inform Assoc 2011;18:631–8.

[21] Briones N, Dinu V. BMC Med Genet 2012;13:7.

[22] Cendrowska J. Int J Man-Mach Stud 1987;27:349–70.

[23] Chayama K, Hayes CN, Yoshioka K, Moriwaki H, Okanoue T, Sakisaka S, et al. J Gastroenterol 2011;46:545–55.

[24] Chazard E, Preda C, Merlin B, Ficheur G, PSIP consortium Beuscart R. Stud Health Technol Inform 2009;150:552–6.

[25] Chen L, He ZS, Huang T, Cai YD. Med Chem 2010;6:388–95.

[26] Chen L, Lu L, Feng K, Li W, Song J, Zheng L, et al. J Comput Chem 2009;30:2248–54.

[27] Chen R, Resnick SM, Davatzikos C, Herskovits EH. Neuroimage 2012;59:2330–8.

[28] Cheung LW. Methods Mol Biol 2012;802:73–85.

[29] Chien CW, Lee YC, Ma T, Lee TS, Lin YC, Wang W, et al. Hepato-Gastroenterol 2008;55:1140–5.

[30] Chopra P, Kang J, Yang J, Cho H, Kim HS, Lee MG. BMC Bioinform 2008;9:92.

[31] Clark P, Niblett T. Mach Learn 1987;3:261–83.

[32] Cohen WW. Fast effective rule induction. In: Twelfth international conference on machine learning, 1995; p. 115–23.

[33] Corley CD, Cook DJ, Mikler AR, Singh KP. Int J Environ Res Public Health 2010;7:596–615. [electronic resource]

[34] Couderc JP. J Electrocardiol 2010;43:595–600.

[35] Cui J, Liu Q, Puett D, Xu Y. Bioinformatics 2008;24:2370–5.

[36] Daemen A, Timmerman D, Van den Bosch T, Bottomley C, Kirk E, Van HC, et al. Artif Intell Med 2012;54:103–14.

[37] Dahabiah A, Puentes J, Solaiman B. In: Conference proceedings: annual international conference of the IEEE engineering in medicine and biology society; 2007 p. 4528–31.

[38] de Castro LN, Timmis J. Artificial immune systems: a new computational intelligence approach. Berlin: Springer-Verlag; 2002.

[39] De BT, Tranchevent LC, van Oeffelen LM, Moreau Y. Bioinformatics 2007;23:i125–32.

[40] De LL, Geurts P, Baele G, Castro-Giner F, Kogevinas M, Van SK. Eur J Human Genet 2010;18:1127–32.

[41] Delen D, Walker G, Kadam A. Artif Intell Med 2005;34:113–27.

[42] Deshmukh S, Khaitan S, Das D, Gupta M, Wangikar PP. Protein Peptide Lett 2007;14:647–57.

[43] Dixon S, Yu X-H. Bioinformatics data mining using artificial immune systems and neural networks. In: 2010 IEEE international conference on information and automation, 2010

[44] Dorigo M, Manniezzo V, Colomi A. IEEE Trans Syst Man Cybernet – Part B 1996;26:29–41.

[45] Dudek G. IEEE Trans Evol Comput 2012;16:847–60.

[46] DuMouchel W, Fram D, Yang X, Mahmoud RA, Grogg AL, Engelhart L, et al. Ann Clin Psych 2008;20:21–31.

[47] DuMouchel W, Smith ET, Beasley R, Nelson H, Yang X, Fram D, et al. Clin Therapeut 2004;26:1092–104.

[48] Exarchos TP, Tzallas AT, Baga D, Chaloglou D, Fotiadis DI, Tsouli S, et al. Comput Biol Med 2012;42:195–204.

[49] Farmer JD, Packard N, Perelson A. Phys D 1986;2:187–204.

[50] Frank A, Asuncion A. UCI machine learning repository. Irvine, CA: University of California, School of Information and Computer Science; 2010 [online source]

[51] Fung DC, Lo A, Jankova L, Clarke SJ, Molloy M, Robertson GR, et al. Methods Mol Biol 2011;781:311–36.

[52] Ge G, Wong GW. BMC Bioinform 2008;9:275.

[53] Gopalakrishnan V, Lustgarten JL, Visweswaran S, Cooper GF. Bioinformatics 2010;26:668–75.

[54] Hakenberg J, Schmeier S, Kowald A, Klipp E, Leser U. Omics J Integr Biol 2004;8:131–52.

[55] Hall M. Correlation-based feature selection for machine learning. Hamilton. New Zealand: The University of Waikoto; 1999;4-1-2013.

[56] Hammann F, Drewe J. Exp Opin Drug Disc 2012;7:341–52.

[57] Harpaz R, Perez H, Chase HS, Rabadan R, Hripcsak G, Friedman C. Clin Pharm Therapeut 2011;89:243–50.

[58] Heinze DT, Morsch ML, Holbrook J. In: Proc/AMIA annual symposium, 2001 p. 254–8.

[59] Holland JH. Adaptation in natural and artificial systems. Cambridge, MA: MIT Press; 1992.

[60] Holmes JH, Durbin DR, Winston FK. In: Proceedings/AMIA annual symposium; 2000 p. 359–63.

[61] Holmes JH, Durbin DR, Winston FK. Artif Intell Med 2000;19:53–74.

[62] Holte RC. Mach Learn 1993;11:63–91.

[63] Hosseinzadeh F, Ebrahimi M, Goliaei B, Shamabadi N. PLoS ONE 2012;7:e40017. [electronic resource]

[64] Huang ML, Hung YH, Chen WY. J Med Syst 2010;34:865–73.

[65] Ilgen MA, Downing K, Zivin K, Hoggatt KJ, Kim HM, Ganoczy D, et al. J Clin Psych 2009;70:1495–500.

[66] Jin H, Wong ML, Leung KS. IEEE Trans Pattern Anal Mach Intell 2005;27:1710–9.

[67] Jupiter DC, VanBuren V. PLoS ONE 2008;3:e1717. [electronic resource]

[68] Kaimakamis E, Bratsas C, Sichletidis L, Karvounis C, Maglaveras N. In: Conference proceedings: annual international conference of the IEEE engineering in medicine and biology society, 2009 p. 3465–9.

[69] Karaolis MA, Moutiris JA, Hadjipanayi D, Pattichis CS. IEEE Trans Inf Technol Biomed 2010;14:559–66.

[70] Kim S, Yoon J, Yang J. Bioinformatics 2008;24:118–26.

[71] Kitsos CM, Bhamidipati P, Melnikova I, Cash EP, McNulty C, Furman J, et al. Cytometry – Part A: J Int Soc Anal Cytol 2007;71:16–27.

[72] Klement W, Wilk S, Michalowski W, Farion KJ, Osmond MH, Verter V. Artif Intell Med 2012;54:163–70.

[73] Ko GM, Reddy AS, Kumar S, Bailey BA, Garg R. J Chem Inf Model 2010;50:1759–71.

[74] Kolekar P, Kale M, Kulkarni-Kale U. Mol Phylogenet Evol 2012;65:510–22.

[75] Kowald A, Schmeier S. Methods Mol Biol 2011;696:305–18.

[76] Koza J. Genetic programming: on the programming of computers by means of natural selection. Cambridge, MA: MIT Press; 1992.

[77] Kozak K, Csucs G. RNA Biol 2010;7:615–20.

[78] Kuo WJ, Chang RF, Moon WK, Lee CC, Chen DR. Acad Radiol 2002;9:793–9.

[79] Le VL, Bloch G, Lauer F. IEEE Trans Neural Networks 2011;22:2398–405.

[80] Lee CH, Chen JC, Tseng VS. Comput Methods Programs Biomed 2011;101:44–61.

[81] Lee YC, Lee WJ, Lin YC, Liew PL, Lee CK, Lin SC, et al. Hepato-Gastroenterology 2009;56:1745–9.

[82] Li L, Tang H, Wu Z, Gong J, Gruidl M, Zou J, et al. Artif Intell Med 2004;32:71–83.

[83] Li L, Wang J, Leung H, Zhao S. Risk Anal 2012;32:1072–92.

[84] Lillo-Le LA, Toussaint Y, Villerd J. Stud Health Technol Inform 2010;160:2–73.

[85] Lin Y, Li W, Chen K, Liu Y. J Am Med Inform Assoc 2007;14:651–61.

[86] Liu B, Abbass HA, McKay B. IEEE Comput Intell Bull 2004;3:31–5.

[87] Liu J, Li Z, Hu X, Chen Y, Park EK. BMC Genomics 2011;12(Suppl 2):S11.

[88] Livingstone DJ, Browne A, Crichton R, Hudson BD, Whitley DC, Ford MG. Methods Mol Biol 2008;458:231–48.

[89] Luk JM, Lam BY, Lee NP, Ho DW, Sham PC, Chen L, et al. Biochem Biophys Res Commun 2007;361:68–73.

[90] Mailund T, Besenbacher S, Schierup MH. BMC Bioinform 2006;7:454.

[91] Manilich EA, Ozsoyoglu ZM, Trubachev V, Radivoyevitch T. J Bioinform Comput Biol 2011;9:251–67.

[92] Marin OR, Ruiz D, Soriano A, Delgado FJ. In: Conference proceedings: annual international conference of the IEEE engineering in medicine and biology society, 2010 p. 1162–5.

[93] Marsolo K, Twa M, Bullimore MA, Parthasarathy S. IEEE Trans Inf Technol Biomed 2007;11:203–12.

[94] Mballo C, Makarenkov V. Combin Chem High Throughput Screen 2010;13:430–41.

[95] McKenzie K, Scott DA, Campbell MA, McClure RJ. Accid Anal Prev 2010;42:354–63.

[96] Megalooikonomou V, Barnathan M, Kontos D, Bakic PR, Maidment AD. IEEE Trans Med Imag 2009;28:487–93.

[97] Michalski RS. In: Michalski RS, , Carbonell J, Mitchell T, editors. Machine learning. An articial intelligence approach, 1983. San Mateo: Morgan Kaufmann; 1983. p. 83–134.

[98] Monmarché N. In: Frietas A, editor. Data mining with evolutionary algorithms, Research directions – papers from the AAAI workshop, 1999. Menlo Park: AAAI Press; 1999. p. 23–6.

[99] Nakayama N, Oketani M, Kawamura Y, Inao M, Nagoshi S, Fujiwara K, et al. J Gastroenterol 2012;47:664–77.

[100] Nasibov E, Kandemir-Cavas C. Comput Biol Chem 2009;33:461–4.

[101] Newcomer SR, Steiner JF, Bayliss EA. Am J Manag Care 2011;17:e324–32.

[102] Ng T, Chew L, Yap CW. J Palliative Med 2012;15:863–9.

[103] Oh JH, Gao J. BMC Bioinform 2009;10(Suppl 4):S7.

[104] Ozgur A, Vu T, Erkan G, Radev DR. Bioinformatics 2008;24:i277–85.

[105] Oztekin A, Delen D, Kong ZJ. Int J Med Inform 2009;78:e84–96.

[106] Pakhomov S, Bjornsen S, Hanson P, Smith S. Med Decis Mak 2008;28:462–70.

[107] Pan Y, Pylatuik JD, Ouyang J, Famili AF, Fobert PR. J Bioinform Comput Biol 2004;2:639–55.

[108] Pearl A, Bar-Or R, Bar-Or D. Stud Health Technol Inform 2008;136:253–8.

[109] Peltola T, Marttinen P, Jula A, Salomaa V, Perola M, Vehtari A. PLoS ONE 2012;7:e29115. [electronic resource]

[110] Peng S, Zeng X, Li X, Peng X, Chen L. J Genet Genomics 2009;36:409–16.

[111] Piroozznia M, Seifuddin F, Judy J, Mahon PB, Bipolar Genome Study (BiGS) Consortium Potash JB, Zandi PP. Psychiatr Genet 2012;22:55–61.

[112] Plyusnin I, Evans AR, Karme A, Gionis A, Jernvall J. PLoS ONE 2008;3:e1742. [electronic resource]

[113] Quinlan JR. Mach Learn 1990;5:239–66.

[114] Raghuraj R, Lakshminarayanan S. Comput Biol Chem 2008;32:302–6.

[115] Rink B, Harabagiu S, Roberts K. J Am Med Inform Assoc 2011;18:594–600.

[116] Rodin A, Mosley JrTH, Clark AG, Sing CF, Boerwinkle E. J Comput Biol 2005;12:1–11.

[117] Rodin AS, Boerwinkle E. Bioinformatics 2005;21:3273–8.

[118] Rosenblatt F. Psychol Rev 1958;65:386–408.

[119] Sabbagh A, Darlu P. Human Hered 2006;62:119–34.

[120] Sakaeda T, Kadoyama K, Okuno Y. Int J Med Sci 2011;8:487–91.

[121] Sakaeda T, Kadoyama K, Okuno Y. PLoS ONE 2011;6:e28124. [electronic resource]

[122] Sbordone L, Sbordone C, Filice N, Menchini-Fabris G, Baldoni M, Toti P. J Periodontol 2009;80:1998–2009.

[123] Schaefers K, Ribeiro D. Stud Health Technol Inform 2012;177:237–41.

[124] Seomun GA, Chang SO, Lee SJ, Kim IA, Park SA. Stud Health Technol Inform 2006;122:899.

[125] Silver H, Shmoish M. Psych Res 2008;159:167–79.

[126] Skinner BT, Nguyen HT, Liu DK. In: Conference proceedings: annual international conference of the IEEE engineering in medicine and biology society; 2007. p. 3120–3.

[127] Slade BA, Leidel L, Vellozzi C, Woo EJ, Hua W, Sutherland A, et al. JAMA 2009;302:750–7.

[128] Smalter A, Huan JL, Jia Y, Lushington G. IEEE/ACM Trans Comput Biol Bioinform 2010;7:197–207.

[129] Sohn SY, Shin H. Ergonomics 2001;44:107–17.

[130] Spasic I, Ananiadou S, McNaught J, Kumar A. Brief Bioinform 2005;6:239–51.

[131] Sree SV, Ng EY, Acharya UR. Technol Cancer Res Treat 2010;9:95–106.

[132] Su CT, Wang PC, Chen YC, Chen LF. J Med Syst 2012;36:2387–99.

[133] Sun P, Yao X. IEEE Trans Neural Networks 2010;21:883–94.

[134] Sundstrom A, Hallberg P. Drug Safety 2009;32:419–27.

[135] Talley EM, Newman D, Mimno D, Herr BW, Wallach HM, Burns GA, et al. Nature Methods 2011;8:443–4.

[136] Tamura T, Sakaeda T, Kadoyama K, Okuno Y. Int J Med Sci 2012;9:441–6.

[137] Tatsunami S, Kuwabara R, Hiroi T, Matsui H, Fukutake K, Mimaya U, et al. Stud Health Technol Inform 2001;84:1–60.

[138] Tikk D, Thomas P, Palaga P, Hakenberg J, Leser U. PLoS Comput Biol 2010;6:e1000837.

[139] Ting HW, Wu JT, Chan CL, Lin SL, Chen MH. J Chin Med Assoc 2010;73:401–6.

[140] Tuana G, Volpato V, Ricciardi-Castagnoli P, Zolezzi F, Stella F, Foti M. BMC Immunol 2011;12:50.

[141] Ubeyli ED, Dogdu E. J Med Syst 2010;34:179–84.

[142] Vasina EN, Paszek E, Nicolau JrDV, Nicolau DV. Lab Chip 2009;9:891–900.

[143] Visweswaran S, Wong AK, Barmada MM. In: AMIA: annual symposium proceedings/AMIA symposium; 2009 p. 673–7.

[144] Wang XS, Tang H, Golbraikh A, Tropsha A. J Chem Inf Model 2008;48:997–1013.

[145] Warrer P, Hansen EH, Juhl-Jensen L, Aagaard L. Br J Clin Pharmacol 2012;73:674–84.

[146] Wilson SW. Knowledge growth in an artificial animal. In: Greffenstette JJ, editor. International conference on genetic algorithms and their applications, 1985. Hillsdale, NJK: Lawrence Erlbaum Associates; 1985. p. 16–23.

[147] Worachartcheewan A, Nantasenamat C, Isarankura-Na-Ayudhya C, Pidetcha P, Prachayasittikul V. Diab Res Clin Pract 2010;90:e15–8.

[148] Wu JL, Yu LC, Chang PC. BMC Med Inform Decis Mak 2012;12:72.

[149] Yang Z, Tang N, Zhang X, Lin H, Li Y, Yang Z. Artif Intell Med 2011;51:163–73.

[150] Yang ZR. Methods Mol Biol 2010;609:197–222.

[151] Yang ZR, Hamer R. Curr Pharm Des 2007;13:1403–13.

[152] Yildirim P, Ceken C, Hassanpour R, Tolun MR. J Med Syst 2012;36:1485–90.

[153] Zhang L, Wang L, Lin W. IEEE Trans Syst Man Cybernet – Part B: Cybernet 2012;42:282–90.

[154] Zhang Y, Lin H, Yang Z, Wang J, Li Y. IEEE/ACM Trans Comput Biol Bioinform 2012;9:1190–202.

[155] Zhao X, Zhang S. Sensors 2011;11:9573–88.

[156] Zhou G, Zhang J, Su J, Shen D, Tan C. Bioinformatics 2004;20:1178–90.

[157] Zmiri D, Shahar Y, Taieb-Maimon M. J Eval Clin Pract 2012;18:378–88.

Bayesian Methods in Biomedical Data Analysis

Hsun-Hsien Chang[a] and Gil Alterovitz[a, b, c]

[a]*Children's Hospital Informatics Program at Harvard-MIT Division of Health Science, Boston, MA, USA*
[b]*Center for Biomedical Informatics, Harvard Medical School, Boston, MA, USA*
[c]*Computer Science and Artificial Intelligence Laboratory, Department of Electrical Engineering and Computer Science, MIT, Cambridge, MA, USA*

8.1 INTRODUCTION

The technologies for designing modern biomedical tools have advanced significantly, which enables the collection of more detailed information of biological systems at higher rates than previously possible. For example, modern gene expression microarrays can reveal the abundance of mRNA quantities in a given gene; or, high-resolution imaging systems can delineate organ structures at the cellular level. The successful technology improvements allow a single biomedical study to generate a large volume of data. In addition, with the increasing capacities of data storage, more samples can be collected in snapshot or time-series studies. The availability of such larger sized datasets implies that we need systematic analyses to extract crucial information from the raw data.

Biological systems are complex systems where cells and biomolecules interact dynamically and adaptively. The way that biological systems function and respond to their environments is a series of interplay of biomolecules and/or cells. For instance, the respiratory function of a lung cell results from a series of biomolecular interactions. The role of a cell has been encoded in DNA molecules, whose interplay produces mRNA that interacts with ribosomes to synthesize proteins. The 3D conformations of proteins collectively determine the cell's function. When there is a mutation in DNA, a cell may exhibit abnormal regulation functions, resulting in diseases such as lung cancer. Another example is the nervous system that controls the movements of our limbs. When we see an apple and want to grab it, the brain triggers a signal that travels through a series of neurons until the neurons at the hand muscle, which then stretches out and grasps the apple.

The operations of biological systems are complicated, and their detailed mechanisms are still poorly understood. One major difficulty is that a system involves a tremendous number of biomolecules and cells whose interplay cannot be easily observed by traditional experimental methods. Therefore, we need a systematic tool to describe the interplay. A popular and powerful approach to infer the causal biological interactions is based on the Bayesian methods, which is grounded in Bayesian statistics. The main feature of Bayesian methods is the inclusion of prior knowledge in the data analysis. When the data are not reliable, we can find a balance between prior knowledge and biomedical data in order to infer the relations among variables. This chapter will address the exploitation of Bayesian statistics to analyze biomedical data.

8.2 FUNDAMENTALS OF BAYESIAN METHODS

Investigating how biological systems function is difficult. Besides the intrinsic complicacy in the biological systems, the difficulty is compounded by biological variability and technical variability. The biological variability stems from the variations in the subjects of a cohort. For instance, some ethnic groups are susceptible to specific diseases; different environments will induce different mutations in DNA structures; consumers eating more healthy foods will maintain a higher level of immunity against flu. On the other hand, the source of technical variability is from the instruments that are used to collect biomedical data. The underlying physical or chemical signals of biomedical data are subject to thermal noise. Therefore, the measured signals are close to the true states.

The ideal method to account for both biological variability and technical variability in biomedical data is to consider all the possible factors in the world. However, this way is not realistic. In the example of identifying biomarkers to lung cancer diagnosis, we could utilize quantum mechanics to delineate how an electron collides with other electrons and protons and how the collision influences inequilibrium of nucleotides, which in turn induces a series of changes in physical and chemical interactions in lung cells. Such descriptions are too detailed to be included in analyzing biological systems. Instead, we can simply focus on the biological states of crucial biomolecules (e.g., DNA, RNA, proteins) and the conditions of environmental factors (e.g., smoking, alcoholism, gender, education). Then, we model these variables as random variables. For example, we can consider disease states (e.g., the stages of cancer tissues) as multinomial random variables, and gene expression intensities in microarray data as Gaussian variables. The use of probabilistic description will capture the biological variability and technical variability without worrying about extremely detailed deterministic descriptions.

8.2.1 **Bayes' Theorem**

Bayes' theorem is named for Thomas Bayes, who first suggested using the theorem to update beliefs. The theorem is the key to many approaches for extracting information from data where one aims to account for background influences on observed phenomena. The rationale of Bayes' theorem works backward from measured data to deduce what might have caused them. For an event, we have an existing belief, or prior knowledge, before seeing the data. Once the data are collected, we can adjust our belief along with the observed data to describe the model in a more faithful way.

Bayes' theorem lays the foundation for our later model building and testing. We use capital letters to denote variables, and lower cases to denote their values. Therefore, assuming that A and B are two random variables, the mathematical description of Bayes' theorem is as follows:

$$p(b|a) = \frac{p(a|b)p(b)}{p(a)} = \frac{p(a|b)p(b)}{\sum_{b'} p(a|b')p(b')}, \qquad (8.1)$$

where a, b, b' are values of the random variables A and B, and the second equality utilizes total probability in the denominator. The theorem relates inverse representations of the probabilities concerning two events A and B; i.e., conditional probability $p(b|a)$ can be reversed to $p(a|b)$ with a factor $\frac{p(b)}{p(a)}$.

Consider an example in lung cancer study. Let A denote the smoking status $p(A = \text{smoker}) = 0.2$ and $p(A = \text{nonsmoker}) = 0.8$; and B denote presence/absence of lung cancer with $p(B = \text{presence}) = 0.1$ and $p(B = \text{absence}) = 0.9$. To evaluate the probability of smokers obtaining lung cancer is equivalent to computing $p(B = \text{presence}|A = \text{smoker})$. From clinical observations, we note that 85% of lung cancer cases are smokers. Then, we can calculate

$$p(B = \text{presence}|A = \text{smoker}) = \frac{0.85 \times 0.1}{0.2} = 0.425. \qquad (8.2)$$

Similarly, we can infer the probability of nonsmokers suffering from lung cancer is

$$p(B = \text{presence}|A = \text{nonsmoker}) = \frac{0.15 \times 0.1}{0.8} = 0.01875. \qquad (8.3)$$

Thanks to Bayes' theorem helping us inferring the probabilities in this example, we can easily see that smokers have a much higher chance of getting lung cancer than nonsmokers. If we did not utilize the data, which is the information of smoking status of the patient, we only can rely on the information of prevalence of lung cancer $p(B)$. Since the probability of getting lung cancer is much lower than that of not getting lung cancer, the decision that neglects data will be prone to wrong interpretation.

8.2.2 Model Selection

In biomedical data analysis, a task is to determine which model best fits with the data. This task is called model selection. The problem of model selection is to select a model from a set of candidate models that can best describe the data generated from experiments. In the above lung cancer example, there are two candidate models: if lung cancer is dependent on smoking or independent of smoking, given the data that collects the patients' cancer/healthy status and smoking/non-smoking history. Another example in genomic microarray analysis is to identify which genes are associated with the disease progression, where different sets of genes are candidate models and we need to pick the best set fitting the data.

Model selection is important. When a model is incorrectly selected, we will give wrong interpretation on the data, leading to a catastrophe. Let us again consider the lung cancer example described above. When a patient has lung cancer but our model diagnoses him as healthy, the patient will lose the treatment opportunities to extend his life. In contrast, when the patient is truly healthy but our model detects cancer in his lung, he will undergo unnecessary surgery that wastes the medical resources.

Now, let us discuss the mathematics of model selection. We can replace variables A and B in Eq. (8.1) with new names in Bayes' theorem and get

$$p(\text{model}|\text{data}) = \frac{p(\text{data}|\text{model})p(\text{model})}{p(\text{data})}. \tag{8.4}$$

The left hand side, $p(\text{model}|\text{data})$, is called posterior probability, which tells us the probability that each of the models is true, given that we've seen a particular value of the data under our particular experimental conditions. When there are a number of candidate models and that the data could take on various values, the term $p(\text{model}|\text{data})$ actually stands for a whole array of related numbers: one probability for each combination of model and data. The term $p(\text{data}|\text{model})$ on the right-hand side of Eq. (8.4) means that: when a certain model is true, how likely the data are generated from our experimental conditions. Using the lung cancer example, the model is presence/absence of lung cancer and data are smoking/nonsmoking.

In Eq. (8.4), the second term $p(\text{model})$ in the numerator is the probability that a particular model is true regardless of our experimental conditions. Since this probability does not depend on the data, it must be the probability that the model was true before the data was generated. This is called the prior probability, which in other words is the belief, or initial guess, that the data analyst already possesses in his mind before running the experiment. This belief will impact the computed posterior probability $p(\text{model}|\text{data})$. However, when the sample size in the data is large, the impact of belief $p(\text{model})$ on $p(\text{model}|\text{data})$ becomes less important and eventually will diminish. A special case occurs when the analyst has no bias toward a particular model, so $p(\text{model})$ is set equal for all candidate models and it can be dropped. The denominator $p(\text{data})$ in Eq. (8.4) is simply the probability of data that occur in our experiment, which does not change at all when we attempt to evaluate the posterior probability of candidate models. Therefore, the data term $p(\text{data})$ can be discarded.

In the model selection problem, we are given multiple candidate models and have to pick the best model from the candidates. In Eq. (8.4), we can add subscripts to denote the models and use the equation to compute the probabilities of all candidate models: $p(\text{model}_1|\text{data})$, $p(\text{model}_2|\text{data})$, ...$p(\text{model}_K|\text{data})$.

Now let us revisit the lung cancer example. We now consider two models. One model considers that the lung cancer is dependent on smoking, and the other considers that lung cancer and smoking are independent. The data are the patients' lung tissue status (i.e., cancer or normal) and smoking history (i.e., yes or no). Mathematically, we want to evaluate the quantities of the following equations:

$$p(\text{cancer dependent on smoking}|\text{tissue status and smoking history}), \tag{8.5}$$

$$p(\text{cancer independent of smoking}|\text{tissue status and smoking history}). \tag{8.6}$$

The model where lung cancer depends on smoking is captured by conditional probability $p(\text{cancer}|\text{smoking})$, and the model where lung cancer and smoking are independent is described by $p(\text{cancer})p(\text{smoking})$. Our task now is to compute the probabilities of the two models and pick the model with a higher probability. Using the numbers given the lung cancer example presented in the previous section, we obtain $p(\text{cancer}|\text{smoking}) = 0.425$ from Eq. (8.2), and $p(\text{cancer})p(\text{smoking}) = 0.1 \times 0.2 = 0.02$. The comparison of these two models concludes that lung cancer is dependent on smoking.

8.2.3 Parameter Estimation

Mathematical models are powerful tools that can be used for the study and exploration of complex biological dynamics. However, bringing theoretical models in agreement with experimental observations relies on properly addressing uncertainty intrinsic to the theoretical development or experimental variations. For instance, the genes BRCA1 and BRCA2 are known to be associated with breast cancer. Their function is to repair damaged DNA. When the expression of BRCA1 is low, the risk of getting breast cancer is higher. However, how low the expression of BRCA1 needs to be to induce breast cancer is not deterministic. Some patients suffer from breast cancer when BRCA1 is expressed 50% lower than the normal level, while in some cases the BRCA1 needs to be almost exhausted. Such biological uncertainty can be described by a probability distribution that is characterized by some parameters. Although the parameters are unknown, we can estimate them in the models to allow more faithful theoretical representations of real biological systems.

There are several methods to estimate parameters. Using Bayes' theorem we can perform parameter estimation in a more reliable way. In Eq. (8.1), we can substitute *parameters* and *data* for A and B, respectively, leading to

$$p(\text{parameters}|\text{data}) = \frac{p(\text{data}|\text{parameters})p(\text{parameters})}{p(\text{data})}. \tag{8.7}$$

Mathematically, we use Θ to denote a random vector that collects all the parameters to be estimated, and Δ to denote the observed data. The equation turns out to be:

$$p(\theta|\Delta) = \frac{p(\Delta|\theta)p(\theta)}{p(\Delta)} = \frac{p(\Delta|\theta)p(\theta)}{\int p(\Delta|\theta')p(\theta')d\theta'}. \tag{8.8}$$

In most studies, what is of greatest interest is the most probable value of Θ, rather than the probability distribution of Θ given the data. The determination of the optimal quantity $\hat{\theta}$ is equivalent to looking for the arguments maximizing $p(\theta|\Delta)$. With reference to Eq. (8.7),

$$\hat{\theta} = \arg\max p(\theta|\Delta) = \arg\max \frac{p(\Delta|\theta)p(\theta)}{p(\Delta)} = \arg\max p(\Delta|\theta)p(\theta). \tag{8.9}$$

The maximization problem can be solved after taking logarithm on the posterior probability, because maximum is preserved under logarithm which is a homogeneous function; that is,

$$\hat{\theta} = \arg\max \log(p(\theta|\Delta)) = \arg\max \left[\log(p(\Delta|\theta)) + \log(p(\theta))\right]. \tag{8.10}$$

Let us now consider univariate Gaussian case. Assume that the data are following Gaussian distribution with unknown mean μ and known variance σ^2. The estimation task is to find the optimal $\hat{\mu}$ based on observed data $\Delta = \{y_1, \ldots, y_N\}$. Then, the likelihood is $p(\Delta|\mu) \sim N(\mu, \sigma^2)$ and prior distribution of μ is assumed Gaussian $p(\mu) \sim N(\mu_0, \sigma_0^2)$. Assume that the N samples in the dataset are independent, the likelihood can be written as:

$$p(\Delta|\mu) = c \sum_{n=1}^{N} p(y_n|\mu). \tag{8.11}$$

Note that likelihood $p(\Delta|\mu)$ and prior $p(\mu)$ are Gaussian, so the posterior distribution $p(\mu|\Delta)$ is also a Gaussian. Since Gaussian distributions are characterized by mean and variance, we can find μ_N and σ_N^2 that parameterize $p(\mu|\Delta) \sim N(\mu_N, \sigma_N^2)$:

$$\mu_N = \left(\frac{N\sigma_0^2}{N\sigma_0^2 + \sigma^2}\right) \bar{\mu}_N + \frac{\sigma^2}{N\sigma_0^2 + \sigma^2}\mu_0, \tag{8.12}$$

$$\sigma_N^2 = \frac{\sigma^2}{N\sigma_0^2 + \sigma^2}\sigma_0^2, \tag{8.13}$$

where $\bar{\mu}_N$ is the sample mean. In this example, we learn three crucial lessons:

i. Since μ_N gives rise to the maximum probability $p(\mu|\Delta)$, the optimal estimate $\widehat{\mu} = \mu_N$.

ii. The linear combination of sample mean $\bar{\mu}_N$ and prior mean μ_0 shown in Eq. (8.8) indicates that the optimal estimate is a balance between the sample mean and prior mean.

iii. When the sample size N is large, the optimal estimate approximates to the sample mean. Moreover, the variance σ_N^2 approaches 0 meaning that there is high confidence to consider the sample mean as the optimal estimate.

Now we can utilize parameter estimation technique to describe the BRCA1 expression level that causes breast cancer. Assume that the normal level of BRCA1 is around 100. When its expression drops down to the range between 0 and 50, physicians frequently observe the occurrence of breast cancer. The clinical observations allow us to draw a tentative belief that the expression level of mutated BRCA1 follows Gaussian distribution with mean $\mu_0 = 25$ and variance $\sigma_0^2 = 10$. In another breast cancer study, we want to extend this prior knowledge to estimate the BRCA1 distribution in the new cohort with 65 patients. We assume that the cohort has a more diversified racial background and hence a wider variance $\sigma^2 = 20$. The measured mean value of BRCA1 in this cohort is $\bar{\mu}_N = 35$. Substituting these numbers into Eq. (8.12) results in

$$\mu_N = \left(\frac{65 \times 10}{65 \times 10 + 20}\right) \times 35 + \frac{20}{65 \times 10 + 20} \times 25 = 34.7, \tag{8.14}$$

$$\sigma_N^2 = \frac{20}{65 \times 10 + 20} \times 10 = 0.29. \tag{8.15}$$

If the experimentalist faced a difficulty in collecting the samples of all 65 patients but got only two samples, the mean and variance become:

$$\mu_N = \left(\frac{2 \times 10}{2 \times 10 + 20}\right) \times 35 + \frac{20}{2 \times 10 + 20} \times 25 = 30, \tag{8.16}$$

$$\sigma_N^2 = \frac{20}{2 \times 10 + 20} \times 10 = 5. \tag{8.17}$$

From this experiment, we can see how the sample size impacts the inferred mean and variance. When there are a number of samples available, the estimated posterior mean is close to the sample mean, and the variance of the estimation is low. In contrast, small sample size means weak data information; the estimated mean is a balance between sample mean and prior information, and its variance widens.

8.3 **BAYESIAN NETWORK ANALYSIS**

A growing demand in biomedical analysis is the need to identify the interconnection among variables. For example, processing neuroimages can display how neurons connect to form the nervous system; analysis of genomic profiles can reverse-engineer how genes control each other. Therefore, there is a need to develop technologies to infer the biological networks.

Various approaches have been proposed to reverse-engineer variable interactions over time, e.g., temporal gene-gene interplay. The approaches range from highly detailed models, such as differential equations [1], to highly abstract models, such as Boolean networks [2]. The former describes the molecular kinetic reactions taking place in a cell, and the latter quantizes expression levels as binary variables that are linked to each other through logical relationships. The framework of Bayesian networks (BNs) has merits over these approaches thanks to its capability of handling data variability, describing variables by probabilistic models, and making predictions based on the inferred networks [3–5].

The lung cancer example presented in the introduction of Bayes' theorem can correspond to a simple Bayesian network, where smoking status interacts with lung cancer. Besides smoking, exposure to radon was reported as a risk factor of lung cancer [6]. Moreover, alcoholism has been found as a source that induces lung cancer [7]. In fact, people with alcoholism are usually heavy smokers, so they are prone to lung cancer. Moreover, these people usually have low income, leading them to living in low-priced houses

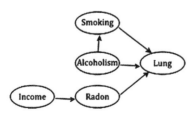

■ **FIGURE. 8.1** Graphical representations of risk factors inducing lung cancer.

that contain higher radon concentrations. These risk factors (i.e., smoking, alcoholism, and radon exposure) at the first glance are independent, but profound thinking can be used to reason about their linkage to lung cancer. The logical reasoning is described in Figure 8.1.

Nowadays biomedical researches collect more types of data in a single study, including demographic information, environmental observations, genomic microarrays, and medical images. While the data are becoming larger, it is extremely difficult to reason the causal networks purely based on human thinking. As such, the framework of Bayesian networks provides a wonderful tool to assist the logic reasoning.

8.3.1 **Inference of Dependence Relations**

Bayes' theorem lays the foundation for inferring dependence relations among variables. Consider random variables A and B. When the two variables are independent, meaning that the occurrence of one does not affect the probability of the other, their joint probability is the product of their probabilities:

$$p(A, B) = p(A)p(B). \tag{8.18}$$

Using conditional probability, it follows that

$$p(A) = \frac{p(A, B)}{p(B)} = p(A|B), \tag{8.19}$$

$$p(B) = \frac{p(A, B)}{p(A)} = p(B|A). \tag{8.20}$$

In contrast, when two variables are dependent,

$$p(A, B) \neq p(A)p(B), p(A) \neq p(A|B), p(B) \neq p(B|A). \tag{8.21}$$

We can also use graphs to depict the dependence relation.

With reference to Figure 8.2, we use a node to represent a variable, and a link to represent the dependence relation. When there is no link, the two variables are independent.

Bayes' theorem can be applied to infer the dependent relation between variables. When we observe a set of data, we can utilize Eq. (8.4) to examine if the dependence relation between two variables is valid. The two posterior probabilities are:

$$p(\text{dependent}|\text{data}) \propto p(\text{data}|\text{dependent})p(\text{dependent}). \tag{8.22}$$

$$p(\text{independent}|\text{data}) \propto p(\text{data}|\text{independent})p(\text{independent}). \tag{8.23}$$

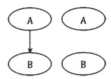

■ **FIGURE. 8.2** Graphical representations of dependent and independent variables.

Assuming that our prior beliefs on the two models are equal, we only have to compare $p(\text{data}|\text{dependent})$ and $p(\text{data}|\text{independent})$ to determine which model is more likely to explain the observed data. The lung cancer example in the section of model selection addressed this topic.

8.3.2 **Bayesian Networks**

Biomedical data often contain a large number of variables, which present a number of challenges for their study. An additional complication is that in many cases a given variable may be dependent on more than one variable. The example shown in Figure 8.3 illustrates that D is dependent on A, B and C. For example, A, B, C, D are smoking, alcoholism, radon exposure, and lung cancer, respectively.

In terms of graphical representation, directed links indicate that the target (child) nodes are dependent on the source (parent) nodes. The joint probability distribution in Figure 8.3 can be written as

$$p(A, B, C, D) = p(A)p(B)p(C)p(D|A, B, C). \tag{8.24}$$

Furthermore, the higher level parent variables, called "upstream variables," may be dependent on other variables. Aggregating all the variables

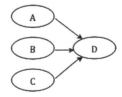

■ **FIGURE. 8.3** Graphical representations of multivariate network.

and their dependence links to the upstream nodes will result in a network. Such networks are frequently called dependence networks because the links represent the dependence relations.

We can now formally introduce Bayesian networks. Bayesian networks are directed acyclic graphs whose nodes represent random variables in the Bayesian sense: they may be observable quantities, latent variables, unknown parameters, or hypotheses. With reference to Figure 8.1, we identify observed risk factors of lung cancer are smoking, alcoholism, and radon exposure. The income level can be a latent variable because it impacts the affordable home prices, although it does not directly induce lung cancer. However, how many cigarettes and how much wine consumed per day will trigger lung cancer are unknown parameters.

The links between pairs of variables represent conditional dependencies; nodes that are not connected represent variables that are conditionally independent of each other. Each node is associated with a probability function that takes as input a particular set of values for the node's parent variables and gives the probability of the variable represented by the node. When the data consist of N variables, there are 2^N candidate network models, and we can use Bayes' theorem to select the best model fitting given data.

8.3.3 Linear Gaussian Model

Many variables in data can be modeled as Gaussian variables. The relations between child node and parent nodes can be modeled as linear regression. Therefore, this chapter focuses on linear Gaussian model for constructing Bayesian networks. Let $Y_1, Y_2, \ldots, Y_N$ be Gaussian random variables representing the continuous measurements of variables $1, 2, \ldots, N$. The biomedical data under consideration now are represented as $\Delta = \{y_1, \ldots, y_N\}$. For each variable n, the task is to find which other variables modulate Y_n with the highest likelihood. The network is achieved once we find out the parents of all variables. In the framework of Bayesian networks, our objective is to learn from a set of candidate network models $\Omega = \{M_1, M_2, \ldots, M_K\}$ the optimal network $\hat{M}$ fit best to the data Δ. Equivalently, we look for the highest posterior probability $p(M_k|\Delta)$. Applying Bayes' theorem to $p(M_k|\Delta)$ results in

$$p(M_k|\Delta) \propto p(M_k)p(\Delta|M_k), \tag{8.25}$$

where $p(M_k)$ is the prior probability of network model M_k and $p(\Delta|M_k)$ is the marginal likelihood. The assumption of first-order Markov chain further leads the marginal likelihood to $p(\Delta|M_k) = p(\Delta|M_k)$. The computation of $p(\Delta|M_k)$ is to average out parameters θ_k from the likelihood function $p(\Delta|M_k, \theta_k)$, where θ_k is the value of the random vector Θ_k parameterizing the joint probability distribution of $Y_1, ..., Y_N$ conditional on M_k. We can exploit the local Markov properties encoded by the network M_k to rewrite the joint probability $p(\Delta|M_k, \theta_k)$ as

$$p(\Delta|M_k, \theta_k) = \prod_{n=1}^{N} p(y_n|pa_{y_n}, \theta_{kn}), \qquad (8.26)$$

where pa_x denotes the values of the parents Pa_X of random variable X, and θ_{kx} is the subset of parameters used to describe the dependence of variable X on its parents.

We further can assume the J subjects in the database are independent. The likelihood function becomes

$$p(\Delta|M_k, \theta_k) = \prod_{n=1}^{N} \prod_{j=1}^{J} p(y_{nj}|pa_{y_{nj}}, \theta_{kn}), \qquad (8.27)$$

where the subscript j indicates the jth subject. The marginal likelihood function is the solution of the integral

$$p(\Delta|M_k) = \int p(\Delta|M_k, \theta_k) p(\theta_k) d\theta_k$$
$$= \int p(\Delta|M_k, \theta_k) p(\theta_k) d\theta_k. \qquad (8.28)$$

Finally, the determination of the best network model is $\hat{M} = \arg\max_k p(M_k) p(\Delta|M_k)$. When we assume that the prior knowledge on the network models is equally probable, the solution to the network is $\hat{M} = \arg\max_k p(\Delta|M_k)$. We next detail the algorithm to compute the network inference.

8.3.3.1 Distributed Computation of Network Inference

A careful examination of Eq. (8.27) reveals that the network inference can be computed in parallel. The inference of the parent variables Pa_{Y_n} of variable n is independent of inferring parents of another variable $n|$. Hence, we can distribute the computational tasks of $p(\Delta|M_k, \theta_k)$ into N computing nodes, where each node takes data y_n and Δ to search which set of variables will maximize likelihood $L_{kn} = \prod_{j=1}^{J} p(y_{nj}|pa_{y_{nj}}, \theta_{kn})$, illustrated in Figure 8.4. In other words, the likelihood function $p(\Delta|M_k, \theta_k)$ of a candidate network M_k is the sum of individual likelihoods L_{kn} calculated at all computing nodes, and the optimal network $\hat{M}$ that maximizes $p(\Delta|M_k)$ is equivalent to finding the maximum $\hat{L}_{kn}$ at each computing node.

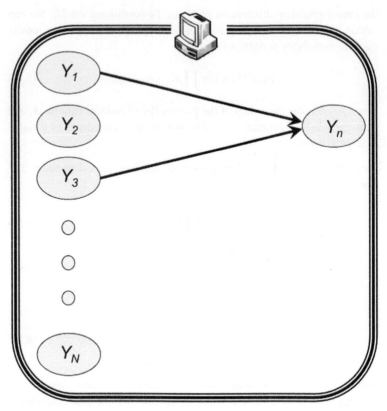

■ FIGURE. 8.4 We can distribute the inference of gene network into N computing nodes. Each computing node takes data of variables and then, in this example, infers that the optimal parents of Y_n are Y_1, Y_3.

The task of evaluating $\hat{L}_{kn}$ at each computing node is analogous to running a regression analysis with independent variables $Y_1, \ldots, Y_N$ and dependent variable Y_n. The likelihood L_{kn} can be derived using linear Gaussian model [5]:

$$L_{kn} = \prod_{j=1}^{J} \left(\frac{\tau_{kn}}{2\pi}\right)^{1/2} \exp\left(-\frac{(y_{nj} - \mu_{knj})^2}{2/\tau_{kn}}\right), \qquad (8.29)$$

where τ_{kn} is the precision and

$$\mu_{knj} = \beta_{kn0} + \sum_{r=1}^{R} \beta_{knr} h_{nrj} \qquad (8.30)$$

is the conditional mean obtained by a first order linear regression where R is the number of parents of Y_n and $H_{nrj} \in \{Y_1,...,Y_N\}$ is the rth parent. By introducing matrix notations,

$$\mathbf{y}_n = [y_{n1}, \ldots, y_{nJ}]^T, \tag{8.31}$$

$$\mathbf{h}_n = \begin{bmatrix} 1, h_{n11}, \ldots, h_{nR1} \\ \vdots \\ 1, h_{n1J}, \ldots, h_{nRJ} \end{bmatrix}, \tag{8.32}$$

$$\mathbf{b}_{kn} = [\beta_{kn0}, \beta_{kn1}, \ldots, \beta_{knR}]^T, \tag{8.33}$$

we can rewrite Eq. (8.29) as

$$L_{kn} = \left(\frac{\tau_{kn}}{2\pi}\right)^{J/2} \exp\left(-\frac{(\mathbf{y}_n - \mathbf{h}_n\mathbf{b}_{kn})^T (\mathbf{y}_n - \mathbf{h}_n\mathbf{b}_{kn})}{2/\tau_{kn}}\right). \tag{8.34}$$

Unlike most existing works that use maximum likelihood, we use Bayesian statistics to robustly estimate parameters τ_{kn} and $\mathbf{b}_{kn}$ [8]. By marginalizing the parameters, we can compute L_{kn} using a closed form [8].

8.3.3.2 *Search for the Optimal Network*

The task of searching for the global optimal network can be decomposed into looking for the optimal parents of individual nodes. The way to find the local optimal network from candidate networks $\Omega = \{M_1, M_2,..., M_k,..., M_K\}$ is equivalent to maximizing L_{kn} over k. The parents of each variable Y_n might be any combination of other variables, so the best set of parents is one of the $K = 2^N$ possible combinations. When N is large, evaluating L_{kn} over all k is computationally expensive. To avoid computational burden, the optimization can be achieved by recursively looking for the best solution at each step, called greedy search methods. We consider a stepwise forward-selection-backward-elimination algorithm to search the optimal network. Let $\Psi \in \{Y_1,...,Y_N\}$, and Pa_{Y_n} be the parent set of Y_n. The steps of the algorithm are as follows.

Step 1: Initialize the parent set Pa_{Y_n} to be empty. Use Eq. (8.34) to compute likelihood L_{kn} based on the current Pa_{Y_n}. Note that when Pa_{Y_n} is empty, Eq. (8.34) is calculated with $\mathbf{h}_n = [1,...,1]^T$ and $\mathbf{b}_{kn} = \beta_{kn0}$.

Step 2: This step performs forward selection. Among all the genes in Ψ/Pa_{Y_n}, select the variable whose addition to Pa_{Y_n} increases likelihood L_{kn} by the greatest amount. If we can find such a gene, the combination of Pa_{Y_n} and the gene assembles a better parent set; hence we replace Pa_{Y_n} with the union of Pa_{Y_n} and the variable, update L_{kn} by the new parent set, and move to Step 3. Otherwise if there exists no variable increasing likelihood L_{kn}, the current parent set Pa_{Y_n} is the optimal and we terminate the algorithm.

Step 3: This step performs backward-elimination. Among all the genes in Pa_{Y_n}, select the variable whose removal from Pa_{Y_n} increases likelihood L_{kn} by the greatest amount. If there exists such a variable, remove it out of Pa_{Y_n}, update L_{kn} by the new parent set, and go back to Step 2.

8.4 BIOMEDICAL APPLICATIONS

The methods introduced in this chapter can be used to solve a number of biomedical questions. In this section, we present some real examples where Bayesian methods and Bayesian networks are used.

8.4.1 Molecular Response of Yellow Fever Vaccination

The yellow fever vaccine (YF-17D) is one of the most effective vaccines ever made. A single dose of YF-17D can give rise to a broad spectrum of immune responses that can persist for up to three decades. Although the vaccine is successful, little is known about the mechanisms by which YF-17D induces the effective, longstanding immune responses [9]. To decipher this mechanism, gene expression profiling is a useful vehicle to monitor the gene networking after vaccination. We inferred the gene network from YF-17D vaccination data, which is available on Gene Expression Omnibus [10] with Accession No. GSE13485. The data contain 15 healthy vaccinated subjects, whose expression microarrays were sampled on days 0, 1, 3, 7, and 21 after vaccination. There were many missing samples on day 1, so we discarded the data at this time point in our network analysis.

For each pair of consecutive times, the gene-gene interaction at the earlier time will cause the changes in expression levels collected at the later time. Therefore, the interaction pattern can be described by Bayesian network method. We let $Y_1, Y_2, ..., Y_N$ be Gaussian random variables representing the gene expression levels. Following the inference algorithm presented in the previous section, we can obtain the gene networks.

Once the networks are inferred, we can use Bayes' theorem to compute the most likely quantities of child nodes from the data of parent nodes. To evaluate

Table 8.1 Predictive and forecast accuracy in the study of yellow fever vaccination.

	Prediction		Forecast	
	Fitted Validation	**Cross Validation**	**Fitted Validation**	**Cross Validation**
Adaptive model (this research)	98.42%	97.38%	97.59%	96.28%
Stationary model	96.05%	95.06%	94.93%	93.71%

the accuracy of our inferred gene network, we measured the prediction and forecast performance. The prediction performance was evaluated as follows: We used the data at $t=1, ..., T-1$ to predict expression patterns at the next times $t=2, ..., T$, respectively; the predicted gene expression levels were compared with the true quantities by mean error rate. The forecast performance was evaluated in the following: We used the initial data at $t=1$ to forecast the longitudinal expression patterns from $t=2$ to $t=T$, and compare the forecasted results with the ground truth by mean error rate (MER). Table 8.1 reports the performance. The accuracy is defined as 1-MER. The predictive accuracy of fitted validation was 98.42% and the forecast accuracy was 97.59%.

We further evaluated the robustness of our method by cross-validation. One trial of cross-validation involves partitioning the whole data into two complementary subsets, performing the analysis on one subset, and evaluating the accuracy on the other subset. To reduce variability, multiple trials of cross-validation are performed using different partitions, and the validation results are averaged over the all trials. In this study, we adopt leave-one-out cross-validation, where each trial of cross-validation takes a single sample for the validation purpose, and the process repeats until every sample has been used as a validation sample. This validation method gives rise to predictive and forecast accuracy of 97.38% and 96.28%, respectively. The results show that our approach achieves accurate performance. In addition, prediction and forecast have close performance, explaining that the network model can be used in either case.

To show how much our adaptive model improves from the stationary models, we applied the same algorithm but enforced the stationary assumption [4]. In terms of accuracy, the stationary model resulted in 96.05% predictive accuracy and 94.93% forecast accuracy; in terms of robustness, the stationary model generated 95.06% predictive accuracy and 93.71% forecast accuracy.

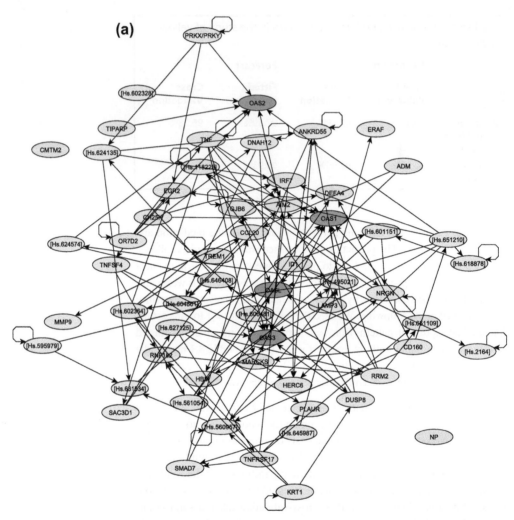

■ **FIGURE. 8.5** The evolution of the gene network centered at genes *OAS1, OAS2, OAS3, OASL* (colored in green) in the study of yellow fever vaccination. (a) day 0 to day 3, (b) day 3 to day 7, and (c) day 7 to day 21. The genes in gray indicate that they are isolated in that transition network. (For interpretation of the references to color in this figure legend, the reader is referred to the web version of this book.)

The improvement from stationary to dynamic models was statistically significant ($p < 0.05$).

The inferred gene network can further help explain the biology of YF-17D vaccination. Genes *OAS1*, *OAS2*, *OAS3*, *OASL* are in the 2–5A synthetase family; they are essential in the innate immune response to viral infection.

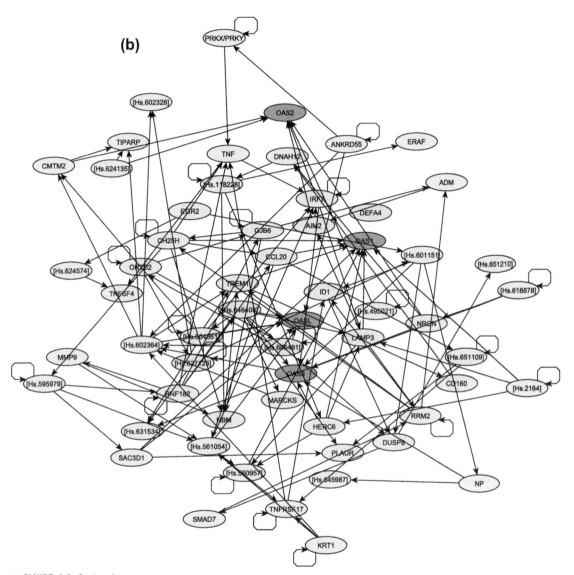

■ **FIGURE. 8.5** Continued

These genes were found elevated expression after YF-17D vaccination [9].
Figure 8.5 visualizes how this *OAS* family interacts with other genes after
patients were vaccinated. The network modulating the *OAS* genes consists of
59 genes, which are summarized in Table 8.2. In addition to the *OSA* genes,
other genes in the 59-gene signature able to induce innate immunity include
AIM2, *IRF7*, and *TNF*. To understand in an organized fashion the functions

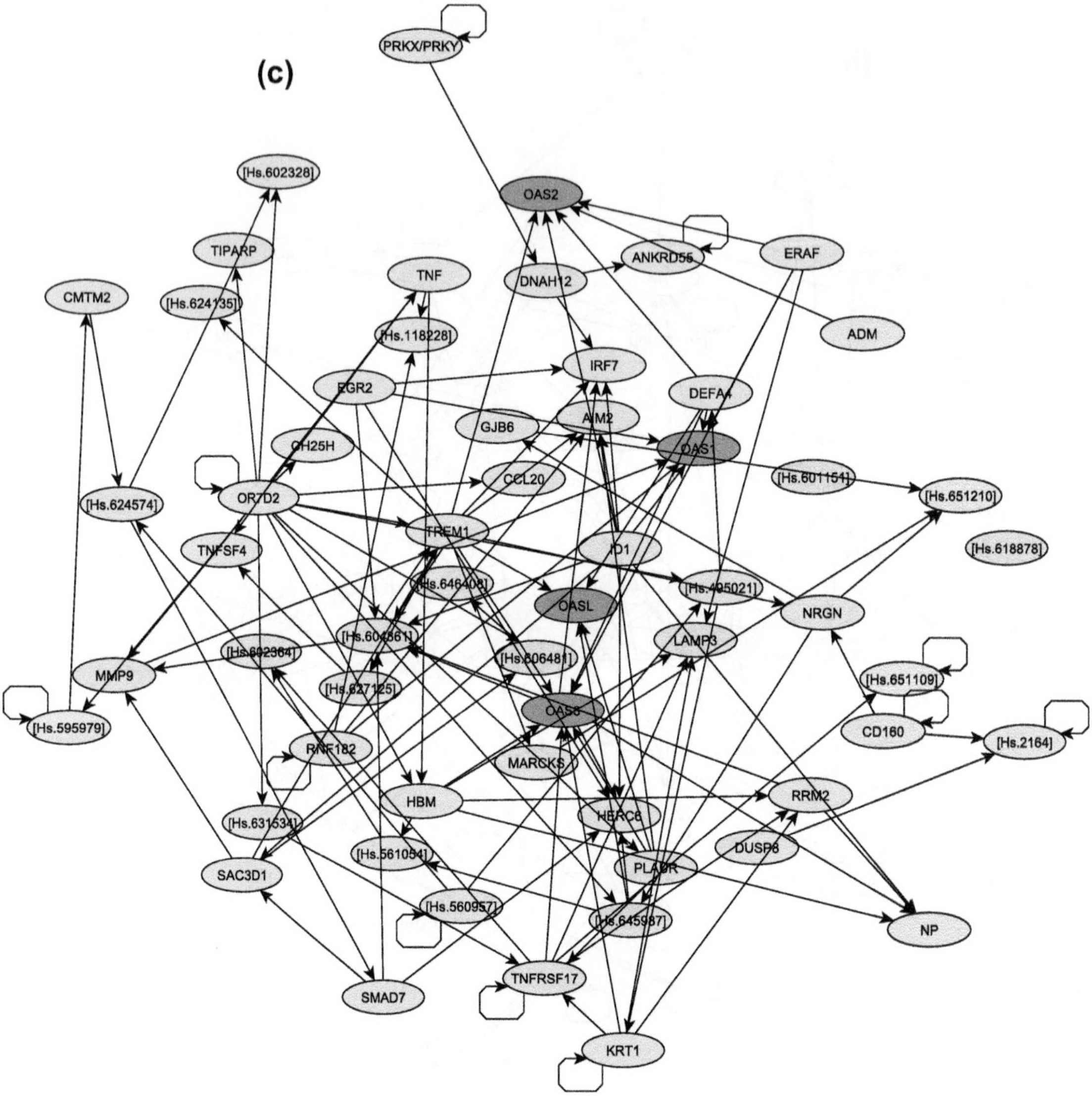

(c)

■ **FIGURE. 8.5** Continued

of this signature driving *OAS* family, we ran pathway analysis by DAVID Bioinformatics Database [11]. Two pathways significantly appeared in this signature: immune response ($p < 10^{-5}$), and response to external stimulus ($p < 0.009$). This finding is not surprising. The aim of YF-17D is to induce the minimum degree of viral infection, so the innate immune response can be

Table 8.2   The 59 genes modulating *OAS* family after yellow fever vaccination. The nameless genes are presented by their UniGene IDs within brackets.

ADM	*AIM2*	*ANKRD55*	*CCL20*	*CD160*	*CH25H*	*CMTM2*
DEFA4	*DNAH12*	*DUSP8*	*EGR2*	*ERAF*	*GJB6*	*HBM*
HERC6	*ID1*	*IRF7*	*KRT1*	*LAMP3*	*MARCKS*	*MMP9*
NP	*NRGN*	*OAS1*	*OAS2*	*OAS3*	*OASL*	*OR7D2*
PLAUR	*PRKX/PRKY*	*RNF182*	*RRM2*	*SAC3D1*	*SMAD7*	*TIPARP*
TNF	*TNFRSF17*	*TNFSF4*	*TREM1*	*[Hs.118228]*	*[Hs.2164]*	*[Hs.495021]*
[Hs.560957]	*[Hs.561054]*	*[Hs.595979]*	*[Hs.601151]*	*[Hs.602328]*	*[Hs.602364]*	*[Hs.604861]*
[Hs.606481]	*[Hs.618878]*	*[Hs.624135]*	*[Hs.624574]*	*[Hs.627125]*	*[Hs.631534]*	*[Hs.645987]*
[Hs.646408]	*[Hs.651109]*	*[Hs.651210]*				

activated to protect the host for a long period. The pathway analysis perfectly supports this fact: the gene signature responds to external stimulus (i.e., vaccine) and triggers innate immunity to provide longstanding protection for the hosts.

8.4.2 Alcoholism by Integrated Genomic and Demographic Analysis

Alcohol dependence is characterized by increasing tolerance to and consumption of alcohol, even in the face of adverse effects [12]. Almost 14% of alcohol consumers in the United States meet the criteria for alcohol dependence at some point in their lifetimes [13]. The consequences of alcohol dependence are severe. Overconsumption of alcohol is a known contributing factor to more than 60 diseases, including mental disorders, cancers, and cardiovascular diseases, and accounts for approximately 2.5 million deaths each year.

There have been several association studies that have sought to identify a small number of susceptible genetic loci for alcoholism [14]. However, complex traits like alcoholism are commonly underpinned by numerous factors, genetic as well as demographic, each of which has a small effect size [15]. Thus, many genome-wide association studies (GWAS) on alcoholism have struggled to pinpoint individual single nucleotide polymorphisms (SNPs) that can only explain a portion of the variation in the phenotype. A study [13] suggests that a new way to integrate both genetic and demographic information will be a new approach to study alcoholism. In this chapter, we utilize Bayesian networks framework to infer the SNP-SNP interactions and the SNP-environment interplay associated with alcoholism.

We used two data sets, COGA (1395 total samples, 918,009 SNPs) and COGEND (1367 total samples, 918,009 SNPs), in this analysis, both of

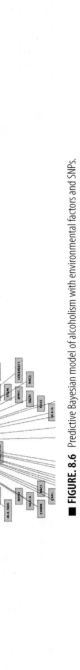

■ **FIGURE. 8.6** Predictive Bayesian model of alcoholism with environmental factors and SNPs.

which are part of the Study of Addiction: Genetics and Environment (SAGE) data superset.

We first removed any SNPs out of Hardy-Weinberg equilibrium (P <0.0001). Hardy-Weinberg equilibrium tests were run separately on self-reported "Blacks" and "Whites" in order to ensure identification of any SNPs common only in one race out of equilibrium. SNPs with minor allele frequency (MAF) below 0.01 or call rate below 98% were also removed from consideration, leaving a total of 934,128 SNPs.

The framework of Bayesian networks was used to capture the interplay of genetic and demographic information. The inferred network is shown in Figure 8.6. We further use this network to classify alcoholic or non-alcoholic. The network achieves 90% accuracy. The demographic-genetic classifier systematically confirms the frequent assertion that alcoholism is a byproduct of genetic and demographic factors. The classifier provides a means to accurately determine a person's risk for alcohol dependence given demographic and genetic information.

8.5 SUMMARY

This chapter systematically introduced Bayesian methods for biomedical data analysis. The unique feature of Bayesian approaches is its inclusion of prior belief in the data modeling. By bringing the belief, or prior knowledge, one can exploit Bayes' theorem to update data or information (e.g., parameters, models) needed for testing a given hypothesis and then analyze the data in a more reliable way.

The size of modern biomedical data is large and many variables in a given dataset may have dependency relationships. Bayesian networks can be used to capture dependence and causal relationships. As the number of variables becomes larger, the algorithms of inferring Bayesian networks are further useful in facilitating the logic reasoning and reverse-engineer the dependence relations. The real-world examples presented in this chapter demonstrate the power of Bayesian methods for biomedical analysis.

REFERENCES

[1] Finkenstadt B, Heron EA, Komorowski M, et al. Reconstruction of transcriptional dynamics from gene reporter data using differential equations. Bioinformatics Dec 15, 2008;24(24):2901–7.
[2] Kim H, Lee JK, Park T. Boolean networks using the chi-square test for inferring large-scale gene regulatory networks. BMC Bioinformatics 2007;8:37.
[3] Kim S, Kim J, Cho KH. Inferring gene regulatory networks from temporal expression profiles under time-delay and noise. Comput Biol Chem Aug, 2007;31(4):239–45.

[4] Zou M, Conzen SD. A new dynamic Bayesian network (DBN) approach for identifying gene regulatory networks from time course microarray data. Bioinformatics Jan 1, 2005;21(1):71–9.

[5] Ferrazzi F, Sebastiani P, Ramoni MF, et al. Bayesian approaches to reverse engineer cellular systems: a simulation study on nonlinear Gaussian networks. BMC Bioinformatics 2007;8(5):S2.

[6] Darby S, Hill D, Auvinen A, et al. Radon in homes and risk of lung cancer: collaborative analysis of individual data from 13 European case-control studies. BMJ Jan 29, 2005;330(7485):223.

[7] Bagnardi V, Randi G, Lubin J, et al. Alcohol consumption and lung cancer risk in the Environment and Genetics in Lung Cancer Etiology (EAGLE) study. Am J Epidemiol Jan 1, 2010;171(1):36–44.

[8] Chang HH, Ramoni MF. Robust cross-race gene expression analysis. In: Proceedings IEEE international conference on acoustics, speech, and signal processing p. 505–8.

[9] Querec TD, Akondy RS, Lee EK, et al. Systems biology approach predicts immunogenicity of the yellow fever vaccine in humans. Nat Immunol Jan, 2009;10(1):116–25.

[10] Edgar R, Domrachev M, Lash AE. Gene Expression Omnibus: NCBI gene expression and hybridization array data repository. Nucleic Acids Res Jan 1, 2002;30(1):207–10.

[11] Huang da W, Sherman BT, Lempicki RA. Systematic and integrative analysis of large gene lists using DAVID bioinformatics resources. Nat Protoc 2009;4(1):44–57.

[12] Li TK, Hewitt BG, Grant BF. The Alcohol Dependence Syndrome, 30 years later: a commentary. the 2006 H. David Archibald lecture. Addiction Oct, 2007;102(10):1522–30.

[13] Bierut LJ, Agrawal A, Bucholz KK, et al. A genome-wide association study of alcohol dependence. Proc Natl Acad Sci USA Mar 16, 2010;107(11):5082–7.

[14] Edenberg HJ, Koller DL, Xuei X, et al. Genome-wide association study of alcohol dependence implicates a region on chromosome 11. Alcohol Clin Exp Res May, 2010;34(5):840–52.

[15] Zondervan KT, Cardon LR. The complex interplay among factors that influence allelic association. Nat Rev Genet Feb, 2004;5(2):89–100.

Learning Classifier Systems: The Rise of Genetics-Based Machine Learning in Biomedical Data Mining

Ryan J. Urbanowicz and Jason H. Moore

Dartmouth College Department of Genetics, Hanover, NH, USA

CHAPTER OUTLINE

9.1 **INTRODUCTION**

9.1.1 **The Biomedical Beast**

While researchers continue to debate the true nature of common disease etiology, and seek out the underlying biology, the daunting magnitude and complexity of the problem has become clear. As is often said, "the more we learn, the less we know." This often seems to be true of biomedical studies where technology has paved the way for the age of the "–omes" [1], and a massive explosion of data collection that, to date, has not proportionally yielded all that much in terms of etiological understanding [2]. Research approaches in the "big data" era present us with an additional set of challenges, including: data management, analysis, and accessibility [3]. Throughout the history of science, having the correct perspective has often proven itself to be the determining factor in our ability to uncover truth. From the shape of the earth, to the cause of infectious disease, having effective tools and an open mind are key to gaining an appropriate perspective.

Technology is largely responsible for paving new avenues to approach the common problem of disease etiology. Starting with genomics [4], modern biomedical research has expanded to include a variety of data-rich landscapes, including: proteomics [5], epigenetics [6], transcriptomics [7], interferomics [8], phenomics [9], metabolomics [10], microbiomics [11], and exposomics [12]. Looking to the future, systems biology is an emerging research perspective seeking to connect these intersecting and interacting avenues using a more interdisciplinary and holistic set of methodologies [13]. However, while we may be getting closer to collecting the majority of the puzzle pieces, biomedical research has given proportionately far less attention to the development of analytical tools and methodologies that are responsible for figuring out how to put the pieces together. It is certainly not to say that the application of traditional analytical strategies, such as linear regression, has been without utility. Before sequencing of the human genome [4] and the completion of the human haplotype mapping project [14], linkage studies yielded many notable successes in characterizing rare Mendelian disease phenotypes, but more so, these works suggested that complex diseases could not be explained by a small number of rare variants with large effects [15]. With the arrival of commercial "SNP-Chips," genome-wide association studies (GWAS) examining single nucleotide polymorphisms (SNPs) became popular, hypothesizing that alleles that were common in the population would explain much of the heritability of common diseases [16]. To date, the failure of GWAS studies to explain "missing heritability" has been taken to suggest that complex disease cannot be explained by a limited number of common variants of moderate effect [17]. Missing heritability is the unexplained portion of phenotypic variance in a population attributable to inherited genetic factors. A number of explanations for this deficit exist, including: (1) poorly captured epigenetic, structural, and/or rare variants (i.e., missing puzzle pieces), (2) gene or environment interaction effects and/or genetic heterogeneity (i.e., understanding how the pieces interact or relate to one another), and (3) inaccurate or missapplied estimates of heritability (i.e., over- or underestimating heritability to begin with) [17–19].

As a result of this perceived failure, interest in SNP-based GWAS has started to wane, and a new wave of popular research is emerging with the development of next-generation sequencing technology, which aims to provide affordable whole genome sequencing and thus allow for the detection of hundreds of thousands of rare variants per individual [20]. While this new vein of genomic investigation is promising, we should be cautious about what we expect the technology alone to uncover, as we learned with GWAS.

Probably the least assuming hypothesis regarding the nature of complex disease is that the etiology of a given disease is likely to include some combination of common variants of small effect, rare variants of large effect, epigenetic factors, and environmental factors [21,22]. Additionally, we should certainly not expect the type or number of these contributing factors to be similar from one disease to another. Considering the unknown scale and complexity of the problem, where should the focus of biomedical informatics lie? While logistical concerns, such as data management and accessibility, are certainly important, in this chapter we concern ourselves with the analytical challenges, answering the call for new tools and methodologies [23,24] to deal with the assembly of the puzzle pieces that we already have, in addition to the ones we will uncover with future technologies and research.

While traditional statistical and analytical methodologies have proven successful for the characterization of simple linear patterns of association, they have yielded limited success when applied to common disease [17,25]. For instance, most GWAS studies have used a single-locus analysis strategy, in which each variant is tested individually for association with a given phenotype. Thornton-Wells et al. [23] reviewed and discussed a variety of phenomena that have been recognized to complicate the epidemiological mapping of genotype to phenotype include epistasis, gene-environment interaction, phenocopy, epigenetics, phenotypic heterogeneity, trait heterogeneity, and genetic heterogeneity. An important challenge for computational biologists is the development of strategies to achieve classification and data mining in the context of these complicating phenomena. While no computational methodology can overcome missing pieces of the puzzle, the quality and availability of the pieces we do have, along with the belief that technological advancement and continued scientific investigation will uncover the rest, makes the statistical detection of non-linear interaction and heterogeneity attractive targets for bioinformatics development.

9.1.2 Complicating Phenomena

Non-linear interaction encompasses the phenomena of epistasis (i.e., gene-gene interaction) as well as gene-environment interaction. The term *epistasis* was first coined by Bateson to describe a genetic masking effect, originally viewed as a multi-locus extension of the dominance phenomenon where a variant at one locus prevents the variant at another locus from manifesting its effect [26]. This definition was in line with a physical and biological interpretation of the phenomena, while in the present discussion we consider a strictly statistical one. Statistical epistasis is traditionally defined as a deviation from additivity in a mathematical model summarizing the relationship between multi-locus genotypes and phenotypic variation in a population [27]. A complete discussion of biological and statistical epistasis has been done previously [28]. It is worth noting that the detection of statistical epistasis does not necessarily translate into biological epistasis. To illustrate the inherent difficulty posed by epistasis, consider the following simple example of statistical epistasis in the form of a SNP-based penetrance function. Penetrance is simply the probability (P) of disease (D) given a particular combination of genotypes (G) that were inherited (i.e., P[D|G]). A single genotype is determined by one allele (i.e., a specific DNA base pair) inherited from either parent. For most SNPs, only two alleles (encoded by *A* or *a*) exist in the biological population. Therefore, because the order of the alleles is unimportant, a genotype can have one of three values: *AA*, *Aa*, or *aa*. The model illustrated in Figure 9.1 is an extreme example of epistasis, also known as pure epistasis [29]. The loci in such models could be viewed as "fully masked" in that no predictive information is gained until all *k* loci are considered in concert. The penetrance for each individual genotype (i.e., marginal penetrance) in this model is 0.5 and is computed by summing the products of the genotype frequencies and penetrance values. Thus, in this model there is no difference in disease risk for each single SNP alone.

	Genotype	SNP 2 BB(.25)	SNP 2 Bb (.5)	SNP 2 bb(.25)	Marginal Penetrance
	AA(.25)	0	1	0	.5
SNP 1	Aa (.5)	1	0	1	.5
	aa(.25)	0	1	0	.5
	Marginal Penetrance	.5	.5	.5	$K = .5$

■ **FIGURE 9.1** A 2-locus purely epistatic penetrance function.

In this model, the heritability is the maximum possible (i.e., 1.0), because the probability of disease is completely determined by the genotypes at these two DNA sequence variations. All of the heritability in this model is due to epistasis. Epistatic associations with disease could occur at any k-way order of interaction.

The meaning of the term *heterogeneity* is context dependent. In the context of admixture, heterogeneity simply refers to genetic differences in population structure [30]. In genetic modeling, a heterogeneous model describes the independent effect of some number of factors [24]. Similarly, in the context of association studies, heterogeneity references an independence effect observed in three different phenomena: allelic heterogeneity, locus heterogeneity, and phenocopy [23]. Allelic heterogeneity occurs when two or more alleles of a single locus are independently associated with the same trait, while locus heterogeneity occurs when two or more DNA sequence variations at distinct loci are independently associated with the same trait. Heterogeneity, typically classified as either genetic (locus and allelic) or environmental (i.e., phenocopy), occurs when individual, or a set of, factors are independently predictive of the same phenotype. Phenocopy occurs when an environmental condition mimics a trait or phenotype produced by a gene. Additionally, trait heterogeneity occurs when a trait or disease has been defined with insufficient specificity such that it is actually two or more distinct underlying traits [23]. Ultimately, in the context of mining genetic and environmental patterns within an association study, there is no practical distinction between genetic heterogeneity, trait heterogeneity, and phenocopy, since these phenomena manifest the same type of independent associations. From a computer science perspective, the problem of heterogeneity is similar to a latent or "hidden" class problem. While the disease status (case or control) of each patient is already known, the individuals making up either class would be more accurately subgrouped into two or more "hidden" classes, each characterized by an independent predictive model of disease. A simple example of heterogeneity is given in Figure 9.2.

9.1.3 **The State of Analytical Informatics**

Traditional modeling strategies such as linear, multiple, or logistic regression are often noted as being inadequate to properly address the complicating phenomena previously discussed [31]. Specifically, parametric statistical methods such as logistic regression often fail to converge on accurate parameter estimates when multiple variables and their interactions are being modeled. Furthermore, the exhaustive evaluation of all possible combinations of genetic variants ranges from computationally expensive to entirely

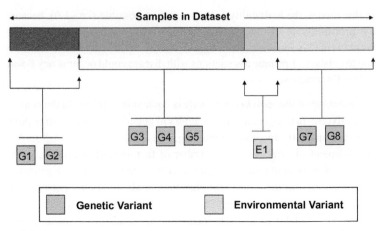

■ FIGURE 9.2   A simple illustration of heterogeneity. Note how a different variant, or set of variants are predictive of disease in an independently subset of the dataset.

intractable. Consider that when studying k-way interactions among n variables, the computational cost is on the order of n^k. This high cost remains a barrier to investigating large values of k [32].

Numerous strategies have been developed and applied to the detection of epistasis in population-based studies of human disease. Separately, the problem of heterogeneity has received much less attention especially in the context of modeling. While a complete review of such strategies is well beyond the scope of this chapter, we will highlight some select examples that emphasize the current state of analytical informatics.

The phrases *machine learning* and *data mining* reference two sides of the same coin. Machine learning describes any methodology that is focused on making a prediction based on known properties learned from training data. Alternatively, data mining is used to label methodologies that seek to discover unknown properties in data. In the present context of biomedical informatics, we concern ourselves with the task of constructing predictive models to be used for classification and knowledge discovery. In line with machine learning, *classification* seeks to categorize a new subject (for instance, by predicting whether or not it is likely to have or develop a specific disease phenotype) based on a training set of observed subjects. In line with data mining, *knowledge discovery* seeks to identify novel, potentially useful, and comprehensible patterns in the data [33]. An emphasis on knowledge discovery is intended to direct the translation of statistical associations into biological understanding. Ultimately all of the strategies discussed herein could be applied as machine learning or data mining algorithms, which is likely why these phrases are often used interchangeably. For simplicity, throughout the remainder of this chapter we will use "machine learning" to cover both phrases since our goals are one in the same.

Machine learning strategies can be *exhaustive* (involving a systematic examination of all possible solution candidates) or they can take a guided or stochastic route in an attempt to more efficiently explore the greater search space. Such strategies may also differ in whether they try to fit a single pre-specified model (i.e., parametric) or are effectively model-free (i.e., non-parametric). For instance, when comparing two exhaustive strategies (a given regression-based method vs. multi-factor dimensionality reduction [MDR] [34]), the regression-based method requires the estimation of model parameters, while MDR does not. MDR has proven to be a particularly successful and popular approach for modeling main effects (e.g., single-locus associations), purely epistatic effects, and combinations of the two [35]. MDR is essentially an attribute construction algorithm that creates a new variable or attribute by pooling genotypes from multiple SNPs.

While exhaustive algorithms may be able to confidently identify the best model within the constraints of a restricted search space, they cannot be scaled to allow for analysis of large numbers of predictor variables, or larger *k*-orders of interaction [34]. This explains much of the interest in non-exhaustive machine learning. Both McKinney et al. [36] and Cordell [31] have reviewed non-exhaustive strategies to detect epistatic interactions associated with disease. Examples include random forests [37], neural networks [38], cellular automata [39], Bayesian model selection [40], computational evolution system (CES) [41], genetic algorithms [42], genetic programming [43], swarm algorithms [44], and artificial immune systems [45].

However, the daunting number of potentially predictive variables in GWAS as well as the unknown order of the true underlying interactions also calls for supplemental algorithms to either filter out variables less likely to be predictive, or to weight the search in favor of those that are more predictive. Examples of such algorithms include ReliefF [46], Tuned ReliefF (TuRF) [47], SURF [48], and evaporative cooling. The combination of such algorithms with machine learning strategies will likely be the key to successful modeling.

As mentioned earlier, there have been far fewer proposed strategies to deal with heterogeneity, a critical component of the modern day conceptualization of complex human disease. Most of the aforementioned machine learning strategies neglect to consider the impact of heterogeneity on the effectiveness of a given algorithm. One notable exception to this is observed in an evaluation of MDR that demonstrated that simulated heterogeneity dramatically hinders MDR's power to detect all underlying modeled factors [49]. Statistical approaches such as the admixture test [50], M test [51], and β test [52] are specific to family-based data and can only identify the *existence* of heterogeneity rather than its characterization. The most common approach to heterogeneity is to try and remove its confounding effect through data stratification. This has been addressed using strategies such as ordered subset analysis [53], latent class analysis [54,55], tree-based recursive partitioning [56], and clustering [57,58]. These methods pre-process a given dataset based on genetic risk factors, demographic data, phenotypic data, or endophenotypes in order to form more homogeneous subsets of subjects. This is in line with the standard epidemiological paradigm that seeks to find a single best disease model within a given homogeneous sample. The obvious drawback of these types of methods is that their success completely relies on the availability, quality, and relevance of these covariates. Additionally, stratification represents a relative reduction in sample size, leading to an inevitable loss in power to detect associations within these homogeneous subsets.

Only a few strategies have been considered that concurrently examine the problems of epistasis and heterogeneity without resorting to some form of stratification. These include MDR [49,59], random forests [60], association rule discovery [61], and CHAMBER [62]. While some algorithms have been successful in accommodating the problem of heterogeneity, explicit characterization has remained a major challenge. CHAMBER, an algorithm that uses graph-building, was uniquely the first to jointly consider the characterization of both interaction and heterogeneity. Specifically, heterogeneity was characterized through the identification of groups of individuals, within which different predictive attributes were correlated with disease risk.

Given the apparent complexity of common disease, and the likelihood that multi-locus interactions and heterogeneity are not only present but likely to be ubiquitous components of disease risk [63], it is critical to develop powerful new strategies that concurrently address these phenomena. Strategies that make assumptions about the nature, number, or source of underlying factors will inevitably be susceptible to complicating phenomena. For the rest of this chapter we will discuss a machine learning strategy that breaks from the traditional modeling paradigm, wherein an individual best model is sought. Algorithms described as genetics-based machine learning strategies (GBML), also include learning classifier systems (LCSs). This class of algorithm evolves a compendium of rules, where each covers a subset of the problem space. In effect, patterns learned from the dataset are distributed over a population of rules, making LCS well suited to concurrently model both interaction and heterogeneity without the need for data stratification.

In the following sections, we will introduce LCSs and describe our own application of this type of algorithm to explicitly address the biomedical informatics challenge of modeling both epistasis and heterogeneity. This collective work constitutes a new pathway for the identification of predictive features and the nature of their association with a disease phenotype in the face of noisy data and unknown complexity.

9.2 LEARNING CLASSIFIER SYSTEMS

9.2.1 The Basics

Learning classifier systems (LCSs) [64] are a rule-based class of algorithms that combine machine learning with evolutionary computing and other heuristics to produce an adaptive system. LCSs belong to a greater category of algorithms referred to as genetics-based machine learning (GBML) algorithms. LCSs represent solutions as sets of rules, affording them the ability to learn iteratively, form niches, and adapt. These multifaceted algorithms have evolved in the cradle of evolutionary biology and artificial intelligence. Figure 9.3 illustrates the hierarchy of fields that found the LCS algorithm concept.

Since their advent, the LCS concept has inspired a multitude of implementations adapted to manage the different problem domains to which they have been applied (e.g., autonomous robotics, function approximation, classification, knowledge discovery, and game strategy). LCSs were originally developed to model behavior in complex systems (e.g., stock market behavior [65]),

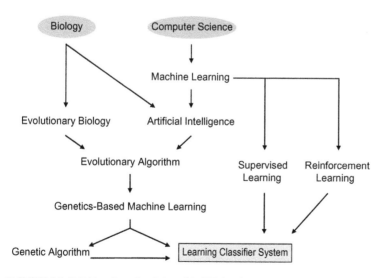

■ **FIGURE 9.3** Field hierarchy—foundations of the LCS algorithm.

as well as to handle multi-step problems (e.g., maze navigation [66]). However, the unique manner in which patterns are learned and stored lends itself well to single-step problems such as classification and data mining, where reward for making correct decisions is not delayed during learning [67].

We begin a brief overview of some of the basic elements of an LCS. It has been said that "LCSs employ two biological metaphors; evolution and learning... [where] learning guides the evolutionary component to move toward a better set of rules" [68]. These concepts are respectively embodied by two mechanisms: (1) the genetic algorithm and (2) a learning mechanism appropriate for the given problem. Both mechanisms rely on what is referred to as the *environment* of the system. In the context of data mining, the environment is simply the training data presented to the algorithm. The rules of an LCS algorithm (sometimes referred to as "agents" or classifiers) are typically represented in the form of "IF *condition* THEN *action*." Using the biological metaphor of an immune system, antibody "agents" possess hypervariable regions in their protein structure, which allows them to bind to specific targets known as antigens. In this way, the immune system has a way to identify and neutralize foreign objects such as bacteria and viruses. Given this example, the behavior of a specific antibody might be represented by rules such as "IF *the antigen-binding site fits the antigen* THEN *bind to the antigen*," or "*IF the antigen-binding site does not fit the antigen* THEN *do not bind to the antigen*." Rules such as these in the context of an LCS use information from the system's environment to make decisions. For classification and data mining problems, the action is instead a class. In other words, a rule speculates that "IF *a given set of attributes in the dataset each have a specific state*, THEN *that individual belongs to a specific class*." Notably, in the context of LCS, an individual rule does not constitute a model, since it will only apply to a subset of the instances in the data.

While many different LCS implementations exist, Holmes et al. [69] outlined four practically universal components: (1) a finite population of rules that, as a set, collectively capture patterns identified from the environment, (2) a performance component, which regulates interaction between the environment and classifier population, (3) a credit assignment component, which either distributes reward or updates rule accuracy, and (4) a discovery component which uses various operators to discover better rules and improve existing ones. Together, these components represent a basic framework upon which a number of novel alterations to the LCS algorithm have been proposed.

While the four components described above represent an algorithmic framework, two primary mechanisms are responsible for driving the algorithm.

These include discovery (generally by means of a genetic algorithm—described shortly), and learning. Discovery refers to "rule discovery," or the introduction of rules that do not currently exist in the population. Ideally, the discovery mechanism will identify better rules over time. The most common discovery mechanism applied in LCS algorithms is a genetic algorithm (GA) [70]. A GA is a computational search technique that manipulates ("evolves") a population of individuals ("rules"), each having an associated "fitness" value. The GA, as a major component of the first conceptualized LCS [71], has completely surpassed LCS in terms of notoriety and common usage. A GA is founded on ideas borrowed from nature. Inspired by the Neo-Darwinist theory of natural selection, the evolution of rules is modeled after the evolution of organisms using four biological analogies: (1) a code is used to represent the genotype/genome (condition), (2) a class (or phenotype) representation is associated with that genotype, (3) a selection process (survival of the fittest), where the fittest organism (rule) has a greater chance of surviving and reproducing to pass its "genetic" information onto the next generation, and (4) genetic operators are used to allow simple transformations of the genome in search of fitter organisms (rules) [72]. Variation in a genome (rule) is typically generated by two genetic operators: mutation and crossover (recombination). Mutation operators randomly modify an element (attribute) in the genotype (condition) of an individual (rule). Crossover operators create new genotypes by recombining the genotypes (conditions) of "parent" individuals (rules). The selection pressure that drives "better" organisms (rules) to reproduce more often is dependent on the fitness function. The fitness function quantifies the optimality of a given rule, allowing that rule to be ranked against all others in the population. In a classification problem, a fitness function proportional to accuracy is typically used. Running a genetic algorithm requires looping through a series of steps for some number of iterations (generations). Also needed is a user-specified population size limit (N) and the desired number of learning iterations. Additionally, a GA requires some strategy to initialize the rule population, such that it broadly covers the range of possible solutions (the search space). The following steps describe a single iteration of a standard genetic algorithm:

1. Update the fitness of all rules in the current population.
2. Select two "parent" rules from the population (with probability proportional to fitness).
3. Crossover or mutate "parent" rules to form "offspring" rules.
4. Add "offspring" rules to the population.
5. If required, delete (kill) enough rules from the next generation (with probability inversely proportional to fitness) to restore the number of rules to N.

The learning component of LCS has traditionally taken the form of reinforcement learning. Since we are dealing with single-step problems, and typically know the phenotype status of subjects, we focus on supervised learning. This is a far simpler learning mechanism that just updates a rule's accuracy. Another notable difference between LCSs and most other machine learning strategies is that they typically adopt what is called *online* or *incremental learning*, where training instances are presented to the learner one at a time. Assuming that training is being done on a finite dataset, once the algorithm has iterated through each instance in the dataset, goes back and goes through the dataset again and again until the user specified maximum number of learning iterations is reached. This is a major part of what makes these systems adaptive and efficient learners. Alternatively, *offline* or *batch learning* implies that all training instances are presented simultaneously to the learner. While most LCS algorithms use online learning, batch learning is standard both in a standalone GA, as well as most other machine learning algorithms. Batch learning is in line with the traditional paradigm of seeking a single best model of disease. The fitness of the model is determined by evaluating it across all instances in the dataset. For the typical LCS, a model is actually an assembly of rules that each only apply to a subset of the data. Therefore learning can take place once instance at a time with fitness updates only taking place in rules that are relevant to the current instance.

9.2.2 **A Historical View**

The LCS concept, now over three decades old, was originally formalized by Holland [73], based around his more well-known invention, the GA [71]. The infancy of LCS research saw the emergence of two founding classes of LCSs, referred to as the Michigan and Pittsburgh styles. The Michigan-style algorithm architecture was originally developed at the University of Michigan [74]. A Michigan-style LCS (M-LCSs) is typically characterized by (1) online learning, (2) a population of rules wherein the GA operates at the level of individual rules, and (3) the "model" or solution is represented collectively by the population of rules. Alternatively, Pittsburgh-style LCSs (P-LCSs) originated at the University of Pittsburgh [75]. P-LCSs are typically characterized by (1) offline learning, (2) a population of variable length "rule-sets" (where each rule-set is a potential "model" or solution), and (3) the GA operates at the level of a single rule-set (each rule-set has its own fitness, rather than each rule). Figure 9.4 illustrates the architectural difference between the Michigan and Pittsburgh styles. Of the two styles, the M-LCS approach has drawn the most attention as it can be applied to a broader range of problems and larger, more complex tasks. As such, it has largely become what many consider to be the standard LCS framework.

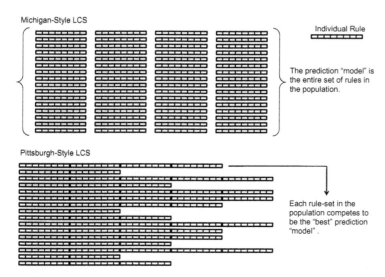

Michigan-Style LCS

Individual Rule

The prediction "model" is the entire set of rules in the population.

Pittsburgh-Style LCS

Each rule-set in the population competes to be the "best" prediction "model".

■ **FIGURE 9.4** Michigan vs. Pittsburgh-style algorithm rule populations.

Indeed, in the following sections of this chapter we will focus on applying the Michigan-style to our problems of interaction and heterogeneity.

Early LCS algorithms were criticized for their inherent complexity and delicate reliability. In the mid-1990s, Wilson introduced an eXtended Classifier System (XCS) [66], that has largely been credited for reinvigorating the research and development of LCS algorithms. XCS represents a parsimonious reimagining of the LCS algorithm architecture that was both general enough to be applicable to many problem domains, and simple enough to obtain consistent results. As a result, XCS has become the most popular LCS implementation to date, leading to the development of many new LCS algorithms based directly, or heavily upon its architecture. One such offshoot of XCS is the sUpervised Classifier System (UCS) [67] which replaced the reinforcement learning component of XCS with a far simpler supervised learning mechanism. This was done to create a system specifically well suited for single-step, supervised learning problems, such as the ones we are interested in here. We mention UCS specifically here, since the work described in the following sections is largely based around the UCS algorithm architecture. A more complete LCS introduction and review has been published previously [64].

While not originally their intended application, LCS literature has intermittently explored applications in biomedical classification since the mid-1990s. Interestingly, one of the earliest attempts to apply an LCS algorithm to such a problem involved classification in common disease research [76].

Soon after, Holmes (author of Chapter 7 of this text) initiated a lineage of LCSs designed for epidemiological surveillance and knowledge discovery that included BOOLE++ [77], EpiCS [78], and EpiXCS [79]. A number of similar applications were developed [80–86], all of which examined the Wisconsin breast cancer data taken from the UCI repository [87]. LCSs have also been applied to protein structure prediction [88–91], diagnostic image classification [92,93], promoter region identification [94], predicting protein functions [95], and microarray data analysis [96,97]. BIOHEL [98] is another prominent LCS algorithm with strong ties to the P-LCS architecture designed to handle large-scale bioinformatics datasets. Clearly LCS algorithms are not new to biomedical applications, but to date, very few biomedical researchers are even aware of their existence.

9.2.3 **An Algorithmic Walkthrough**

The working LCS algorithm is a relatively complex assembly of interacting mechanisms operating in an iterative fashion. The best way to understand how it works is to walk through an iteration of the algorithm. For clarity and relevance to later sections, we will focus on a simplified version of UCS [67]. Should the reader be interested in learning the specific functionality of other LCS algorithms, this example offers an accessible starting point from which to better understand more complex implementations. In this example, we assume a dataset that contains the genotypes for four unique SNPs in a sample of subjects that are either classified as cases or controls. Within the dataset, cases are encoded as "1" and controls as "0." Since SNPs are typically bi-allelic, a given SNP can have any of the three generic allele combinations (genotypes): *AA*, *Aa*, or *aa*, encoded here as "0," "1," or "2." As a result, we adopt a quaternary rule representation, which means that the condition of an LCS rule will be comprised of a string of the following four characters: "0," "1," "2," or "#." The pound sign ("#") acts as a wildcard, such that a rule condition "10#0" would match the attribute inputs "1000," "1010," and "1020." Figure 9.5 illustrates how this quaternary representation may be used to evolve concise, interpretable rules. Ideally, an LCS would evolve rules which specify genotype combinations that best discriminate between cases and controls.

Figure 9.6 outlines the UCS algorithm. Next, we examine each step involved in a learning iteration, as labeled in Figure 9.6:

Step 1: UCS learns iteratively. It samples one instance at a time, learns from it, and then moves on to the next. The algorithm begins by selecting one training instance in the dataset without replacement, such that the algorithm views every instance in the dataset with equal frequency.

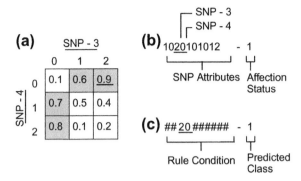

(a)

	SNP - 3		
	0	1	2
SNP - 4 0	0.1	0.6	<u>0.9</u>
1	0.7	0.5	0.4
2	0.8	0.1	0.2

(b) ┌ SNP - 3
         │ ┌ SNP - 4
        10<u>20</u>101012 - 1
        └——————┘   └┘
        SNP Attributes Affection
                        Status

(c) ## <u>20</u> ###### - 1
        └——————┘   └┘
        Rule Condition Predicted
                        Class

■ **FIGURE 9.5** A quaternary rule representation: (a) An example penetrance table modeling an epistatic interaction between SNPs 3 and 4 within a dataset comprised of 10 SNPs. Shaded cells indicate genotypes with high penetrance (probability of disease). (b) An example training instance from a dataset generated using the disease model in (a). (c) An example rule utilizing the quaternary representation. Notice how the LCS rule illustrated here has evolved to identify the "high-risk" geno-type (SNP3 = 2 and SNP4 = 0) underlined in (a).

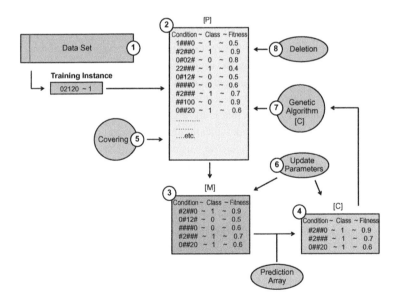

■ **FIGURE 9.6** Simplified UCS algorithm—an example learning iteration.

Step 2: This training instance is passed to the population of rules [P], which has a maximum size of N rules. Each rule in [P] is made up of a condition, a classification, and an associated fitness parameter {F}. In the present example, a rule's fitness {F} is equal to its accuracy {A} (which will be defined later). Initially, [P] is empty.

Step 3: A match set [M] is formed, which includes any rule in [P] that has a condition matching the attribute states of the instance.

Step 4: A correct set [C] is formed, which includes any rule in [M] which specifies the correct class of the training instance. If we want to test the current predictive ability of the current [P] of rules, instead of forming [C] we would instead form a prediction array. The prediction array examines all rules in [M] and sums up the fitness values for rules representative of each class. In this way, all rules within [M] get a fitness and numerosity weighted vote in how the current instance should be classified. The prediction array is also used any time we want to apply the collective LCS "model" to the task of prediction. The prediction array is not required for supervised learning, which is why it is not included as a learning step.

Step 5: If in Step 3 or Step 4, either [M] or [C] turns out to be empty (because no such rules yet exist in [P]), randomly generate a rule that both matches the condition and class of the training instance and add it to [P], [M], and [C]. This covering mechanism is responsible for initializing the rule population, and partially responsible for exploring new areas of the search space. The number of wildcards incorporated into the new rule condition is dependent on the rate (p#) set by the user.

Step 6: Update the rule parameters of rules found in [M] and [C]. In this example, we will only describe update fitness, the most important parameter. Be aware, that in most LCS implementations, a number of other parameters are typically tracked to better direct learning. These include parameters such as numerosity (how many copies of that rule are currently maintained in the population), the age of a rule, and the last time the GA was applied to it. As previously mentioned, here we set $\{F\} = \{A\}$. Accuracy is defined as the number of times a rule has been included in a correct set (since it was added to [P]) divided by the number of times it has been included in a match set. In this example, the fitness of a rule reflects its predictive accuracy only within the dataset instances to which it applies (and not to the dataset as a whole).

Step 7: The GA uses a roulette wheel selection process to probabilistically select two parent rules from [C] proportional to the rule fitness. Offspring rules are generated from parent rules as previously described, with the probability of crossover set to (χ), and the probability of mutation set to (μ). Notably, earlier LCS algorithms selected parent rules from [P] or [M] rather than [C].

Step 8: Whenever the number of rules in [P] becomes greater than the user-specified maximum population size (N), a deletion mechanism removes rules from [P] until this number is reached. Rules are selected for deletion with a probability inversely proportional to fitness. Notably, N is calculated by summing the rule numerosities for all rules in [P]. In other words, if there are N rules in the population, there are not necessarily N unique rules. Rule numerosity is often used as an indication of the importance of a rule, based on the premise, that if a rule is valuable for making good predictions, the M-LCS will continue to find and maintain copies of it.

9.2.4 **Limitations with Solutions**

While M-LCS algorithms are inherently flexible and powerful, offering the many advantages we have already discussed, they classically exhibit a number of drawbacks that are each a target for future improvement. These include scalability, run time, interpretability, ease of use (which includes the number of run parameters that must be specified by the user), accessibility (there very few implementations of user-friendly LCS software available), and performance optimization. While many of these have already been, and continue to be addressed in the literature, in this chapter we discuss our work in addressing three limitations which we identified to be particularly critical to our problem of interest.

Previously, we explored the application of different LCS algorithms to the detection and modeling of simulated epistatic and heterogeneous genetic disease associations and demonstrated their ability to successfully detect predictive factors in the presence of heterogeneity, and pure epistasis [99,100]. These proof of principle analyses identified M-LCSs rather than P-LCSs to be the more promising style for our particularly complex, noisy problem domain. Additionally this initial work helped us to prioritize our efforts in adapting an M-LCS algorithm to our problem.

The most glaring concern was the problem of interpretability, a crucial component in data mining. Similar to algorithms such as neural networks or random forests, M-LCS solutions have often been characterized as a "black box." While each has proven very successful at classification, extracting knowledge about how those decisions were made is often time consuming and unreliable. In the context of an M-LCS, knowledge discovery has traditionally involved rule sorting combined with manual rule inspection. While this approach may be sufficient for simpler problems, the complicating influence of noise and the need to discriminate between predictive and non-predictive attributes calls for novel strategies. In the forthcoming section titled "Interpretability and Knowledge Discovery," we discuss our work for developing an analysis pipeline with visualization-guided knowledge discovery to address this obstacle. In addition to significance testing (previously lacking in most LCS analyses), the pipeline presents subjective visualization strategies for inferring patterns of attribute interaction and heterogeneity from the rule-set [101].

The issue of scalability refers to how rapidly the learning time or system size grows as the problem complexity increases. Previously, we discussed how many machine learning strategies have benefitted from attribute filtering or weighting to reduce problem complexity and improve algorithm performance. In the forthcoming section titled "Aiding Scalability with Expert Knowledge," we discuss our work in applying expert knowledge to guide the covering and mutation operators within an M-LCS algorithm [102].

Lastly, while our previous work [99] has indicated that an M-LCS successfully performs the task of classification even in the presence of heterogeneity, there still lacked a mechanism for explicitly identifying heterogeneity and linking instances in the dataset to respective heterogeneous subgroups. In the forthcoming section titled "Characterizing Heterogeneity," we discuss our work developing AF-UCS [103]. This extension of the UCS algorithm introduces attribute tracking and feedback as novel mechanisms to address this problem, and improve learning and generalization in supervised M-LCS algorithms.

In the following sections, we review these efforts aimed at making M-LCSs not just a viable option for biomedical data mining, but a uniquely appealing one.

9.3 FACING THE CHALLENGES
9.3.1 Interpretability and Knowledge Discovery

Knowledge discovery has been described as the "non-trivial process of identifying valid, novel, potentially useful, and ultimately understandable patterns in data" [33]. Efforts to improve knowledge discovery in P-LCSs or similar GBML algorithms are synonymous with improving overall performance (e.g., as quantified by accuracy, generality, speed, and solution compactness), since these algorithms explicitly strive to evolve a concise rule-set that can be directly inspected and interpreted [98,104,105]. As in P-LCSs, knowledge discovery in M-LCS is traditionally achieved through manual inspection of rules. Manual inspection simply involves an examination of the best rules in the population in order to determine which attributes with specific states are predictive of a particular class. Due to the number of rules in M-LCS solutions, it has been suggested to rank rules by numerosity (number of rule copies in the population) and then inspecting those with the highest numerosities in order to identify key parts of the solution [66].

A largely ubiquitous goal for both LCS styles is to simultaneously optimize both accuracy and rule generality. However, these goals can be at odds with one another—especially in the presence of noise. For example, in typical M-LCSs, despite implicit generalization pressures, fitness is ultimately determined by rule accuracy. Thus, as long as some non-predictive attribute confers a slight accuracy advantage in the training set, a rule that includes it will be chosen over a more appropriately generalized rule. This is the driving force behind overfitting. Overfitting often indicates that the system is learning structure that is idiosyncratic to the training set and therefore generalization is occurring suboptimally. Without prior knowledge of the problem complexity or structure, achieving the ideal balance between accuracy and generalization may be impractical or even impossible. With that in mind, it seems unreasonable to expect M-LCSs to automatically evolve optimal individual rules for interpretation. The task then becomes one that aims to address the query: what reliable attribute patterns can we derive from the rule population as a whole?

For M-LCSs, existing strategies aimed at facilitating knowledge discovery focus on reducing the size of the rule population using rule compaction [106–109] or condensation [110,111], or alternatively, by modifying the rule representation [111,112]. These strategies are all in line with the classic paradigm of knowledge discovery wherein the goal is to identify explicit rules for interpretation that are accurate, and maximally general.

Kharbat et al. took a somewhat different approach to M-LCS rule compaction (rule-dependent as opposed to data-dependent) in order to extract minimal and representative rules from the original rule-set [113,115]. Rules were clustered based on similarity and these clusters were used to generate aggregate average rules and aggregate definite rules presenting the common characteristics of the cluster. These resulting aggregate rules are then interpreted by an expert in the field seeking knowledge discovery. This strategy reflected a more global perspective of rule-set evaluation looking for common patterns in a large population of rules. In the remainder of this section, we describe our strategy for extending this line of global thinking [101].

Specifically, the goals for applying a M-LCS to noisy single-step data mining problems include: (1) distinguishing predictive from non-predictive attributes with statistical confidence, (2) identifying optimally generalized and accurate rule association patterns, and (3) facilitating the identification of, and discrimination between, interaction and heterogeneity. These goals are critical for making M-LCS a viable data mining tool for our bioinformatics problem of interest. To address these goals, we developed a globally minded analysis pipeline that introduces novel statistics, a strategy for significance testing, and the application of visualizations to guide knowledge discovery in M-LCSs. We have successfully applied this pipeline to a complex simulated genetic association dataset embedded with heterogeneity and epistasis [101]. Unique to gene association studies, we demonstrated that this analysis pipeline facilitates the identification and characterization of heterogeneity and epistasis.

In this section and those that follow, complex simulated datasets which concurrently model both epistasis and heterogeneity were generated using GAMETES [29,116]. GAMETES is a freely available piece of software for generating purely epistatic disease models. For the purposes of the analysis pipeline discussion, a dataset was used with two separate two-locus purely epistatic models [101]. In total, the dataset contained four predictive attributes, where only two attributes were predictive within a respective subset of the data. Additionally, the dataset contained 16 randomly generated nonpredictive attributes. Minor allele frequencies of all four predictive attributes were 0.2, heritabilities for both underlying models was 0.4, the ratio of samples representative of either model was 50:50, and the dataset sample size was 1600.

To highlight the need for such an analysis pipeline, we begin with an example of manual inspection within the rule population evolved by UCS on a noisy simulated dataset. Table 9.1 displays the top 10 rules identified by UCS after 200,000 learning iterations. Half the samples in the dataset were generated with a predictive epistatic interaction between attributes "X0" and "X1," while the other half were generated with a different epistatic interaction between attributes "X2" and "X3." All other attributes were randomly simulated as non-predictive. Optimally generalized rules would strictly specify one of these two pairs of attributes (i.e., X0, X1 or X2, X3), but no others. Examining the top 10 rules in Table 9.1, we can see that this is never the case. We do see that the correct attribute pairs often occur together in these top rules, but one or two other non-predictive attributes tend to be specified as well. Specification of these non-predictive attributes affords the rule higher accuracy in the training data (all top rules in Table 9.1 have 100% accuracy). Scanning down the complete ordered list of rules, we finally observed an optimally generalized rule 43rd down on the list; however, without already knowing the true association pattern we would have no way of identifying that rule as optimal. So how do we separate the attributes that are reliable, and those which are the product of overfitting in a noisy environment?

Our proposed analysis pipeline includes the following steps: (1) run the M-LCS algorithm with 10-fold cross-validation (CV) on the dataset, (2) run

Table 9.1 Manual rule inspection of a UCS rule population. Rules (R's) are ordered by decreasing numerosity (Num.). To save space, we have left out SNPs (X's) which were generalized in each of these top 10 rules. The accuracy of each rule listed in the table was 100%.

	X0	X1	X2	X3	X4	X6	X7	X8	X10	X11	X15	X18	CLASS	NUM.
R1	#	#	0	1	#	#	1	#	#	#	#	1	1	10
R2	1	0	1	0	#	#	#	#	#	#	#	#	1	9
R3	#	0	1	1	#	#	#	#	0	#	1	#	0	9
R4	2	1	#	#	#	#	1	#	#	#	#	#	1	6
R5	1	1	#	#	2	#	#	#	#	0	#	#	0	6
R6	0	1	0	1	#	#	#	#	#	#	#	#	1	6
R7	#	#	1	0	#	0	#	#	0	#	1	#	1	6
R8	1	0	#	#	#	#	#	2	#	#	#	#	1	5
R9	#	#	1	1	#	0	#	#	0	#	#	1	0	5
R10	#	#	1	1	#	#	#	#	0	#	2	#	0	5

a permutation test with 1000 permutations, (3) confirm significance of testing accuracy, (4) identify significant attributes and significantly co-occurring pairs of attributes, (5) train the M-LCS algorithm on the entire dataset, (6) generate a clustered heat map of the rule population, (7) generate a network depicting attribute co-occurrence, and (8) combine statistical results with visualizations to interpret and generate hypothesis for further exploration and validation. This pipeline could be expanded to knowledge discovery in any M-LCS applied to a single-step data mining problem.

9.3.1.1 *Run the M-LCS*

This subsection details Steps 1 and 2. First, we employed a 10 fold CV strategy in order to determine average testing accuracy and account for overfitting. The dataset is randomly partitioned into 10 equal parts and UCS is run 10 separate times during which 9/10ths of the data is used to train the algorithm, and a different 1/10th is set aside for testing. We averaged training and testing accuracies over these 10 runs. Next, we set up our permutation test. A permutation test involves repeating the analysis on variations of the dataset (with class status shuffled) in order to determine the likelihood that the observed result could have occurred by chance. We chose to use the permutation test since we do not know the chance distribution of our statistics ahead of time. We generated 1000 permuted versions of the original dataset by randomly permuting the affection status (class) of all samples, while preserving the number of cases and controls. For each permuted dataset we ran UCS using 10 fold CV. In total, permutation testing requires 10,000 runs of UCS.

9.3.1.2 *Significance Testing of M-LCS Statistics*

This subsection details Steps 3 and 4. First, and foremost, we confirmed that our average testing accuracy from Step 1 is significantly higher than those obtained by random chance. We utilized a typical one-tailed permutation test with a significance threshold of $p < 0.05$. To determine p for a test statistic (in this case average testing accuracy) calculate the test statistic for each of the 1000 permuted, CV analyses. If the true test statistic from Step 1 is greater than 95% of the 1000 permuted runs, you can reject the null hypothesis at $p < 0.05$. Here, the null hypothesis is: the observed value of the statistic could have likely occurred by chance. If the true test statistic is greater than all of the 1000 permuted runs, a minimum p of 0.001 is achieved. Our analysis on the aforementioned dataset yielded a significant testing accuracy of 0.701 ($p = 0.001$).

If average testing accuracy is not significantly high, this suggests that M-LCS was unable to learn any useful generalizations from the data, and there is little reason to progress with the rest of this analysis pathway. Failure to obtain a significant testing accuracy suggests either the absence of a useful generalization within the data, or that the run settings for the M-LCS were inappropriate for the detection of an existing generalization (e.g., a larger population size or greater number of learning iterations may be required).

Once a significant testing accuracy is confirmed, we used the permutation test analysis to identify attributes in the dataset that show significant importance in making accurate classification. Here we describe novel population state metrics (test statistics describing the state of the rule population) for making such an inference from the rule population: (1) Specificity Sum (SpS) and (2) Accuracy Weighted Specificity Sum (AWSpS). The SpS is identical in principle to our previously described power estimation strategy [99]. The premise for this statistic states that if an M-LCS is learning useful generalizations while training on the data, attributes that are important for making correct classifications will tend to be specified more frequently within rules of the population. Alternatively, attributes that are not useful for making correct classifications will tend to be generalized ("#"/"don't care" symbol used). SpS is calculated separately for each attribute, and is simply the number of rules in the population that specifies a value for that attribute (as opposed to having a "#"). This calculation takes rule numerosity into account, since numerosity represents the number of copies of that rule presently in the population. As an alternative to SpS, we also consider AWSpS, which simply weights the SpS by the respective rule accuracies. Like SpS, AWSpS is calculated separately for each attribute and takes numerosity into account. Table 9.2 gives a simple example in which both SpS and AWSpS are calculated from a hypothetical population consisting of four rules. Notice how SpS and AWSpS scores for attributes "X1" and "X4" stand out from the rest.

The intuition behind using AWSpS vs. SpS is based on the idea that: at any given learning iteration, it is possible for a non-predictive attribute to be specified frequently in rules of the population just by chance. Consider the hypothetical situation in which a predictive attribute and non-predictive attribute happen to be specified with equal frequency. We would expect that, overall, rules specifying the predictive attribute would tend to have higher accuracies than rules with the non-predictive attribute. Therefore, by weighting specification frequency by accuracy, we would be more likely to correctly favor the predictive attribute as important to classification and avoid false positives. Conversely, by chance, non-predictive attributes could be specified along with predictive attributes in a highly accurate rule. In this case, the non-predictive attributes might receive a parasitic boost from the overall high accuracy of the rule, potentially encouraging a false positive. Because of this dilemma we considered both statistics.

Table 9.2 Example calculation of SpS and AWSpS within unordered hypothetical rules.

	X1	X2	X3	X4	CLASS	NUMEROSITY	ACCURACY
R1	2	#	#	1	0	5	0.73
R2	#	0	#	2	1	1	0.51
R3	2	0	#	1	0	2	0.88
R4	#	0	1	#	1	1	0.62
SpS	7	4	1	8			
AWSpS	5.41	2.89	0.62	5.92			

Again, we used permutation testing to determine the significance of attributes using the SpS and AWSpS metrics. For each attribute, we separately calculated SpS and AWSpS over the 10 CV rule populations trained in Step 1. We also compared this sum for each attribute to the 1000 respective sums from permutation testing to determine whether the true SpS or AWSpS is significantly higher than we would expect by chance. Significance values are calculated as previously described for each attribute. This step provides us with a statistically justified strategy for discriminating between predictive and non-predictive attributes in an M-LCS rule population.

Our previous work [101] has shown that the SpS and AWSpS for our four predictive attributes (i.e., X0, X1, X2, X3) are significantly higher than would be expected by chance with sums dramatically larger than non-predictive attributes.

The last population state metric we introduced considered pairwise attribute co-occurrence within rules. We considered this statistic in order to evaluate attribute interactions as well as help discriminate between interactions and heterogeneity. We calculated co-occurrence for every non-redundant pair-wise combination of attributes in the dataset. For a dataset with 20 attributes (such as the one we examined in [101]), we calculated 190 co-occurrence values. We calculated co-occurrence as follows: for every pair of attributes we go through each of the 10 CV rule populations and sum the number of times that both attributes are concurrently specified in a given rule. In the example from Table 9.2 the Co-occurrence Sum (CoS) for the attribute pair (X1, X2) would be two since the pair only co-occurs in Rule 3, and the rule has a numerosity of two. The significance of co-occurrence scores is determined as before using the results of permutation testing for each pair of attributes.

Our study [101] showed that epistatic pairs of predictive attributes yielded the two highest CoSs. Below these two pairs, there was an immediate drop-off in the magnitude of observed CoS (almost halved). These results suggest that attribute pairs $(X0, X1)$, and $(X2, X3)$ each represent an interacting pair. But, since the four other pairwise combinations of these attributes have about half the co-occurrence, we might suspect heterogeneity as opposed to a three- or four-way interaction. In a later subsection, we will discuss a visualization strategy for these co-occurrence results. In practice, this co-occurrence analysis could be extended to higher order co-occurrence between all three-way combinations of attributes (or beyond).

9.3.1.3 *A Heat Map Visualization*

As previously suggested [117], the "visualization of classification models can create understanding and trust in data mining models." While visualization strategies are not entirely new to the LCS field, to date they have been applied only to track learning progress within the search space [118,119]. The key difference here is that visualization is applied directly to knowledge discovery for the identification of global attribute generalizations.

This subsection details Steps 5 and 6. All M-LCS runs described up to this point have been dedicated to obtaining test statistics and making statistical inferences. The first step toward visualization is to train the M-LCS on the entire dataset. M-LCS algorithms are typically very adaptive with a tendency to maintain some level of diversity in the population as it attempts to search for better and better rules. As a result, we would expect that some proportion of the rules to be poor classifiers with useless generalizations. As previously mentioned, rule compaction and condensation algorithms offer a method of eliminating useless rules and reducing the size of the rule population. While beyond the scope of the present discussion, such an algorithm could be used at this point in the analysis pipeline in an attempt to remove some of these useless, "noisy" rules. However, based on preliminary observations that explored rule compaction algorithms, we would caution the reader that a dramatic reduction in the size of the rule population may be counterproductive to successfully identifying global patterns.

The next step includes re-encoding of the rule population. The objective of the heat map visualization is to discriminate predictive attributes from nonpredictive attributes and to look for patterns of attribute interaction and heterogeneity. Therefore, we encoded each rule such that any specified attribute is coded as a 1 while a "#" is coded as a 0. Additionally, we expanded our rule population such that there are N copies of each rule reflecting respective numerosities. Similar to ordering by rule numerosity within manual inspection, this step draws greater attention to attribute patterns within rules having a higher numerosity. The last processing step before visualization is to apply a clustering algorithm to the coded and expanded rule population.

Kharbat et al. pioneered the clustering a population of M-LCS rules for rule compaction [114,115]. In our previously published study [101], we employed agglomerative hierarchical clustering using hamming distance as the distance metric. Clustering was performed on both axes (i.e., across rules and attributes). Both clustering and 2D heat map visualization were performed in R using the *hclust* and *gplots* packages, respectively.

Lastly, we applied 2D heat maps to highlight global attribute patterns for knowledge discovery in M-LCSs. Figure 9.7 gives an example of 2D heat maps visualizing the rule population. In Figure 9.7a, the only clearly discernible pattern is the relative high specification of the four modeled attributes (X0, X1, X2, and X3) on the left. These four columns stand out as having more yellow[1] color than the others. After clustering, the utility of this visualization becomes much more apparent. While portions of Figure 9.7b are relatively noisy, we see two dominant rule patterns emerge, one involving attributes X0 and X1, and the other involving attributes X2 and X3. Note how hierarchical clustering separates these independent epistatic models, suggesting the presence of a heterogeneity vs. higher order interactions. If a four-way interaction was present, we would instead expect all four attributes to cluster together.

9.3.1.4 *A Co-Occurrence Network*

This subsection details Step 7. A network visualization may be generated using either the M-LCS run from Step 5, or from the 10 CV runs from Step 1. We use the 10 CV runs, since they include statistical analysis and summation over multiple runs. To generate the co-occurrence network we used Gephi (http://gephi.org/) an open source graph visualization software. Using the 190 CoSs calculated in our previously published study [101], we generated an adjacency matrix in a format consistent with Gephi requirements. Using Gephi, we generated a fully connected, undirected network, where nodes represent individual attributes, the diameter of a node is the SpS for that attribute, edges represent co-occurrence, and the thickness of an edge is the respective CoS. Additionally, Gephi offers a built-in function to filter edges from the network based on edge weight. Users can progressively filter out edges representing smaller CoSs in order to identify dominant patterns.

Figure 9.8 gives the co-occurrence network illustrating the 190 previously calculated CoSs. Filtering the network is a largely subjective process since the ideal filter threshold to capture the true underlying pattern is not known ahead of time. However, by adjusting the filter threshold the investigator can isolate dominant patterns and exclude those less likely to be of interest. In Figure

---

[1] For interpretation of color in Figure 9.7, the reader is referred to the web version of this book.

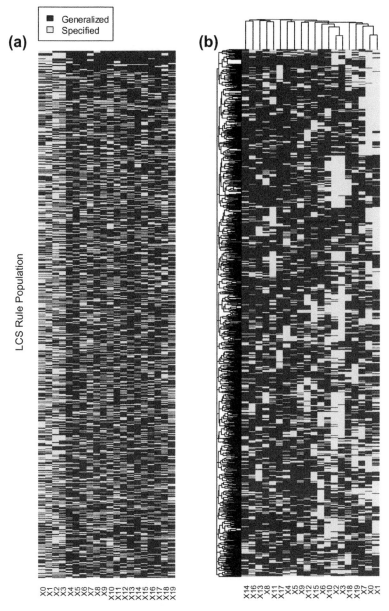

■ **FIGURE 9.7** Heat-map visualizations of the evolved M-LCS rule population. (a) Illustrates the raw rule population after encoding and expansion. Each row in the heat-map is 1 of 2000 rules comprising the population. Each column is one of the 20 attributes. Four of these (X0, X1, X2, and X3) were modeled as predictive attributes. (b) Illustrates the same population after hierarchical clustering on both axes. According to the attribute dendrogram, each pair of interacting attributes (X0, X1) and (X2, X3) modeled in this data, cluster together best of all attributes.

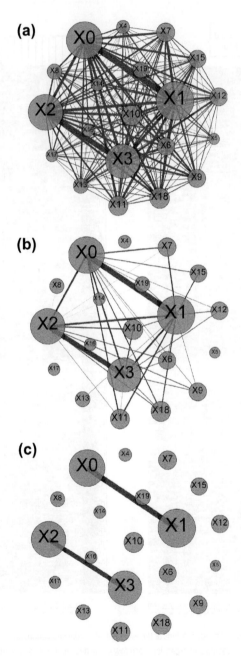

■ **FIGURE 9.8** Co-occurrence networks—(a) Illustrates the fully connected network before any filtering is applied. The diameter of a node is the SpS for that attribute, edges represent co-occurrence, and the thickness of an edge is the respective CoS. (b) The network after filtering out all CoSs that did not meet the significance cut-off. (c) The network after filtering out all but the two highest CoSs.

9.8, images (a) through (b) show the network with a progressively more stringent edge weight filter. In each, the strong co-occurrence between $(X0, X1)$ as well as between $(X2, X3)$ can be observed, illustrating the interaction between these respective attribute pairs. In addition, the diameter of the nodes draws attention to the same four predictive attributes. Figure 9.8c accurately captured the underlying relationships modeled in that simulated dataset. More specifically, we observed interaction between pairs $(X0, X1)$ and $(X2, X3)$ but independence between the pairs, as would be expected given the embedded heterogeneity. Notice the relationship between Figures 9.7 and 9.8. The network visualization efficiently summarizes the key features of the heat map.

9.3.1.5 *Guided Knowledge Discovery*

This subsection details Step 8. The final step in our analysis pipeline involves the merging of all empirical and subjective observations made thus far in order to characterize useful rule generalizations, and generate hypotheses for further investigation. Up to this point, the pipeline analysis previously described [101] had: (1) successfully identified our four predictive attributes, significantly differentiated them from "noise" attributes, (2) identified strong, significant co-occurrence between both epistatic attribute pairs, but observed a dramatic drop in co-occurrence for other pairwise combinations of the four predictive attributes (evidence against a higher order interaction), (3) observed separate clustering of the significant attribute pairs in the 2D heat map (evidence of heterogeneity), and (4) observed two dominant attribute co-occurrence pairs (evidence of interaction within each pair, and heterogeneity between them). Together, these observations correctly reflect the predictive attributes, interactions, and heterogeneity embedded in this complex simulated data. If only manual inspection had been used, we would have several additional irrelevant attributes to consider as candidates, we would lack statistical confidence to back up our claims, and it would be difficult or impossible to get a clear picture of the true underlying patterns of association (see Table 9.1).

In this section, we have reviewed work in which we have: (1) introduced novel population state metrics (SpS, AWSpS, and CoS) for global rule-population characterization, (2) adapted significance testing to M-LCS evaluation, and (3) adapted visualization strategies to facilitate the identification of rule patterns [101]. This work was applied successfully to a challenging genetic association problem involving epistasis and heterogeneity. We demonstrated that this approach could be used to discriminate between predictive and non-predictive attributes, characterize interactions, and make observations which correctly point to underlying heterogeneous patterns. To the best of our knowledge, this was the first attempt to apply significance testing to knowledge discovery in LCSs.

While this pipeline offers a promising pathway for interpretation, this type of analysis is limited by substantial computational expense in running the M-LCS algorithm along with the necessary permutations and cross-validation. Given current computational technology, this makes analysis of large-scale genetic datasets impractical. M-LCSs and the analysis pipeline introduced here would be better suited to candidate studies with a refined set of potentially predictive attributes. Beyond UCS and the bioinformatic problem considered in this work, this pipeline has the potential for application to any M-LCS tasked with a single-step data mining problem. Even if the proposed pathway as a whole is not applicable or practical for all problem domains we expect that certain components, such as our visualizations, will be more universally relatable.

9.3.2 Aiding Scalability with Expert Knowledge

In this section, we shift back to the challenge of addressing scalability and learning speed. As discussed earlier, we have approached this problem by applying expert knowledge to the covering and mutation operators of an M-LCS algorithm [102]. To achieve this goal, we discuss how to: (1) derive expert knowledge from Spatially Uniform ReliefF (SURF) [48], (2) adopt a logistic function to reliably transform any set of expert knowledge scores into a set of attribute respective probabilities, and (3) utilize these probabilities to intelligently guide covering and mutation operators within M-LCS toward regions of the problem domain most likely to be of interest.

9.3.2.1 *Expert Knowledge from SURF*

Expert knowledge (EK) is an external source of information providing, in this context, a measure of attribute quality. In this example the external measure is statistical, but it could just as easily be biological. The usefulness of EK is entirely dependent on its quality. There are many statistical and computational methods for determining the quality of attributes. In previous work [102], we selected a method that is capable of identifying attributes that predict class primarily through dependencies or interactions with other attributes. To this end, we selected SURF [48] as the source of EK. SURF estimates the quality of attributes through a nearest neighbor algorithm that selects neighbors (case or control instances) within an automatically determined distance threshold. Weights, or quality estimates, for each attribute are estimated based on whether the nearest neighbor (nearest hit) of a randomly selected instance from the same class and the nearest neighbor from the other class (nearest miss) have the same or different values. In addition to SURF, Greene et al. [48] also evaluated Tuned ReliefF (TuRF) [47], which was designed for human genetics application. TuRF systematically removes attributes that have low quality estimates so that the ReliefF values of the remaining attributes can be re-estimated. SURF and TuRF could be combined in future work to derive EK-scores, but in our study [102] we exclusively utilized SURF to generate EK-scores for each evaluated dataset. Note that the SURF run time is negligible compared to that of UCS: requiring a matter of seconds to run.

9.3.2.2 *Transformation of EK into Probabilities*

This subsection reviews our application of the logistic function in order to transform raw EK scores into normalized probability values. We start with a set of raw EK values (K). We know neither the range nor distribution of the EK values. The only requirement is that greater importance should translate to a larger EK score. Let k_i be the ith score within K.

We use the logistic function to transform the raw values into selection probabilities. Namely,

$$\ell_{\alpha,\beta}(x) = \frac{1}{1 + e^{-(\alpha+\beta x)}}. \tag{9.1}$$

Before applying this function we must determine values for constants α and β. First, the user specifies a range constant d. We have chosen $d=0.4$, which yields an output range of $(0.5 - d = d_l = 0.1, 0.5 + d = d_u = 0.9)$. This range ensures that the attribute with the lowest EK score retains at least a 10% chance to be specified, while the attribute with the highest EK score has no greater than a 90% chance to be specified. Next, the user must specify c, which is the resulting sum of probabilities in the transformed set. This is useful when one wants to guarantee that a selection algorithm, given the set of probabilities, returns a certain number of individuals on average. In our previous study [102], we wanted selection to choose 50% of the attributes during covering, therefore we set $c=10$ since datasets each have 20 attributes. Lastly, the user must specify how many digits of precision (set to 5 here) we use when calculating α in Step 5. EK transformation progresses in five steps as follows:

Step 1: Compute the range $r = max(K) - min(K)$.

Step 2: Shift scores such that the lowest score is at minimum zero. If $min(K)<0$, then add $abs(min(K))$ to every EK score.

Step 3: Compute β such that the logistic function's slope "nicely" occupies the data range, i.e.,

$$\ell_{\alpha,\beta}(-r/2) = d_l \tag{9.2}$$

and

$$\ell_{\alpha,\beta}(r/2) = d_u. \tag{9.3}$$

Since α does not affect slope we set $\alpha=0$ while calculating β. We solve for β after some simple algebra with the following:

$$\beta = 2 \ln \left(\frac{1 - d_l}{d_l} \right) / r. \tag{9.4}$$

Step 4: Compute an initial guess for α such that:

$$\ell_{\alpha,\beta}(min(K)) = d_l. \tag{9.5}$$

Since α simply shifts the function left or right we only need to move the curve such that the minimum EK score is transformed to d_l. We solve for this initial α_o using the following equation derived again with some simple algebra:

$$\alpha_0 = -\beta(min(K) + r/2). \tag{9.6}$$

Step 5: In order to find α such that the transformed probabilities sum to c we iteratively search for an appropriate value of α using the Newton-Raphson method. For our purposes, β is a constant. We applied differential calculus to obtain:

$$\alpha_j = \alpha_{j-1} - \frac{\sum_{i=1}^{n} \ell_{\alpha,\beta}(k_i) - c}{\sum_{i=1}^{n} \ell'_{\alpha,\beta}(k_i)}. \tag{9.7}$$

We iterate this equation until $\alpha_j=\alpha_{j-1}$ with respect to the digits of precision. At this point, applying the logistic function to the input scores (K) using the computed parameters, α, β, will produce a set of probabilities that sum to the desired c.

9.3.2.3 *Applying EK to Covering and Mutation*

Once EK-based probabilities have been generated for all attributes, we can incorporate these as weights to guide LCS learning. To achieve this, we apply these probabilities to both covering and mutation operators within M-LCS. As discussed, the covering operator is responsible for population initialization, as well as ensuring that a matching rule exists for a given data instance within each learning iteration. Previously, EK has been successfully applied to population initialization in genetic programming [120].

In the context of M-LCS, EK probabilities drive the specialization (state is important) or generalization (state is not important) of attributes within rules. Having chosen a c of 10, rules generated via covering will tend to have half of the 20 attributes specified, and half generalized. A traditional covering mechanism would thus give each attribute a 50% chance of being specialized. With the incorporation of EK, attributes with higher EK-scores (likely to be useful) will have a higher probability of being specified, and vice versa.

As mentioned earlier, the mutation mechanism is a discovery component of the M-LCS. When activated, mutation traditionally randomly permutes an element of the rule such that if it had been specified it becomes generalized and vice versa. Previously, EK has been successfully applied to mutation in genetic programming [121]. Here, we apply EK probabilities to mutation, such that if an attribute is selected for "possible" mutation, the probability of mutation is equal to the EK probability for that attribute. Specified attributes with high EK scores will be less likely to be generalized while generalized attribute with high EK scores will more likely to be flipped to specified. The opposite is true for attribute with low EK scores.

Our work [102] examined four algorithmic implementations: (1) UCS algorithm without EK, (2) UCS with EK applied to covering only, (3) UCS with EK applied to mutation only, and (4) UCS with EK applied to both covering and mutation. The results of this work indicated that EK could be successfully applied to an M-LCS algorithm to improve learning efficiency, and thus ameliorate the problem of scalability and run time. In particular, EK applied to covering was able to significantly improve learning without interfering in the detection of patterns of epistasis or heterogeneity. This work supports the overall conclusion of related studies examining EK in the context of evolutionary algorithms [120–122]: that EK can be effective at pointing the algorithm toward attributes of greatest interest therefore facilitating the algorithm's ability to find "the genetic needle in the genomic haystack." This work suggests that future implementations of such an M-LCS could benefit from a smart EK-guided cover mechanism, which will initialize the algorithm to begin exploring areas of the search space more likely to be of value.

9.3.3 **Characterizing Heterogeneity**

In this section, we return to the particularly unique problem of dealing with heterogeneous patterns of association. We have developed AF-UCS as an expansion of the UCS algorithm to allow for the explicit characterization of heterogeneity, as well as to improve efficient generalization and learning in the M-LCS [103]. This work introduced attribute tracking, a mechanism akin to memory, for supervised learning in M-LCS. Additionally, we introduced attribute feedback and applied it to the mutation and crossover mechanisms, probabilistically directing rule generalization based on an instance's tracking scores. Lastly, we demonstrated how the clustering of subjects based on these tracking scores may be used to characterize heterogeneity, as well as to suggest how they may be used to identify individuals belonging to etiologically heterogeneous subgroups (or disease sub types).

The concept of adding memory to LCSs has been previously explored [123–125]. However, in previous studies, this form of memory was both temporary and designed to improve performance on non-Markov, multi-step problems by preserving limited information regarding a previous state. Alternatively, *attribute tracking* is a collective form of memory designed to be applied to single-step supervised learning problems. Essentially this mechanism learns which attributes are most important to the accurate classification of each individual instance, storing and accumulating this knowledge independent of the rule population. This mechanism is driven by incremental learning and therefore is specific to M-LCSs rather than P-LCSs.

We begin here by describing our algorithm AT-UCS, which combines attribute tracking alone with UCS. Figure 9.9 illustrates attribute tracking as it is incorporated into UCS. Attribute tracking is stored as a vector of summed accuracy scores that accumulate over learning iterations. Each instance in the dataset has its own unique vector with length equal to the number of attributes. Therefore AT-UCS will maintain a matrix of attribute tracking scores with the same dimensions as the training data. Tracking scores for a given instance are only updated during learning iterations in which that instance are called. Following the typical formation of the match and correct sets (described as the rules of the correct set that are passed to the environment where the attribute tracking vectors are stored [67]). For each rule in the correct set, we do the following: (1) check each attribute in the rule to see if it has been specified (i.e., not "#"), then, if so, (2) update the attribute tracking score for that attribute by adding the accuracy of the rule.

After learning is complete, normalization, clustering, and visualization can be applied to attribute tracking scores. In noisy data, some instances will be easier to classify than others. These instances will tend to accumulate higher attribute tracking scores making comparisons between instances more challenging. To overcome this, we normalize attribute tracking scores within each instance such that they lie between 0 and 1. Normalization is achieved here by dividing each tracking score by the sum of all tracking scores for that instance.

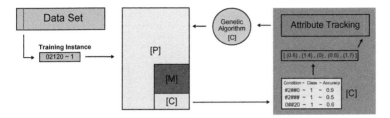

■ **FIGURE 9.9** Attribute tracking in the context of a UCS learning iteration. Only the steps relevant to attribute tracking are included. Notice how attribute tracking scores are updated each iteration only for the current training instance, and based on what attributes had been specified in the rules of the current [C]. The list of values in the purple box is added to the current instance's tracking scores. (For interpretation of the references to color in this figure legend, the reader is referred to the web version of this book.)

Our visualization strategy began with agglomerative hierarchical clustering of the attribute tracking matrix in R. Clustering was performed on both axes (i.e., across instances and attributes). Next, we visualized the clustered scores in a heat map. Figure 9.10 illustrates an example of our attribute tracking score visualization using the same dataset described in the section on "Interpretability and Knowledge Discovery." As described previously [101], for the purposes of visualization we train AT-UCS on the entire dataset (no CV). The attribute scores from Figure 9.10 were obtained over the course of 200,000 learning iterations, followed by normalization. With normalization, an attribute's tracking score is given with respect to the other scores for an instance as opposed to all scores in the dataset. Normalization removes overall magnitude bias from clustering, allowing us to better compare attribute patterns between instances. We would expect some instances to obtain higher overall attribute tracking magnitudes during training, since certain niches of the underlying problem may be solved sooner than others (by chance or because they were easier to find). When this occurs, instances representative of that niche will match rules with higher accuracy for a greater number of epochs (i.e., cycles through the dataset), resulting in a larger accumulation of attribute tracking scores. Given that the patterns recognized in Figure 9.10 quite accurately reflect the heterogeneity and interactions modeled in the given dataset, we propose that similar analysis and visualization of attribute tracking scores can also serve to guide knowledge discovery in M-LCS data mining. It is worth noting that because all our models have a heritability < 1, we expect a certain number of instances to be unreliably classified based on the given set of attributes. Therefore, we expect a certain amount of noise in our attribute tracking scores. Attribute tracking can be run either on its own or in concert with attribute feedback.

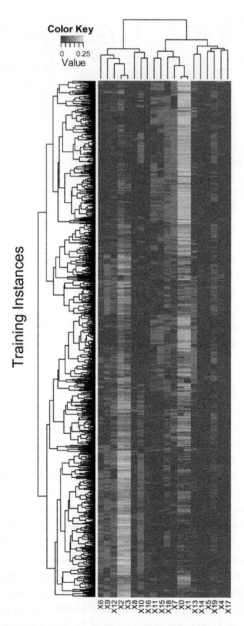

■ **FIGURE 9.10** Heat-map of normalized and clustered attribute tracking scores obtained after running AT-UCS on the simulated dataset previously described in this chapter. Each row in the heat-map is 1 of 1600 instances comprising the training data. Each column is one of 20 attributes in that dataset (X0, X1, X2, and X3 are predictive). Yellow indicates higher normalized tracking scores, while blue indicates lower ones. (For interpretation of the references to color in this figure legend, the reader is referred to the web version of this book.)

Attribute feedback is a heuristic which draws upon the knowledge learned in attribute tracking to promote efficient generalization and improve learning in the presence of noisy, complex, and heterogeneous data. Attribute feedback probabilistically directs generalization pressures in the genetic algorithm (GA) based on relative attribute tracking scores. Specifically, we implement attribute feedback into both mutation and uniform crossover mechanisms.

Attribute feedback converts the attribute tracking scores into probabilities that in turn are used to direct the GA mechanisms. The premise behind attribute feedback is to apply collective experience, specific to a given instance, to pressure the GA into focusing on attributes likely to be valuable for accurate classification, and avoid specifying attributes that are not. Ideally, this will promote efficient generalization and reduce overfitting. Additionally, since this pressure is specific to each instance, it should promote niching and maintain relevant diversity in the rule population.

Another benefit to attribute feedback involves the persistence of the accumulated experience. Typically, knowledge learned by an LCS is contained exclusively in the rule population. Since it is possible for good rules to be deleted by chance, there is the potential for knowledge loss, which in turn can slow down learning. By including a form of persistent memory we can, in some part, preserve experiential knowledge of the rule population that was lost in deletion.

Preliminary analysis indicated that employment of attribute feedback early in the learning process yielded significantly less success. This makes sense since the knowledge accumulated by attribute tracking early on is likely to be poor. Therefore we implement attribute feedback such that at a given iteration it is used with probability equal to the proportion of completed algorithm iterations (*%Complete*). Thus early in learning, it is employed sparingly, while later it is employed frequently.

As mentioned, we implement attribute feedback into both mutation and uniform crossover. Once either mechanism is called, we first decide whether to use the original mechanism, or the respective mechanism with attribute feedback. As mentioned, we used attribute feedback with probability equal to *%Complete*. If attribute feedback is to be used, we begin by calculating the specification probability (*Pspec*) for each attribute in the instance. We obtain these probabilities by transforming the current vector of tracking scores for that instance. First, we subtract the minimum tracking score from all scores in the vector. Next, we find the maximum score (*maxT*) in this new vector and divide each score by $maxT + maxT*0.01$ giving us the desired probabilities. We add 1% of *maxT* to the denominator to ensure that the attribute with the highest track score has less than a 100% of *Pspec*. However, the attribute with the lowest track score will inevitably have a 0% *Pspec*. The choice of 0.01 here is arbitrary and could potentially be varied by the user as a run parameter. If the instance has not yet been involved in a learning iteration ($maxT = 0$), the *Pspec* for each attribute is set at 50%.

The original mutation mechanism permutes attributes in a rule condition to either specify the instance's state, or generalizes it (i.e., add a "#"/don't care symbol). The probability of mutation is equal for each attribute in the condition. Alternatively with attribute feedback, if the attribute is currently generalized, then we only flip to the specified state with a probability of *Pspec*. Here, attributes learned by the attribute tracking that are deemed to be less important to classification are encouraged to remain generalized, and vice versa. If the attribute is currently specified, then we only flip to "#" with a probability of $1 - Pspec$. Here, attributes learned by attribute tracking to be more important to classification are encouraged to remain specified, and vice versa.

The goal of uniform crossover with attribute feedback is to produce an offspring that takes the best from both parents (Schwarz), and put what's left in the other offspring (DeVito) [126]. Again, crossover can only swap the specification of an attribute with generalization. Therefore, for a given attribute, parent rules either agree to specify, agree to generalize, or differ. When they differ, the Schwarz offspring receives the specified attribute with a probability of *Pspec*. Here, attributes learned by the attribute tracking to be important to classification tend to be specified in Schwarz and, by default, generalized in DeVito. The opposite is true for attributes with respectively lower attribute tracking scores.

Evaluation over a spectrum of simulated datasets indicates that attribute feedback can significantly increase testing accuracy, generality, and the power to find all predictive attributes in the data, while decreasing the population size, run time, and the power to find at least one interacting pair of predictive attributes [103]. Attribute tracking and feedback are likely to be valuable in complex, noisy, data mining problems such as the one described in this study, especially when the goal of analysis is the thorough characterization of underlying patterns of interaction and heterogeneity.

9.4 **RISE OF THE MACHINES**

9.4.1 **Conclusions**

In this chapter, we set out to examine an alternate paradigm of epidemiological modeling, one that makes minimal assumptions about underlying associations and one that evolves a solution comprised of many models instead of a single best classifier. The flexible, adaptive nature of LCS algorithms led us to the hypothesis that they would be well suited to discovering complex patterns of disease association, and uniquely well suited to discover patterns of heterogeneity. While Michigan-style LCS (M-LCS) algorithms have proven themselves to be a powerful and flexible machine learning strategy, we have examined a number of drawbacks to these systems in the context of biomedical data mining. In order to make M-LCS an attractive option for this problem, this chapter has discussed a set of recently published solutions addressing the most critical of these drawbacks. These include the development of: (1) simple global metrics to identify predictive attributes within the rule population, (2) strategies evaluating statistical significance in the context of an M-LCS, (3) strategies to improve scalability and learning though the application of expert knowledge, and (4) algorithmic mechanisms to explicitly characterize patterns of heterogeneity and improve learning efficiency (i.e., attribute tracking and feedback). These advances remove some major barriers keeping these versatile algorithms from mainstream use in biomedical data mining. However, there is still a wealth of opportunity for research in the successful development and application of M-LCS algorithms such as the one we have focused on in this chapter. We believe that it is critical for investigators to embrace machine learning strategies which allow the data to speak for itself, without making assumptions about underlying patters of association.

9.4.2 **Future Work**

As we have assembled this chapter, we are in the midst of developing a new M-LCS algorithm that combines what has been learned in the preceding sections and draws upon other advancements made collectively by the LCS research community to address many of the general LCS algorithm drawbacks reviewed earlier. This new algorithm, Extended Supervised Tracking and Classifying System (ExSTraCS), will be freely available for download, user-friendly, and offer all of the advancements discussed in this chapter, along with ability to simultaneously accommodate both discrete attributes (such as SNPs) as well as continuous attributes (such as microarray values), as well as extend from discrete endpoints (such as case vs. control) to quantitative traits (such as height).

9.4.3 **Resources**

To learn more about LCS algorithms, we refer readers to a number of previously published review papers [64,69,127–135]. Additionally, a detailed examination of the design and analysis of LCS algorithms has also been published [136]. For those interested in actively pursuing LCS-based research and development, an LCS and GBML web-based community may be found at http://gbml.org. This site offers postings of recent work, topical discussions, as well as access to freely available LCS algorithms and software. Additionally, an annual international workshop on learning classifier systems (IWLCS) has been held in association with the Genetic and Evolutionary Computation Conference (GECCO) since 2003.

REFERENCES

[1] Myers A. The age of the "ome": genome, transcriptome and proteome data set collection and analysis. Brain Res Bull; 2011.

[2] Shriner D, Vaughan L, Padilla M, Tiwari H. Problems with genome-wide association studies. Science 2007;316(5833):1840–2.

[3] Howe D, Costanzo M, Fey P, Gojobori T, Hannick L, Hide W, et al. Big data: the future of biocuration. Nature 2008;455(7209):47–50.

[4] Collins F, Lander E, Rogers J, Waterston R, Conso I. Finishing the euchromatic sequence of the human genome. Nature 2004;431(7011):931–45.

[5] Bantscheff M, Schirle M, Sweetman G, Rick J, Kuster B. Quantitative mass spectrometry in proteomics: a critical review. Anal Bioanal Chem 2007;389(4):1017–31.

[6] Goldberg A, Allis C, Bernstein E. Epigenetics: a landscape takes shape. Cell 2007;128(4):635.

[7] Betts J. Transcriptomics and proteomics: tools for the identification of novel drug targets and vaccine candidates for tuberculosis. IUBMB Life 2008;53(4–5): 239–42.

[8] Kandpal R, Saviola B, Felton J. The era of 'omics unlimited. Biotechniques 2009;46(5):351–5.

[9] Zbuk K, Eng C. Cancer phenomics: RET and PTEN as illustrative models. Nature Rev Cancer 2006;7:35–45.

[10] Spratlin J, Serkova N, Eckhardt S. Clinical applications of metabolomics in oncology: a review. Clin Cancer Res 2009;15(2):431–40.

[11] Egert M, De Graaf A, Smidt H, De Vos W, Venema K. Beyond diversity: functional microbiomics of the human colon. Trends Microbiol 2006;14(2):86–91.

[12] Wild C. Complementing the genome with an exposome: the outstanding challenge of environmental exposure measurement in molecular epidemiology. Cancer Epidemiol Biomarkers Prev 2005;14(8):1847–50.

[13] Ideker T, Galitski T, Hood L. A new approach to decoding life: systems biology. Ann Rev Genom Human Genet 2001;2:343–72.

[14] Crow J. A haplotype map of the human genome. Nature 2005;427:1299–320.

[15] McClellan J, King M. Genetic heterogeneity in human disease. Cell 2012; 141(2):210–7.

[16] Reich D, Lander E. On the allelic spectrum of human disease. Trends Genet 2001;17(9):502–10.

[17] Manolio T, Collins F, Cox N, Goldstein D, Hindorff L, Hunter D, et al. Finding the missing heritability of complex diseases. Nature 2009;461(7265):747–53.

[18] Van der Sluis S, Verhage M, Posthuma D, Dolan C. Phenotypic complexity, measurement bias, and poor phenotypic resolution contribute to the missing heritability problem in genetic association studies. PLoS One 2010;5(11):e13929.

[19] Queitsch C, Carlson K, Girirajan S. Lessons from model organisms: phenotypic robustness and missing heritability in complex disease. PLoS Genet 2012;8(11):e1003041.

[20] McKernan K, Peckham H, Costa G, McLaughlin S, Fu Y, Tsung E, et al. Sequence and structural variation in a human genome uncovered by short-read, massively parallel ligation sequencing using two-base encoding. Genome Res 2009;19(9):1527–41.

[21] Eichler E, Flint J, Gibson G, Kong A, Leal S, Moore J, et al. Missing heritability and strategies for finding the underlying causes of complex disease. Nature Rev Genet 2010;11(6):446–50.

[22] Gibson G. Rare and common variants: twenty arguments. Nature Rev Genet 2012;13(2):135–45.

[23] Thornton-Wells T, Moore J, Haines J. Genetics, statistics and human disease: analytical retooling for complexity. Trends Genet 2004;20(12):640–7.

[24] Cordell H. Epistasis: what it means, what it doesn't mean, and statistical methods to detect it in humans. Human Mol Genet 2002;11(20):2463–8.

[25] Donnelly P. Progress and challenges in genome-wide association studies in humans. Nature 2008;456(7223):728–31.

[26] Bateson W. Mendel's principles of heredity. Cosimo, Inc.; 2007.

[27] Fisher R. The correlation between relatives on the supposition of Mendelian inheritance. Trans Roy Soc Edinburgh 1919;52(02):399–433.

[28] Moore J, Williams S. Traversing the conceptual divide between biological and statistical epistasis: systems biology and a more modern synthesis. Bioessays 2005;27(6):637–46.

[29] Urbanowicz R, Kiralis J, Sinnott-Armstrong N, Heberling T, Fisher J, Moore J. GAMETES: a fast, direct algorithm for generating pure, strict, epistatic models with random architectures. BioData Mining 2012;5:16.

[30] Long J. The genetic structure of admixed populations. Genetics 1991;127(2):417–28.

[31] Cordell H. Detecting gene-gene interactions that underlie human diseases. Nature Rev Genet 2009;10(6):392–404.

[32] Moore J, Ritchie M. The challenges of whole-genome approaches to common diseases. J Am Med Assoc 2004;291(13):1642–3.

[33] Fayyad U, Piatetsky-Shapiro G, Smyth P, Uthurusamy R. Advances in knowledge discovery and data mining. Cambridge: MIT Press; 1996.

[34] Ritchie M, Hahn L, Roodi N, Bailey L, Dupont W, Parl F, et al. Multifactor-dimensionality reduction reveals high-order interactions among estrogen-metabolism genes in sporadic breast cancer. Am J Human Genet 2001;69:138.

[35] Andrew A, Nelson H, Kelsey K, Moore J, Meng A, Casella D, et al. Concordance of multiple analytical approaches demonstrates a complex relationship between DNA repair gene SNPs, smoking and bladder cancer susceptibility. Carcinogenesis 2006;27(5):1030–7.

[36] McKinney B, Reif D, Ritchie M, Moore J. Machine learning for detecting gene-gene interactions: a review. Appl Bioinform 2006;5(2):77.

[37] Jiang R, Tang W, Wu X, Fu W. A random forest approach to the detection of epistatic interactions in case-control studies. BMC Bioinform 2009;10(Suppl. 1):S65.

[38] Motsinger-Reif A, Dudek S, Hahn L, Ritchie M. Comparison of approaches for machine-learning optimization of neural networks for detecting gene-gene interactions in genetic epidemiology. Genet Epidemiol 2008;32(4):325–40.

[39] Moore J, Hahn L. A cellular automata approach to detecting interactions among single-nucleotide polymorphisms in complex multifactorial diseases. In: Pacific symposium on biocomputing, Vol. 7; 2002. p. 53–64.

[40] Zhang Y, Liu J. Bayesian inference of epistatic interactions in case-control studies. Nature Genet 2007;39(9):1167–73.

[41] Moore J, Hill D, Fisher J, Lavender N, Kidd L. Human-computer interaction in a computational evolution system for the genetic analysis of cancer. Genet Program Theory Practice 2011;IX:153–71.

[42] Carlborg O, Andersson L, Kinghorn B. The use of a genetic algorithm for simultaneous mapping of multiple interacting quantitative trait loci. Genetics 2000;155(4):2003–10.

[43] Urbanowicz R, Barney N, White B, Moore J. Mask functions for the symbolic modeling of epistasis using genetic programming. In: Proceedings of the 10th annual conference on genetic and evolutionary computation. ACM; 2008. p. 339–46.

[44] Greene C, Gilmore J, Kiralis J, Andrews P, Moore J. Optimal use of expert knowledge in ant colony optimization for the analysis of epistasis in human disease. Evolut Comput Mach Learn Data Mining Bioinform 2009:92–103.

[45] Penrod N, Greene C, Granizo-MacKenzie D, Moore J. Artificial immune systems for epistasis analysis in human genetics. Evolut Comput Mach Learn Data Mining Bioinform 2010:194–204.

[46] Kononenko I. Estimating attributes: analysis and extensions of RELIEF. Machine learning: ECML-94. Springer; 1994. p. 171–82.

[47] Moore J, White B. Tuning ReliefF for genome-wide genetic analysis. Evolut Comput Mach Learn Data Mining Bioinform 2007:166–75.

[48] Greene C, Penrod N, Kiralis J, Moore J. Spatially Uniform ReliefF (SURF) for computationally efficient filtering of gene-gene interactions. BioData Mining 2009;2:1–9.

[49] Ritchie M, Hahn L, Moore J. Power of multifactor dimensionality reduction for detecting gene-gene interactions in the presence of genotyping error, missing data, phenocopy, and genetic heterogeneity. Genet Epidemiol 2003;24(2):150–7.

[50] Smith C. Testing for heterogeneity of recombination fraction values in human genetics. Ann Human Genet 1963;27:175.

[51] Morton N. Sequential tests for the detection of linkage. Am J Human Genet 1955;7(3):277.

[52] Risch N. A new statistical test for linkage heterogeneity. Am J Human Genet 1988;42(2):353.

[53] Schmidt S, Scott W, Postel E, Agarwal A, Hauser E, De La Paz M, et al. Ordered subset linkage analysis supports a susceptibility locus for age-related macular degeneration on chromosome 16p12. BMC Genet 2004;5:18.

[54] Shao Y, Cuccaro M, Hauser E, Raiford K, Menold M, Wolpert C, et al. Fine mapping of autistic disorder to chromosome 15q11-q13 by use of phenotypic subtypes. Am J Human Genet 2003;72(3):539–48.

[55] Fenger M, Linneberg A, Werge T, Jorgensen T. Analysis of heterogeneity and epistasis in physiological mixed populations by combined structural equation modelling and latent class analysis. BMC Genet 2008;9:43.

[56] Shannon W, Province M, Rao D. Tree-based recursive partitioning methods for subdividing sibpairs into relatively more homogeneous subgroups. Genet Epidemiol 2001;20(3):293–306.

[57] Thornton-Wells T, Moore J, Haines J. Dissecting trait heterogeneity: a comparison of three clustering methods applied to genotypic data. BMC Bioinform 2006;7:204.

[58] Thornton-Wells T, Moore J, Martin E, Pericak-Vance M, Haines J. Confronting complexity in late-onset Alzheimer disease: application of two-stage analysis approach addressing heterogeneity and epistasis. Genet Epidemiol 2008;32(3):187–203.

[59] Edwards T, Lewis K, Velez D, Dudek S, Ritchie M. Exploring the performance of multifactor dimensionality reduction in large scale SNP studies and in the presence of genetic heterogeneity among epistatic disease models. Human Hered 2009;67(3):183–92.

[60] Lunetta K, Hayward L, Segal J, Van Eerdewegh P. Screening large-scale association study data: exploiting interactions using random forests. BMC Genet 2004;5:32.

[61] Bush W, Thornton-Wells T, Ritchie M. Association rule discovery has the ability to model complex genetic effects. Computational intelligence and data mining, CIDM. IEEE; 2007. p. 624–9.

[62] Mushlin R, Gallagher S, Kershenbaum A, Rebbeck T. Clique-finding for heterogeneity and multidimensionality in biomarker epidemiology research: the chamber algorithm. PloS One 2009;4(3):e4862.

[63] Moore J, Asselbergs F, Williams S. Bioinformatics challenges for genome-wide association studies. Bioinformatics 2010;26(4):445–55.

[64] Urbanowicz R, Moore J. Learning classifier systems: a complete introduction, review, and roadmap. J Artif Evolut Appl 2009;2009:1.

[65] LeBaron B, Arthur W, Palmer R. Time series properties of an artificial stock market. J Econ Dyn Control 1999;23(9):1487–516.

[66] Wilson S. Classifier fitness based on accuracy. Evolut Comput 1995;3(2):149–75.

[67] Bernado-Mansilla E, Garrell-Guiu J. Accuracy-based learning classifier systems: models, analysis and applications to classification tasks. Evolut Comput 2003;11(3):209–38.

[68] Dam H, Abbass H, Lokan C, Yao X. Neural-based learning classier systems. Trans Knowledge Data Eng 2008;20:26–39.

[69] Holmes J, Lanzi P, Stolzmann W, Wilson S. Learning classifier systems: new models, successful applications. Inf Process Lett 2002;82:23–30.

[70] Goldberg D. Genetic algorithms in search, optimization and machine learning. Boston, MA, USA: Addison-Wesley Longman Publishing Co., Inc.; 1989.

[71] Holland J. Adaptation in natural and artificial systems. Ann Arbor: University of Michigan Press; 1975.

[72] Holmes, J. (2000). Learning classifier systems applied to knowledge discovery in clinical research databases. Learning classifier systems, from foundations to applications. p. 243–62.

[73] Holland J. Adaptation. Progr Theor Biol 1976;4:263–93.

[74] Holland J, Reitman J. Cognitive systems based on adaptive agents. In: Waterman DA, Hayes-Roth F, editors. Pattern-directed inference systems; Academic Press, Inc. Orlando, FL, USA; 1978.

[75] Smith S. A learning system based on genetic adaptive algorithms. PhD thesis. University of Pittsburgh; 1980

[76] Congdon C. A comparison of genetic algorithms and other machine learning systems of a complex classification task from common disease research. PhD thesis. University of Michigan; 1995

[77] Holmes J. A genetics-based machine learning approach to knowledge discovery in clinical data. In: AMIA annual symposium; 1996. p. 883.

[78] Holmes J. Discovering risk of disease with a learning classifier system. In: Proceedings of the seventh international conference of genetic algorithms (ICGA97); 1997. p. 426–33.

[79] Holmes J, Sager J. Rule discovery in epidemiologic surveillance data using EpiXCS: an evolutionary computation approach. Lect Notes Comput Sci 2005;3581:444.

[80] Walter D, Mohan C. ClaDia: a fuzzy classifier system for disease diagnosis. In: Proceedings of the 2000 congress on evolutionary computation, Vol. 2; 2000.

[81] Wilson S. Mining oblique data with XCS. Revised papers from the third international workshop on advances in learning classifier systems; 2000. p. 158–76.

[82] Bacardit J, Butz M. Data mining in learning classifier systems: comparing XCS with GAssist. Lect Notes Comput Sci 2007;4399:282.

[83] Gao Y, Huang J, Rong H, Gu D. LCSE: learning classifier system ensemble for incremental medical instances. Lect Notes Comput Sci 2007;4399:93.

[84] Bernado E, Llora X, Garrell J. XCS and GALE: a comparative study of two learning classifier systems with six other learning algorithms on classification tasks. In: Proceedings of the fourth international workshop on learning classifier systems (IWLCS-2001); 2001. p. 337–41.

[85] Kharbat F, Bull L, Odeh M. Mining breast cancer data with XCS. In: Proceedings of the ninth annual conference on genetic and evolutionary computation; 2007. p. 2066–73.

[86] Unold O, Tuszynski K. Mining knowledge from data using anticipatory classifier system. Knowl Based Syst 2008;21(5):363–70.

[87] Blake C, Merz C. UCI repository of machine learning databases; 1998.

[88] Stout M, Bacardit J, Hirst J, Smith R, Krasnogor N. Prediction of topological contacts in proteins using learning classifier systems. Soft Comput — A Fus Found Methodol Appl 2009;13(3):245–58.

[89] Bacardit J, Stout M, Hirst J, Sastry K, Llora X, Krasnogor N. Automated alphabet reduction method with evolutionary algorithms for protein structure prediction. In: Proceedings of the ninth annual conference on genetic and evolutionary computation. New York, NY, USA: ACM Press; 2007. p. 346–53.

[90] Smith R, Jiang M. MILCS: a mutual information learning classifier system. In: Proceedings of the 2007 GECCO conference companion on genetic and evolutionary computation. New York, NY, USA: ACM Press; 2007.

[91] Bacardit J, Widera P, Marquez-Chamorro A, Divina F, Aguilar-Ruiz J, Krasnogor N. Contact map prediction using a large-scale ensemble of rule sets and the fusion of multiple predicted structural features. Bioinformatics 2012

[92] Llora X, Reddy R, Matesic B, Bhargava R. Towards better than human capability in diagnosing prostate cancer using infrared spectroscopic imaging. In: Proceedings of the ninth annual conference on genetic and evolutionary computation. New York, NY, USA: ACM Press; 2007.

[93] Alayon S, Estevez J, Sigut J, Sanchez J, Toledo P. An evolutionary Michigan recurrent fuzzy system for nuclei classification in cytological images using nuclear chromatin distribution. J Biomed Inform 2006;39(6):573–88.

[94] Unold O. Grammar-based classifier system for recognition of promoter regions. Lect Notes Comput Sci 2007;4431:798.

[95] Romao L, Nievola J. Hierarchical classification of gene ontology with learning classifier systems. Adv Artif Intell, IBERAMIA 2012;2012:120–9.

[96] Glaab E, Bacardit J, Garibaldi J, Krasnogor N. Using rule-based machine learning for candidate disease gene prioritization and sample classification of cancer gene expression data. PloS One 2012;7(7):e39932.

[97] Bassel G, Glaab E, Marquez J, Holdsworth M, Bacardit J. Functional network construction in Arabidopsis using rule-based machine learning on large-scale data sets. Plant Cell Online 2011;23(9):3101–16.

[98] Bacardit J, Burke E, Krasnogor N. Improving the scalability of rule-based evolutionary learning. Memetic Comput 2009;1:55–67.

[99] Urbanowicz R, Moore J. The application of Michigan-style learning classier systems to address genetic heterogeneity and epistasis in association studies. In: Proceedings of the 12th annual conference on genetic and evolutionary computation. ACM; 2010. p. 195–202.

[100] Urbanowicz R, Moore J. The application of Pittsburgh-style learning classifier systems to address genetic heterogeneity and epistasis in association studies. In: Parallel problem solving from nature, PPSN XI; 2011. p. 404–13.

[101] Urbanowicz R, Granizo-Mackenzie A, Moore J. An analysis pipeline with statistical and visualization-guided knowledge discovery for Michigan-style learning classifier systems. IEEE Comput Intell Mag 2012;7(4):35–45.

[102] Urbanowicz R, Granizo-Mackenzie D, Moore J. Using expert knowledge to guide covering and mutation in a Michigan style learning classifier system to detect epistasis and heterogeneity. In: Parallel problem solving from nature – PPSN XII; 2012. p. 266–75.

[103] Urbanowicz R, Granizo-Mackenzie A, Moore J. Instance-linked attribute tracking and feedback for Michigan-style supervised learning classifier systems. In: Proceedings of the 14th international conference on genetic and evolutionary computation conference. ACM; 2012. p. 927–34.

[104] Llora X, Reddy R, Matesic B, Bhargava R. Towards better than human capability in diagnosing prostate cancer using infrared spectroscopic imaging. In: Proceedings of the 9th annual conference on genetic and evolutionary computation. ACM; 2007. p. 2098–105.

[105] Bacardit J, Garrell J. Bloat control and generalization pressure using the minimum description length principle for a Pittsburgh approach learning classifier system. Learn Class Syst 2007:59–79.

[106] Wilson S. Compact rulesets from XCSI. Adv Learn Class Syst 2002:65–92.

[107] Fu C, Davis L. A modified classifier system compaction algorithm. In: Proceedings of the genetic and evolutionary computation conference. Morgan Kaufmann Publishers Inc.; 2002. p. 920–5.

[108] Dixon P, Corne D, Oates M. A ruleset reduction algorithm for the XCS learning classifier system. Learn Class Syst 2003:20–9.

[109] Gao Y, Huang J, Wu L. Learning classifier system ensemble and compact rule set. Connect Sci 2007;19(4)

[110] Kovacs T. XCS classifier system reliably evolves accurate, complete and minimal representations for Boolean functions. Cognitive Science Research Papers — University of Birmingham CSRP; 1997.

[111] Lanzi P. Mining interesting knowledge from data with the XCS classifier system. In: Proceedings of the genetic and evolutionary computation conference (GECCO-2001); 2001. p. 7–11.

[112] Butz M, Lanzi P, Llora X, Goldberg D. Knowledge extraction and problem structure identification in XCS. Parallel problem solving from nature – PPSN VIII. Springer; 2004. p. 1051–61.

[113] Kharbat F, Bull L, Odeh M. Mining breast cancer data with XCS. In: Proceedings of the ninth annual conference on genetic and evolutionary computation. ACM; 2007. p. 2066–73.

[114] Kharbat F, Odeh M, Bull L. New approach for extracting knowledge from the XCS learning classifier system. Int J Hybr Intell Syst 2007;4(2):49–62.

[115] Kharbat F, Odeh M, Bull L. Knowledge discovery from medical data: an empirical study with XCS. Learn Class Syst Data Mining 2008:93–121.

[116] Urbanowicz R, Kiralis J, Fisher J, Moore J. Predicting the difficulty of pure, strict, epistatic models: metrics for simulated model selection. BioData Mining 2012;5:15.

[117] Seifert C, Lex E. A novel visualization approach for data-mining-related classification. in information visualization. In: 13th international conference. IEEE; 2009. p. 490–5.

[118] Butz M. Documentation of XCSFJava 1.1 plus visualization. MEDAL Report; 2007.

[119] Smith R, Jiang M. MILCS in protein structure prediction with default hierarchies. In: Proceedings of the first ACM/SIGEVO summit on genetic and evolutionary computation. ACM; 2009. p. 953–6.

[120] Greene C, White B, Moore J. Sensible initialization using expert knowledge for genome-wide analysis of epistasis using genetic programming. Evolutionary Computation, CEC'09. IEEE; 2009. p. 1289–96.

[121] Greene C, White B, Moore J. An expert knowledge-guided mutation operator for genome-wide genetic analysis using genetic programming. Pattern Recogn Bioinform 2007:30–40.

[122] Moore J, White B. Exploiting expert knowledge in genetic programming for genome-wide genetic analysis. In: Parallel problem solving from nature — PPSN IX; 2006. p. 969–77.

[123] Cliff D, Ross S. Adding temporary memory to ZCS. Adap Behav 1994;3(2):101–50.

[124] Lanzi P. Adding memory to XCS. In: Evolutionary computation proceedings, IEEE world congress on computational intelligence; 1998. p. 609–14.

[125] Lanzi P, Wilson S. Toward optimal classifier system performance in non-Markov environments. Evolut Comput 2000;8(4):393–418.

[126] Twins [Dir. Ivan Ritman. Perfs. Arnold Schwarzenegger and Danny DeVito]; 1988.

[127] Wilson S, Goldberg D. A critical review of classifier systems. In: Proceedings of the third international conference on genetic algorithms table of contents; 1989. p. 244–55.

[128] Booker LB, Goldberg DE, Holland JH. Classifier systems and genetic algorithms. Machine learning: paradigms and methods table of contents; 1989. p. 235–82.

[129] Lanzi P, Riolo R. A roadmap to the last decade of learning classifier system research (from 1989 to 1999). Lect Notes Comput Sci 2000;2000:33–61.

[130] Kovacs T. Learning classifier systems resources. Soft Comput — A Fus Found Methodol Appl 2002;6(3):240–3.

[131] Lanzi P, Riolo R. Recent trends in learning classifier systems research. Natural computing series; 2003. p. 955–88.

[132] Bull L, Kovacs T. Foundations of learning classifier systems. Springer; 2005.

[133] Sigaud O, Wilson S. Learning classifier systems: a survey. Soft Comput — A Fus Found Methodol Appl 2007;11(11):1065–78.

[134] Butz M. Combining gradient-based with evolutionary online learning: an introduction to learning classifier systems. In: Seventh international conference on hybrid intelligent systems, HIS 2007; 2007. p. 12–7.

[135] Lanzi P. Learning classifier systems: then and now. Evolut Intell 2008;1:63–82.

[136] Drugowitsch J. Design and analysis of learning classifier systems: a probabilistic approach. Springer; 2008.

Engineering Principles in Biomedical Informatics

Riccardo Bellazzi, Matteo Gabetta, and Giorgio Leonardi

Dipartimento di Ingegneria Industriale e dell'Informazione, Università di Pavia, Pavia, Italy

Scientists study the world as it is; engineers create the world that has never been.

—Theodore von Kármán

10.1 INTRODUCTION

Biomedical informatics is at the intersection of many disciplines [1], carrying the ambition of improving people's health through the leveraging of better use of information. Such a goal relies on many pillars, ranging from

313

basic biomedical and clinical knowledge to organizational aspects, as well as from novel technologies related to human factors.

Since one of the key components of biomedical informatics is the design, development, and deployment of computational solutions, it is evident that the role of engineering and its principles is of utmost importance. As reported in Wikipedia, engineering is "the creative application of scientific principles to design or develop structures, machines, apparatus, or manufacturing processes, or works utilizing them singly or in combination; or to construct or operate the same with full cognizance of their design; or to forecast their behavior under specific operating conditions; all as respects an intended function, economics of operation, or safety to life and property." Therefore "the crucial and unique task of the engineer is to identify, understand, and interpret the constraints on a design in order to produce a successful result" [2].

In a nutshell, engineering principles stand in: (1) studying a system, (2) modeling it, (3) designing an artifact that has predictable behavior, within the limits of the system model when interacting with the system, (4) applying such artifact in reality, and, finally (5) measuring and assessing its real impact, in order to improve modeling and design in an iterative process [3]. Rather interestingly, such an engineering approach can be also effectively used in biomedical informatics and its partial or poor application is often a source of severe failures of biomedical informatics in practice. Of course, the modeling and design task is peculiar and particularly difficult, since it is very difficult to isolate a small part of the reality in such a way that the system to be modeled is easily manageable, and thus the models relatively simple themselves. Moreover, models in biomedicine need to describe a complex environment such as a healthcare system, or, the activities of a single hospital or care provider. Furthermore, the models need to span over a variety of basic modeling approaches, from mathematical modeling to software engineering. The design of tools often requires one to integrate existing solutions and not (only) to develop new ones. Finally, the evaluation requires several layers, including safety, costs, effectiveness, and efficacy.

In this chapter, we will concentrate our attention on the aspects related to modeling, which represents a cornerstone in the engineering process. The chapter will thus provide some examples of modeling tools that can be effectively exploited to design biomedical informatics solutions, with particular reference to information systems at the very heart of biomedical informatics (e.g., computational tools aimed at managing and representing information).

10.2 **BUILDING INNOVATIVE PRODUCTS: IMPLICATIONS FOR BIOMEDICAL INFORMATICS**

Biomedical informatics is inherently related to the development of software tools and solutions designed to be successfully exploited by users (e.g., healthcare practitioners, researchers, patients, citizens). In other words, one of the goals of biomedical informatics is to design and deploy software products and services. For this reason, it is crucial that such products are seen from the perspective of their life cycle, their level of innovation and, thus, that design and deployment strategies follow engineering principles.

By adapting the definition of Rogers as well as from Wikipedia [4,5], innovation is the development of new value for the users by developing solutions that meet new needs, inarticulate needs, or old needs in new ways. This is achieved by new or more effective products, processes, services, and technologies. When an innovative product becomes available, it follows a life cycle that can be described by a curve known as *diffusion* or *s*-curve, which represents the productivity of innovation against time [5]. Such a curve is characterized by three phases. In the first phase, the productivity slowly increases because the innovative product needs time to be diffused and marketed. After some time, the productivity has sudden increases quickly, corresponding to the second phase of market acceptance. If other innovations and investments are added, this phase may last for some time. The last, and third, phase corresponds to a decrease in the productivity rate, which occurs when the product is mature and provides stable revenues. The *s*-curve is grounded on the assumption that the life cycle of a product typically follows five stages described by Raymond Vernon [6]: (1) introduction, (2) growth, (3) maturity, (4) saturation, and (5) decline.

In the case of software products and services, many companies try to avoid the third phase of the *s*-curve, corresponding to the end of the maturity stage, and the following saturation and decline stages, by continuously investing in innovation. As far as biomedical informatics is concerned, the software life cycle typically also includes a quality system, which may lead to software certification. This certification is an essential precondition in the case that software is to be part of a medical device. If a quality system needs to be put in place, it should include, in accordance with FDA regulations, control strategies to deal with Design, Materials, Production & Processes, Equipment & Facilities and, finally, Records and Documents [7]. The aspects related to quality and to design control, as well as the certification theme, are particularly crucial, since they may severely prolong the first phase of the *s*-curve of the innovation life cycle: in case this phase is too long, a product may never reach the fast growth stage.

An engineering approach is a proper, and probably essential, way to deal with the issues mentioned above. Modeling the domain, simulating the processes, and rationally planning the workflow may speed up design and production as well as optimize the costs.

In the case of software development, different engineering design principles may guide the software life cycle [8,9]. In general, all software projects follow the basic steps of planning, implementation-documentation-testing, deployment, training, and maintenance. However, there are many differences in the way these steps are articulated in practice. In general, we can distinguish between several models, as briefly presented below.

The most widely used model is the so-called "waterfall" model, in which developers follow the standard steps sequentially: (1) Requirements specification, (2) Software design, (3) Implementation, (4) Testing, (5) Deployment, and (6) Maintenance. The steps are finished and initiated by project reviews and milestones.

Many authors have criticized the use of the waterfall model for software development, since software needs fast prototyping but allows for product revisions more easily than "hardware" [10]. An alternative approach is known as the spiral model. In this case, a number of prototypes are implemented and tested, following three steps iteratively: (1) determine goals; (2) identify risks; and (3) develop and test the prototypes. Since the system is tested and redesigned several times, such a model requires a much stronger involvement of the users,

A relatively recent evolution of participative design is represented by "agile" approaches, in which the software is iteratively developed following a user-centered approach based on feedback, regular tests, and successive releases of the software [11].

The strategies described above need formal ways to represent users, interactions, processes, and systems. Proper modeling improves the capability of designing and deploying software solutions, thus leading to more principled, efficient, and effective biomedical informatics tools, systems, and services. In the following, we will concentrate on some of the most important modeling tools for software development. We will also focus our attention to the role of high-level modeling in data analysis and data mining.

10.3 MODELING INFORMATION FLOWS FOR SOFTWARE ENGINEERING: THE UNIFIED MODELING LANGUAGE

The Unified Modeling Language (UML) is the predominant standard language for the design of information systems, such as software and databases, but also for business modeling and non-software systems design. Since the main foundation of UML is grounded in the Object-Oriented (O-O) paradigm, the majority of available documentation refers to applications in software design and software engineering. However, the broad concepts of UML make it also amenable to modeling processes and organizations. This is clearly stated in the UML definition [12]:

"UML is a language with a very broad scope that covers a large and diverse set of application domains."

and

"The Unified Modeling Language is a visual language for specifying, constructing, and documenting the artifacts of systems. It is a general-purpose modeling language that can be used with all major object and component methods, and that can be applied to all application domains (e.g., health, finance, telecom, aerospace) and implementation platforms (e.g., J2EE, .NET)."

The Object Management Group (OMG) adopted UML as one of its technologies in 1997 and still manages the specifications of this standard. In recent years, UML has evolved and has been revised many times—the last major revision was UML 2.0 (adopted in 2005).

UML is basically a visual modeling language, so its vocabulary is made by a set of graphical symbols and notations and its semantics are aimed at defining rules to combine available elements; both the vocabulary and the semantics focus on the conceptual and physical representation of the system to be modeled.

The reasons that should drive a system designer to use UML lie mainly in its object-oriented nature that allows one to identify different parts of the system (the objects), their behavior (the methods), and the ways that the system interacts in its environment.

Despite being a modeling language, UML does not provide a method or a process for modeling, it simply provides the language; this makes UML enough flexible and extendable to be used with many different system modeling techniques, in other words: UML is methodology-independent.

UML is a language for visualizing, specifying, constructing, and documenting models with the following features:

- Writing a model in UML allows everyone who knows the vocabulary and the semantics of the language to visualize and understand the project. Providing a less constraining form of communication, despite being more immediate to be used, could penalize the understanding of outsiders, and people new to the project group. Furthermore, a graphical modeling language stands between a completely unstructured form of design and a programming language, so it can be useful to move the ideas in practice with the best efficiency.

- UML allows one to build specific models that are complete, precise, and without ambiguities.
- Models expressed in UML can be directly translated in many programming languages, in order to construct the skeleton for the following implementation phase. It is also possible, with reverse-engineering processes, to reconstruct a model from an implementation back into the UML.
- UML can handle all the details about the documentation of a system, its requirements and tests and the planning and release-management phases.

UML is also a cornerstone in the OMG managed Model-Driven Architecture (MDA), a software design approach that allows the system to be built, in its first instance, as platform-independent model (with a large use of UML) and, in a further phase, to be implemented with a domain-specific language (thanks to a fully or partially automated code generation process). This approach makes possible a platform-independent design with the great advantage of insulating the core of the application from specific technologies.

The UML language provides a set of diagrams, each one suitable to address a specific problem; these diagrams can be divided into three main families: (1) Structure Diagrams, (2) Behavior Diagrams, and (3) Interaction Diagrams (which are actually a subfamily of Behavior Diagrams) (see Figure 10.1):

- Structure Diagrams represent, from different levels of abstraction, the static structure of the model and how its parts are related to each other. The different elements of these diagrams represent important parts of the system. Structure Diagrams include the Class Diagram, Object Diagram, Component Diagram, Composite Structure Diagram, Package Diagram, Profile Diagram, and Deployment Diagram.
- Behavior Diagrams model the dynamic behavior of the system (i.e., its changes of status over time or, to simplify, what happens in the modeled system). Behavior Diagrams include the Use Case Diagram, Activity Diagram, and State Machine Diagram.
- Interaction Diagrams are a subfamily of Behavior Diagrams and represent the flow of the information (both actual and control data) through the modeled system. Interaction Diagrams include the Sequence Diagram, Communication Diagram, Timing Diagram, and Interaction Overview Diagram.

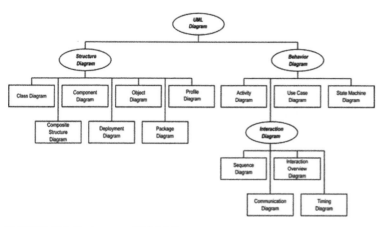

■ **FIGURE 10.1** The taxonomy of UML 2.0 diagrams.

An exhaustive discussion of all the diagram types is out of the scope of this book chapter; in the next part we will briefly describe some of the diagrams that have been used in the real case examples described in the following section.

10.3.1 Class Diagrams

A Class Diagram represents the logical structure of the model, it is a Structure Diagram, and therefore it captures what are the entities of the system, which attributes they have and the relations among each other. Each Class is represented as a box containing: (1) the name of the class, (2) its attributes, and (3) the tasks it can accomplish. Relations occurring between the classes of the diagram are represented with arrows; one arrow connects two Classes and, depending on its shape, it can represent many different types of Relations (e.g., aggregation, composition, dependence, and generalization) that are a cornerstone of the O-O paradigm. Other important notations of the diagram are the Multiplicity Indicators, associated with the relations, and the Visibility Modifiers.

10.3.2 Use Case Diagrams

The Use Case Diagrams, which belong to the Behavior Diagrams family, help represent the actions that the system can accomplish by interacting with one or more external users called Actors. Each action described is considered exclusively as an interaction of the Actors with the boundary of the system and should lead to an observable result for the users of the system or for its stakeholders. The main elements of a Use Case Diagram are: (1) the

System (sometimes omitted) that is represented with an empty square that separates the internal elements from the external; (2) the Actors, portrayed as stick figures, that represent entities (humans, other systems, etc.) that can interact with the System; and (3) Use Cases, drawn as ovals containing a describing name, represent meaningful functions or services offered to one or more Actors. The interaction between the Actors and the Use Cases is represented with arrows.

10.3.3 Activity Diagrams

Activity Diagrams show the flow of control of the modeled system, with particular attention to the conditions that regulate this flow (e.g., one action will occur only when a particular condition is verified). The elements of this diagram are: (1) Activities, represented with a rounded rectangle with a name describing it: they are the main element of this diagram; and (2) a limited number of shapes that represent the control-flow elements (start, end, decisions, etc.) typical of the flowchart diagrams.

10.3.4 Sequence Diagrams

Sequence Diagrams are the most common type of Interaction Diagrams; a Sequence Diagram represents the behavior of the system as a series of sequential steps over time and it is suited to define the workflow, the message passing, and the cooperation of the elements of the system over time in order to achieve a specific goal. The main building blocks of this diagram are: (1) the Lifelines, drawn as vertical lines with a describing box on the top, that represent the object that simultaneously live in the system; and (2) the Messages exchanged between two Lifelines, drawn as horizontal arrows described with some text and characterized by the shape of the arrow. When a Lifeline is active, its vertical line becomes an Activation Box that ends when the Lifeline goes back to inactive. When an object is destroyed its Lifeline terminates with an "X."

10.4 UML APPLICATIONS IN BIOMEDICAL INFORMATICS

In this section, we show some examples of UML adoption to model and design biomedical informatics systems.

Bornberg-Bauer and Paton have described a Conceptual Data Modeling (CDM) approach [13], which concerns the development of precise but implementation-independent models for data, in order to make explicit their structural properties. A crucial advantage of such a modeling technique is to make the data interchange with others easier. Bornberg-Bauer and Paton

[13] describe the techniques on which a CDM process is based and collected some examples within a bioinformatics context where CDM has been
applied with success.

Bornberg-Bauer and Paton underline the need of techniques like CDM
because of the increasing amount of biological data that are presented in
disparate formats that often leave implicit many important features and are
based on different vocabularies coming from different disciplines.

The techniques suitable to apply CDM described in the aforementioned
paper are Entity-Relationship Modeling (ERM) and UML Modeling. As it
concerns UML, in particular, Bornberg-Bauer and Paton analyze two different papers where the Class Diagrams have been used to model the structure
of proteins [14] and genome sequences [15], respectively (see Figure 10.2).
Bornberg-Bauer and Paton underline the potential usefulness of CDM (with
ERM or UML Class Diagrams) in developing, making explicit, and communicating clear and detailed description of data that are available or that
are about to be produced.

Kumarapeli et al. described how UML has been able to model the Primary
Care Data Quality program, a business process designed to improve the
quality of clinical care, in order to enhance its efficiency and predictability
[16]. In the modeling phase, they exploited three types of UML diagrams:

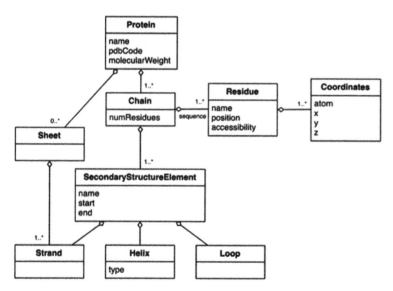

■ **FIGURE 10.2** A simplified version of a Class Diagram (only classes names, attributes and relationships) representing the model for protein structure, as reported in [13].

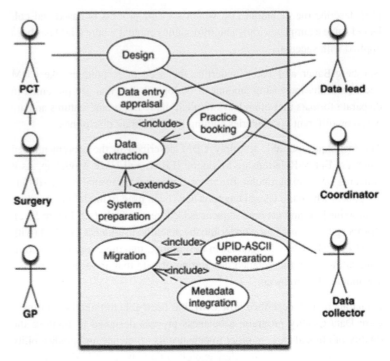

■ **FIGURE 10.3** A detail of the Use Case Diagram reported in [16].

(1) Use Case Diagrams were used, as shown in Figure 10.3, in the preliminary phases, to display the relationships between use cases and actors; (2) Class Diagrams, starting from the use case model, were used to represent a more detailed structural view of the system; and, finally, (3) Class Diagrams indicated which classes were associated with the process-improvement objectives.

Kumarapeli et al. used Activity Diagrams to represent the workflow of each step of the process, to better understand the relationships among the classes and the influence that data from earlier phases have on subsequent stages, as depicted in Figure 10.4. Finally, Kumarapeli et al. used Sequence Diagrams to explain the communication process between software and human agents, their interactions, and the messages exchanged during the process.

Kumarapeli et al. conclude with a number of positive aspects of this novel use of UML in health-business improvement process; in fact, they have been able to identify many critical aspects of the systems analyzed and UML has enabled them to provide insights on how to improve the reliability and predictability of the processing steps of the data routinely collected.

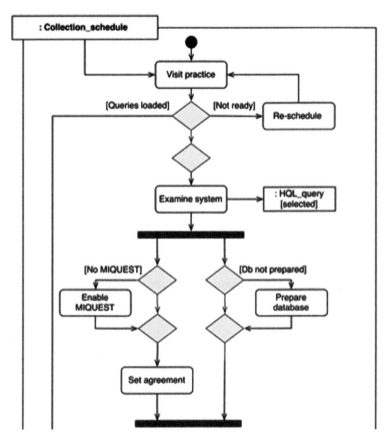

■ **FIGURE 10.4** A detail of the Activity Diagram for the data-extraction stage of [16].

Roux-Rouquie et al. examined the usefulness of UML to describe and specify complex biological systems and processes [17]; this systems biology task is needed in order to allow an unambiguous representation of biological systems. Such a representation makes it possible to translate biological systems knowledge into mathematical and computational formalisms, analyzable, amenable to simulation, and predictable. Roux-Rouquie et al. opted for UML modeling because it provides sharable and documented descriptions in specifying processes, object, and relations; furthermore, UML proved its usefulness in representing the complexity of biological systems.

Boskovic et al. describe how O-O modeling, and in particular UML, could deal with a Real-Time (RT) task, such as the design of an Electrocardiograph system (ECG) [18]. The goal was to minimize the loss of information during the process of modeling (especially taking into account the criticalities due to a RT environment). The O-O design paradigm for this study was implemented in all the stages of the software engineering process, in particular: (1) Use Case Diagrams were used in the requirement analysis stage, in order to define the boundaries and interactions between the system and the external world; (2) the general structure of the system was modeled with Class Diagrams that make explicit which are the main application classes and their relationships; and, finally, (3) the dynamic behavior of the ECG system was designed with Sequence Diagrams, a tool that Boskovic et al. found to be powerful for timely identification of hidden requirements (see Figure 10.5).

Boskovic et al. state that O-O techniques, and UML in particular, can lead to a flexible and extensible design which supports the modeling of different scale RT systems.

Raistrick described the use of UML and, more generally, of the Model-Driven Architecture (MDA) approach in the context of an extension of the processing of clinical data to provide a "patient-based electronic record" for the UK National Health Service [19]. In particular, UML and MDA were used to: (1) model the new access control capabilities for

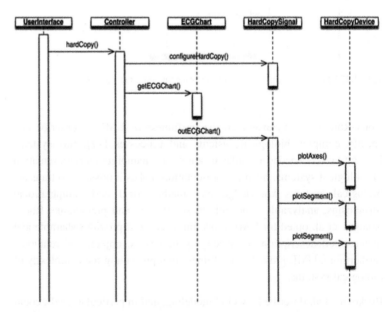

■ **FIGURE 10.5** Sequence Diagram representing the Hardcopy process of an ECG signal, as reported in [18].

the system; (2) specify the characteristics of existing key components, in order to facilitate their integration with new components; and (3) enable automatic code generation without losing platform independency of the model. The use of the MDA approach influenced all the phases of the project: analysis of requirements, modeling, demonstration of the different usage scenarios to the stakeholders and, finally, evaluation of the cost of different platform implementations. Raistrick concludes that MDA and UML provide a powerful solution to problems such as: (1) developing new components to be integrated with legacy systems; (2) porting the new components to multiple platforms with the minimum possible effort; and (3) establishing a stable and agreed set of requirements with the stakeholders.

In summary, the key aspect of the above mentioned studies is that UML, thanks to the different modeling tools it includes, is a very important framework to model, at a conceptual level, complex systems and processes. Use cases, activity diagrams, sequence diagrams, class diagrams provide the level of detail and granularity that is needed in a software project, thus enabling to take into account not only technical aspects, but also the users and the intertwining of roles, competences, and people underlying biomedical scenarios. It is therefore likely that, in the near future, UML will become a reference instrument for biomedical informatics software design.

10.5 FROM MODELING TO SIMULATION: CAREFLOW REPRESENTATION, SIMULATION, AND LEARNING

UML modeling is greatly suited to represent complex systems. Once a model has been created, however, an important engineering principle is to design the artifact to take into account the predictions of the effect that such an artifact will have on the real world. A powerful instrument to perform such predictions in complex environments, characterized by uncertain behavior, is to perform simulation. For example, a Monte Carlo simulation allows for deriving a number of potential scenarios that describe the statistical distribution of the variables of interest (say, for example, a treatment outcome, its costs, or the timing of human resource consumption).

A topic of particular interest for the design of health information systems is the representation and simulation of a "careflow" (i.e., the series of actions performed to care for a patient). A formalized careflow must therefore model medical knowledge to define "what to do," as well as operational and organizational knowledge to define "how" and "who" must perform such actions.

A first attempt to explicitly deal with modeling and simulation steps in health care was performed in 2001 by Quaglini et al. [20], who derived a complete "engineered" pipeline in a scenario where patients were treated based on a clinical guideline.

Evidence-based clinical guidelines are "systematically developed statements to assist practitioner and patient decisions about appropriate health care for specific clinical circumstances" [21]. Designed to improve quality of care by reducing unnecessary practice variation, clinical guidelines are widespread in many clinical contexts. In order to improve the adherence of care provider to guidelines and to make them readily available at the point of care, a noteworthy effort has been devoted to representing them in a computer-interpretable format [22], and different modeling languages have been designed to this task [23]. Referring to the works of Quaglini et al. and Panzarasa et al. [20,24], guidelines were modeled with a system, called GUIDE, which used a slightly modified version of the UML activity diagram to describe the main steps of the guideline.

In order to obtain a computational model, useful for simulation, the activity diagram was then translated into a high-level Petri network (called Petri nets) [25]. This enabled the model to take into account the resources, ranging from personnel to devices, which are needed to deal with modeled cases.

Petri nets have been widely used to simulate workflows, and thus careflows. Briefly, a Petri net is a network made of a finite set of places (P), a finite set of transitions (T), and a finite set of arcs, which connect places to transitions and transition to places; arcs cannot connect nodes of the same type (e.g., places to places and transitions to transitions). A place can contain zero or more tokens (represented in the networks as a black dot). A transition is enabled when all places that are inputs of that transition have a token. An enabled transition may fire from every input place: as a consequence a token is moved to a place that is the output of that transition. Given the initial places of the tokens and specific laws for firing, a Petri net may be effectively used to run simulations.

Classical Petri nets allow modeling important constructs occurring in complex systems made of multiple processes, such as conditions, synchronization, parallelism, choice, and iteration. However, they have been found to be not expressive enough to describe the variety of situations occurring in the real practice of medical care. For this reason, it was proposed to apply the so-called "high level" Petri nets. Such nets also represent "colors," hierarchies, and time [26,27]. The "colors" represent data flows, hierarchies allow defining interrelated sub-networks, while adding time permits the simulation of the time needed for each transition.

Petri nets have been used to represent guidelines and simulate them in the context of a Hospital careflow management system [26]. Thanks to a simple matching algorithm, the UML activity diagram is represented in a colored Petri Net, which is then augmented and quantified on the basis of the data available on the resources of the hospital and their constraints (e.g., number of surgery rooms). Such an "organizational model" is represented into a ontology of the organization. Thanks to this modeling activity, it has been possible to simulate the implementation of a guideline for the management of patients with acute ischemic stroke under different conditions [24].

Even though Petri Nets have been largely used in workflow and careflow modeling, they have been criticized because of three main issues: (1) their limited ability to handle multiple instances of subprocesses at the same time; (2) their limitations in dealing with complex synchronization between subprocesses; (3) the locality of the mechanisms for firing transitions, while in complex behavior there are events that may cause transition regardless of the local situation [27].

For this reason, a new language for workflow modeling and simulation has been proposed by Van der Aalst and colleagues, called YAWL (Yet Another Workflow Language) [27].

YAWL was introduced after a deep study to collect the limitations of existing workflow languages. This study produced a very large set of workflow patterns [28,29], defining the basic and complex constructs, which must be offered by a workflow language, to allow engineers building expressive and efficient workflows. YAWL has been inspired by Petri nets, but it is a completely new language with independent semantics and support for existing workflow patterns. As a language for the specification of control flows, YAWL is highly expressive [30], has a formal semantics, and offers graphical representations for many of its concepts. The graphical representation of the language's modeling elements is shown in Figure 10.6.

A workflow specification in YAWL offers a complete coverage of the workflow execution through four *perspectives*: (1) The *control-flow perspective* (or process perspective) describes tasks and their execution ordering through different constructors; (2) The *data perspective* deals with processing data, such as business documents, variables, and other objects, which flow between activities; (3) The *resource perspective* provides an organizational structure anchor to the workflow in the form of human and device roles responsible for executing tasks; and (4) The *operational perspective* describes the elementary actions executed by tasks, where the actions map into underlying applications.

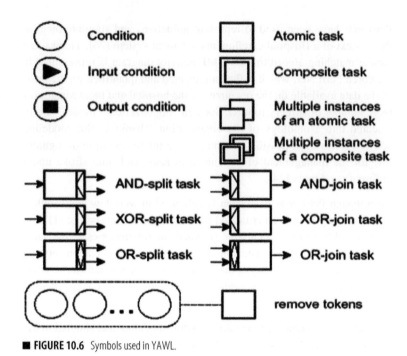

■ **FIGURE 10.6** Symbols used in YAWL.

A YAWL process is defined as a set of extended workflow nets (EWF nets), which form a hierarchical structure. The root of this structure corresponds with the top-level process, while each composite task (or subprocess) refers to a unique EWF net at a lower level in the hierarchy. Every EWF net is composed of tasks and conditions.

Tasks may be atomic tasks or composite tasks representing EWF nets at a lower level in the hierarchical structure. Each task can be instantiated multiple times using the concept of multiple instances for atomic or composite task. Tasks can also be associated with pre- and post-conditions, defining, respectively activation and completion rules.

Conditions can be seen as places of a Petri net. Every process definition starts with a unique input condition and ends with a unique output condition.

Connections are possible between condition-task (and vice versa) and task-task. The latter may be interpreted as an implicit hidden condition between the tasks connected.

AND, XOR, and *OR* splits and joins are natively supported using the corresponding symbols in Figure 10.6. In addition, YAWL allows using the process data to define rules selecting which tasks must be activated after a XOR or an OR split.

Finally, YAWL also provides a notation for *removing tokens* from a specified region denoted by dashed rounded rectangles and lines. The enabling of the task that will perform the cancelation may or may not depend on the tokens within the region to be "canceled." In any case, the moment this task executes, all tokens in this region are removed. This notation allows for various cancelation patterns.

YAWL is supported by the YAWL system, an open source web-based workflow management system, whose execution engine can be connected with external plug-ins to offer additional features such as allowing manipulation of data within external applications, using communication tools (e.g., for sending SMS or emails to workflow users), or exploiting flexibility services.

Leonardi et al. used YAWL to build a serviceflow management system for the management of the care process of chronic patients [31]. The management of this type of patient is a complex process, which requires the cooperation of different agents belonging to several organizations. Patients have to move to different locations to meet different professionals and to access the necessary health services. Leonardi et al. suggested there should be only one organization, a VHCO (Virtual Health Care Organization), which provides both virtual and face-to-face encounters. Towards achieving this goal, they handled the information and communication requirements implementing the care process as a serviceflow: a high-level multi-organizational workflow where each task represents a contact between the patient and the VHCO, and each subprocess implements the operations to be performed for providing the services needed in each contact. The system manages the care process through three components: (1) the model of the care process represented as a Serviceflow; (2) the organizational ontology representing the VHCO; and (3) agreements and commitments between the parties defined in a contract. These components are implemented using the different perspectives of YAWL: the control-flow perspective for the component (1), the organizational perspective for the component (2), and the data perspective for the component (3).

Workflow management systems must also deal with exceptions: unexpected deviations from the standard execution flow that can happen (virtually) at each point of the process. Among the workflow management systems able to manage exceptions natively, it is worth mentioning the work of Reichert et al. [32]. The ADEPT project provides a high level of flexibility through the support of non-trivial *ad hoc* deviations at the process instance level, allowing engineers to introduce control-flow changes during the execution of a process instance. These deviations also allow for quick implementation of process changes through process schema evolution. Van der Aalst has adopted another approach with the integration of the Worklet Service in

YAWL. In particular, the Worklet Dynamic Process Selection Service for YAWL provides the ability to substitute a workitem in a YAWL process with a dynamically selected worklet—a discrete YAWL process that acts as a sub-net for the workitem and so handles one specific task in a larger, composite process activity [33]. An extensible repertoire (or catalog) of worklets is maintained. Each time the service is invoked for a workitem, a choice is made from the repertoire based on the data within the workitem, using a set of rules to determine the most appropriate substitution. The workitem is checked out by the YAWL engine, and then the selected worklet is launched as a separate case.

Careflows are complex processes, and their optimization can help health care organizations to provide better services to patients at a lower cost. An important task for optimizing careflows is the one of finding the gap between what is prescribed to be done (e.g., as defined in clinical guideline recommendations) versus what is actually being done to treat the patients.

Process Mining (PM), introduced by Van der Aalst et al., describes a family of *a posteriori* analysis techniques that exploit the information recorded by the information systems (IS) of health care structures [34]. In particular, this information can be transformed into Process Logs (PL), containing sequences of activities related to particular cases (i.e., patients). Each activity is associated to additional information such as the person executing or initiating the activity, the timestamp of the activity, or data recorded with the event (e.g., the dose of a drug). The goal of PM is to extract process-related information from PL, such as process models, organizational and social nets, and performance indicators such as execution and waiting times and bottlenecks. It is important to mention that the focus of PM is on discovery of models from PL, and that this task is performed even if there is not an *a priori* model.

PM analysis can be performed using ProM: a platform-independent open source framework which supports a wide variety of process mining and data mining techniques, and can be extended by adding new functionalities in the form of plug-ins. The ProM framework can read event logs that are in the MXML format. With the ProM import tool, data from various systems, such as MS Access, can be converted into the MXML format.

Interesting results in the health care domain have been described by Mans et al. [35]. Specifically, Mans et al. analyzed process logs generated by different hospitals of the Lombardia region (Italy), focusing on patients affected by ischemic stroke. Among the results obtained, the authors pointed out differences in the treatment strategy of different hospitals, as shown in

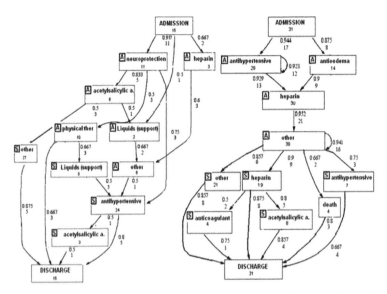

■ **FIGURE 10.7** The treatment processes mined for the two hospitals H1 (left) and H2 (right). With respect to the original output, to facilitate the reader, labels "A" and "S" have been added indicating events belonging to the acute and subacute phases, respectively.

Figure 10.7, applying a mining technique called "Heuristic Miner" to data related to the hospitalization phase of the treatment.

In Figure 10.7, for example, Mans et al. show that hospital 2 performs hypertension therapy earlier and much more intensively than the other hospital. In the domain of ischemic stroke, it is known that antihypertensive treatment is a common practice, although not always justified by scientific evidence. Hospital 1 seems to be more "research-oriented," since it adopts therapeutic protocols such as neuroprotection, and is more compliant with the more recent clinical guidelines, which recommend early physical therapy. These results can be shown to physicians or health care managers to look for motivations behind the differences and behind eventual non-compliance with clinical guidelines. After analyzing these motivations, decisions can be made to improve efficiency and compliance of the actual application of the care processes in the different structures.

Process models can also be translated into colored petri nets and simulated over the real data, to obtain performance indicators and bottlenecks. For example, applying this technique to pre-hospitalizaton data collected through direct interviews with patients, Figure 10.8 has been obtained and explained.

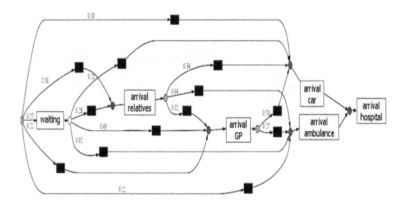

■ **FIGURE 10.8** The Petri net representing the pre-hospital process.

Figure 10.8 shows the discovered Petri net of the pre-hospital process. This analysis returns information and indicators, such as the percentage of patients associated with a particular activity—e.g., average/variance of the total flow time or the time spent between activities. In particular, bottlenecks can be identified by places, which indicate a high waiting time to the next non-hidden transition (i.e., non-black transition). In Figure 10.8, places colored blue, yellow,[1] or purple, respectively, represent a low (<6 h), medium (< 12 h and ⩾ 6 h), and high average waiting time (⩾ 12 h) at that place. Among other conclusions, what can be derived from the picture is that after occurrence of the events "waiting time" (patient stopped waiting), "arrival relatives," and "arrival GP," on average, it still takes considerable time before the next action occurs. Note that the time lag between the stroke onset and the arrival in the hospital is on average 28 h and has a standard deviation of 45 h. This is probably due to a frequent underestimation of stroke symptoms by patients/relatives/general practitioners. At the same time, a great variability among people is shown. This can be derived from the picture which shows the most frequent paths following the occurrence of an event. For example, after stroke onset, 27% of the patients decided to wait instead of calling relatives (18%) or calling a general practitioner (22%).

Clearly, different kind of performance indicators can be obtained for the discovered Petri net. Moreover, once such a Petri net is available, simulations with different parameters can be run to see what are the consequences after the removal of a bottleneck, such as change in throughput time.

---

[1] For interpretation of color in Figure 10.8, the reader is referred to the web version of this book.

10.6 ENGINEERING PRINCIPLES AND IDEAS IN BIOMEDICAL DATA MINING

Since data mining (as described in Chapter 7) is a field that borrows strengths from several disciplines, it is not surprising that engineering principles are quite widely used and applied. In particular, there are two different domains in which engineering approaches have been particularly important and useful: (1) modeling dynamic systems and (2) building and evaluating data mining models.

10.6.1 Modeling and Analyzing Dynamical Systems

Dealing with temporal data is a complex task [36–38], which often includes the combination of advanced models and data analysis methods. Very often, biomedical informatics deals with the collection of time-oriented data, including biomedical signals and time series.

On the one hand, biomedical signals are collected by sensors or by monitoring systems; they are characterized by a fixed and frequent sampling time. For these kinds of data a variety of methods are available to extract clinically interesting features and to provide decision-making instruments to clinicians and researchers [39–45]. On the other hand, time series can be collected during long-term follow-up of patients; such data are usually multivariate and irregularly sampled, with a frequency that is related to the patients' visits. In this latter case, only recently the literature has proposed some interesting methods to analyze the data in the area of temporal data mining [46,47]. Clinical data have been also combined with administrative data. Such data may contain additional information on the process of patients' management, including hospitalization or drug prescription, but do not contain clinical values and rarely reports clinical outcomes [48–50].

An interesting engineering viewpoint of temporal data and dynamical systems is provided by systems theory, which has been applied by the authors of this chapter to provide a unified view of signal and data processing amenable of a Bayesian Network representation [51] (in addition to Chapter 8 of this text, see also the online tutorial http://www.cs.ubc.ca/~murphyk/Bayes/bayes.html). These ideas are shared by many other researchers in the field, who did work in biomedical informatics and physiological modeling [52] and by a recent paper by Lucas and colleagues [53].

Within systems theory [54,55] a dynamic system can be described by a suitable triple: (1) a time domain, (2) a set of state variables, and (3) a state transition function. The state variables are the variables of the problem that are sufficient to model the system evolution, while the state transition function mathematically describes the evolution of the system over time, in dependence of the inputs and of the initial conditions. Often, the system can be measured through a set of output variables, which depend on the state variables. Mining data coming from a dynamical systems means learning the trajectories of the (not measured) state variables from the knowledge of the output variables in a noisy context. This may involve learning the state transition function, too. The state reconstruction problem is then usually divided in systems theory into three sub-problems, called smoothing, filtering, and prediction [51,56]. Smoothing is related to the reconstruction of the entire state trajectory in a certain time interval using all the measurements available in that time interval. Filtering means reconstructing the present state given all data collected in the previous time interval. Finally, prediction is related to forecasting the state in a future time interval on the basis of the data collected in a past interval. In signal processing, Kalman filtering techniques have been applied in a variety of practical applications, and its theoretical results are well known [57]. However, if the state description is not based on continuous variables only, the sampling time is irregular, and the noise affecting the measurement has unknown distribution, it is necessary to deal with more general models, able to describe situations that are more typical in biomedical informatics. An example is represented by Dynamic Bayesian Networks [58,59] (DBNs). DBNs are the time-oriented version of Bayesian Networks, a well-known model of probabilistic environment that represents variables as nodes, their conditional independence relationships through an oriented acyclic graph, quantified by means of conditional probability tables. In DBNs the time domain is discrete, the state space has finite values, and the conditional probability tables describe the probability distribution of the current state given the previous state value; the model is thus Markovian. The state transition function is the joint probability distribution of the next state values given the current ones, computed thanks to the Bayesian networks calculation machinery. The DBNs are therefore able to estimate the state of the system and at the same time to predict its values in the future.

Different generalizations of the DBN framework that are able to deal with time-invariant continuous-time systems (with discrete observations) and discrete-time systems with discrete observations have been presented [51]. In both cases, we have studied how to represent and solve DBNs when the state space is finite (discrete) (see Figure 10.9) and when it is continuous (see Figure 10.10).

A number of pros and cons related to the different modeling choices have been reported in the literature, showing that such kind of representation can

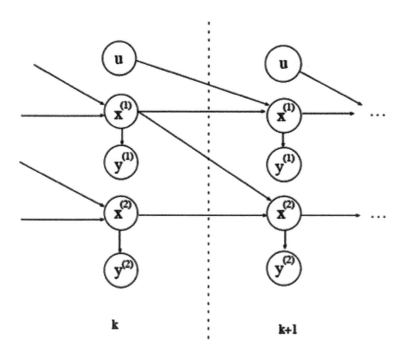

■ **FIGURE 10.9** A DBN with finite state space. State variables are denoted with $x^{(1)}$ and $x^{(2)}$, output variables as $y^{(1)}$ and $y^{(2)}$, while u is the input variable. The network is quantified by means of a set of conditional probability tables: $P(x^{(1)}(k+1)|\,x^{(1)}(k),u)$, $P(x^{(2)}(k+1)|\,x^{(1)}(k),x^{(2)}(k))$, $P(y^{(1)}(k)|\,x^{(1)}(k))$, $P(y^{(2)}(k)|\,x^{(2)}(k))$.

deal with a number of different situations, including irregularly sampled data that can be mapped on a regular grid [56].

However, one limitation of DBNs is represented by the need to deal with discrete time. Many processes are continuous in time, so DBNs force time discretization and, consequently, inference is performed by computing the joint probability distribution at each time step [60]. This limitation of DBN applicability can be a source of computational inefficiency, in particular when the different processes modeled in the network evolve at different time granularities and the data are irregularly sampled.

Recently, a different model has been proposed to overcome such limits, the so-called Continuous time Bayesian networks (CTBNs). They have been used, for example, to model social networks [61], cardiogenic heart failure [62] and, thanks to CTBNs classifiers, stroke rehabilitation [63].

A CTBN is a probabilistic graphical model where nodes are discrete random variables, where state evolves continuously over time, with a probability

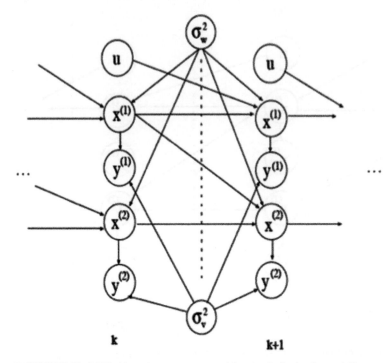

■ **FIGURE 10.10** A DBN with continuous state space and Gaussian distribution. State variables are denoted with $x^{(1)}$ and $x^{(2)}$, output variables as $y^{(1)}$ and $y^{(2)}$, u is the input variable, and σ_w^2 and σ_v^2 are parameters of the xs' and ys' probability distributions (e.g., the variances of Gaussian distributions).

law that depends on the state of their parents in the graph. For each node in the graph, such a probability law is a continuous transition model expressed as a set of conditional intensity matrices—one for each instantiation of the parents' values. Given a node x with s states and an instance of the parents $pa(x)$, the matrix is:

$$
Q^{pa(X)} = \begin{bmatrix} -q_1 & q_{1,2} & \cdots & q_{1,n} \\ q_{2,1} & -q_2 & \cdots & q_{2,n} \\ \cdots & \cdots & \cdots & \cdots \\ q_{s,1} & q_{s,2} & \cdots & -q_s \end{bmatrix},
$$

q_i can be seen as the instantaneous probability to leave the state i, assumed to be equal to $\sum_{j \neq i} q_{i,j}$, while $q_{i,j}$ can be seen as the instantaneous probability to move from x_i to x_j. The probability of staying in the state i for a time span ΔT is $P(i|\,Pa(x)) = 1 - e^{-q_{i,j}\Delta T}$.

An interesting set of CTBNs are the so-called CTBN classifiers, where the output variable Y is a discrete class. In this case "Naïve Bayes-like" or "Augmented Transition Networks-like" models have been proposed [64].

A peculiar aspect of CTBNs is that they allow not only point evidence (e.g., observations sampled at a given time-stamp), but also continuous evidence (e.g., observed values during a given time interval). Continuous evidence is also referred to as an *evidence stream*; evidence streams can be completely or partially observed.

As exact inference in CTBNs is NP-hard, several approximate algorithms have been proposed, including expectation propagation [63] and Markov chain Monte Carlo (MCMC) strategies [65,66].

Finally, CTBNs' structured learning has also been addressed. In this case, the problem is somehow simpler than in the standard DBN case, since the network may have cycles and it is thus possible to learn the local structure of each CTBN node independently.

However, it is worthwhile to note that there are contexts in which such kind of modeling is not applicable, in particular when the description of the system through a state space representation is too difficult (e.g., sparse data on many variables involving a time-variant transition function) and the quantitative knowledge available is not sufficient. In this case, it is useful to resort to other methods, which are able to combine qualitative and quantitative knowledge.

An example is represented by the approaches based on Temporal Abstractions (TAs) [46,67]. TAs are aimed at finding specific qualitative patterns, such as "high temperature" or "blood pressure increasing," in time-stamped data. Such patterns can be multivariate and flexibly composed using the Allen's algebra operators, thus describing complex clinical behaviors. TAs, pioneered by Shahar [46], have been studied by several authors and successfully exploited in many clinical contexts [67–74]. Recently, they have been used as the first step of association rule learning algorithms [67].

10.7 BUILDING AND EVALUATING DATA MINING MODELS

Following an engineering approach, different standards have been proposed to formalize the data mining process. It has been proposed to define some guidelines for predictive data mining in medicine based on one of these standards, CRISP-DM [75]. CRISP-DM was designed in the late 1990s by the Cross-Industry Standard Process for the Data Mining Interest Group (www.crisp-dm.org) [76]. It is made up of six phases, reported in Figure 10.11:

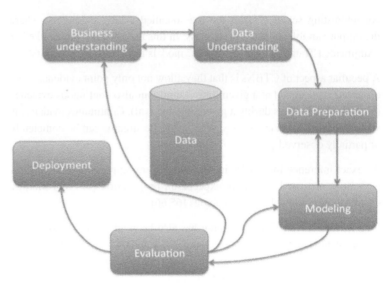

■ **FIGURE 10.11** The CRISP model. The DM process is based on a set of intertwined steps, which can be performed iteratively: business understanding, data understanding, data preparation, modeling, evaluation, and deployment.

(1) business understanding, (2) data understanding, (3) data preparation, (4) modeling, (5) evaluation, and (6) deployment.

Such different phases are orchestrated in an iterative way, such that they can allow for designing, testing, and revising models in a typical engineering process. This standard has inspired Bellazzi and Zupan to define the following guidelines to derive predictive data mining models in medicine [75]. Specifically, they proposed to deal with the "business understanding and data understanding phase" by first defining the specific predictive data mining task and then asking the data miner to answer to a problem-related set of questions. Predictive data mining is defined as the process of deriving the model that finds the best relationships between a number of attributes and an outcome variable on the basis of the available data. The goal of predictive data mining in clinical medicine is seen as the construction of sound and reliable models, able to help health care professionals to take better decisions. Once a data mining activity has been understood, it is important to understand the data. Therefore it is crucial to assess if: (1) the data available are sufficient, (2) the literature has already reported some important relationships among the attributes and between the attributes and the outcomes, and thus (3) it is possible to define new attributes or attributes transformation, which may be effective for the data analysis process. As a next step, it is important to limit the space of the data mining models, by considering other relevant aspects, such as if it is (1) crucial to have transparent, easy to explain, models or (2) the performance is more important than explanation. Moreover, it is also essential to understand if the confidence intervals of predictions and the probabilities of such predictions are needed in the decision process. Finally, taking into account the available knowledge when building the model may improve the quality of the results.

After business and data understanding, the next step is data preparation. Together with data cleaning, data formatting, and normalization, it is important to prepare data for the evaluation phase. A crucial aspect is therefore to define the evaluation strategy and then to split the data accordingly [77]. In the case of cross-validation or bootstrapping, it is necessary to prepare different folds or samples, or in case of hold-out, it is necessary to take out the dataset to be used for the final evaluation of the model.

Once the data are prepared and conveniently split, the models selected in the business and data understanding phase are learned, with particular attention to the issues related to feature ranking and feature selection. Since the evaluation strategy is crucial in model learning, the models are refined in the cross-validation and bootstrap schemes to assess design parameters, too. Predictive models are then evaluated by considering different measures on the test set and by taking into account their comprehensibility. Such evaluation metrics include accuracy, sensitivity, specificity, area under the ROC curve, and Brier score [77]. Comprehensibility can be assessed with specific test studies belonging to the tradition of biomedical informatics [78]. Additional details about evaluation of data mining is given in Chapter 7.

Finally, a crucial, though often unreported step, is related to the deployment and dissemination of such models. This is the real test that a model must pass: being a decision support instrument requires studies reporting the patterns of use by health care professionals or decision makers, and, ultimately, the definition of clear clinical outcomes, including survival, hospitalization rate, costs.

10.8 DISCUSSION

In this chapter, we have focused our attention on the role of engineering principles in biomedical informatics. The core of such principles consists in modeling, designing, and assessing artifacts in an iterative way. We have described some important tools to properly perform such tasks when applied to software design and biomedical informatics problems, ranging from UML modeling, workflow description and simulation, dynamic system representation, and finally evaluation of data mining models.

The application of such principles is unfortunately not widespread enough in the current practice of biomedical informatics. Looking at the reports of failures of health care IT [79–81], there are some situations in which health IT failures or poor management have negatively affected the healthcare process, and have caused increased costs, errors, and delays [82–84]. Recently, the problem has become so important that some researchers have introduced the concept of "Bad Health IT" as "IT that is ill-suited to purpose, hard to use, unreliable, loses data or provides incorrect data, causes cognitive overload, slows rather than facilitates users, lacks appropriate alerts, creates the need for hypervigilance" and "is lacking in security, compromises patient privacy or otherwise demonstrates suboptimal design and/or implementation" [85].

Of course, sensational press headlines related to important failures may easily cause a strong negative impact to biomedical informatics. As is well known, the successes and good reputation built over decades of work can be seriously compromised by a few, but resounding, cases; in the case of biomedical informatics the impact can be to slower the adoption of health IT solutions and may have serious financial costs.

Looking at the profound reasons for Bad Health IT, in the majority of cases the causes of such failures can be grouped in two categories: (1) poor technology design; or (2) organizational and socio-technical problems [86]. Here, we advocate that both categories are in fact related to modeling issues—i.e., the designers have not properly modeled the overall context in which the software solutions had to be put in place. A common feature across the spectrum of Health IT projects is their great complexity, due to the number of processes and systems as well as the number of actors (stakeholders) they have to deal with. Modeling complexity thus remains one of the main challenges of biomedical informatics. The basic methods introduced in this chapter are not only useful to model software products, but also for modeling processes in which humans interact with systems, with a specific attention to time-related aspects.

As reported by Coiera and colleagues [87], it is likely that in the next ten years Health IT will be disseminated at a rate that has not occurred previously. Moreover, it is also likely that the complexity of those systems will increase even further, enlarging the scope and the number of users involved, permeating the society. For this reason, there is an urgent need to explicitly deal with systems safety and risk management. As happened with the airplane industry in the 1950s, a crucial role will need to be taken by modeling and simulation, since the software systems are becoming so complex and safety-critical that they cannot be tested at the full scale before deployment. The implication is that the biomedical informatics community will definitely need to abandon the traditional "clinical trial" scheme for testing new software tools, since IT is not a drug, but rather a socio-technical or organizational intervention. Engineering principles design will therefore become a pillar for dealing with the increasing challenges that the future will bring.

10.9 **CONCLUSIONS**

Engineering widely contributes to biomedical informatics. It provides design principles and instruments, mathematical and software tools and, more than anything else, the product life cycle spirit. Each novel artifact, including an information system, which is used in practice, needs to follow the innovation life cycle that is relevant to its context (e.g., biological or clinical). Its design must be inspired by a user needs analysis, careful modeling and simulation, and its exploitation requires assessment and revision. Finally, it is necessary to continuously monitor its adherence to the user needs, in order to assess when it is necessary to re-engineer the artifact or, finally, to abandon it for a new technology. It is therefore easy to conclude that engineering is a precondition of biomedical informatics, as well as one of its souls. Of course, since the ultimate goal of technology is to improve human life, and, in case of biomedical informatics, to improve clinical care, it is crucial that the engineering push is always counterbalanced by a medical pull and that all disciplines involved, ranging from mathematics and statistics, to public health and business. All these components must work together as parts in a *concerto* where the result is for the benefit of the patient. Modeling techniques, such as those embodied in engineering, provide an approach to understand, and therefore potentially improve, the complex interactions of health care. It is important to note that such an aim to model the complexities of any encounter should never be forgotten in our daily activities.

REFERENCES

[1] Bellazzi R, Diomidous M, Sarkar IN, Takabayashi K, Ziegler A, McCray AT. Data analysis and data mining: current issues in biomedical informatics. Methods Inf Med 2011;50(6):536–44.

[2] <http://en.wikipedia.org/wiki/Engineering>.

[3] Coiera E. Guide to health informatics. London: Arnold; 2003.

[4] <http://en.wikipedia.org/wiki/Innovation> [accessed 27.12.12].

[5] Rogers EM. Diffusion of innovation. New York, NY: Free Press; 1962.

[6] Vernon R. International Investment and International Trade in the Product Cycle, The Quarterly Journal of Economics MIT Press, USA, 1966.

[7] Johnson J. FDA Regulation of medical devices. CRS Report R42130; 2012, <http://www.fas.org/sgp/crs/misc/R42130.pdf>.

[8] <http://en.wikipedia.org/wiki/Software_development_process> [accessed 27.12.12].

[9] Ralph P, Wand Y. A proposal for a formal definition of the design concept. In: Lyytinen K, , Loucopoulos P, , Mylopoulos J, Robinson W, editors. Design requirements engineering: a ten-year perspective. Springer-Verlag; 2009. p. 103–36.

[10] Whitten JL, Bentley LD, Dittman KC. Systems analysis and design methods. 6th ed. McGraw Hill College; 2003.

[11] <http://www.agile-process.org/> [accessed 27.12,12].

[12] OMG Unified Modeling Language (OMG UML) infrastructure—version 2.4.1 (formal/2011-08-05). <http://www.omg.org/spec/UML/2.4.1/Infrastructure>.

[13] Bornberg-Bauer E, Paton NW. Conceptual data modeling for bioinformatics. Brief Bioinform 2002:3166–80.

[14] Gray P, Paton N, Kemp G, Fothergill J. An object-oriented database for protein structure analysis. Protein Eng 1990;4(3):235–43.

[15] Paton N, Khan S, Hayes A, et al. Conceptual modeling of genomic information. Bioinformatics 2000;16(6):548–57.

[16] Kumarapeli P, De Lusignan S, Ellis T, Jones B. Using Unified Modelling Language (UML) as a process-modelling technique for clinical-research process improvement. Med Inform Internet Med 2007;32:51–64.

[17] Roux-Rouquie M et al. Using the Unified Modelling Language (UML) to guide the systemic description of biological processes and systems. Biosystems 2004;75:3–14.

[18] Boskovic D, Besic I, Avdagic Z. Object-oriented integrated approach for the design of scalable ECG systems. Stud Health Technol Inform 2009;150:625–9.

[19] Raistrick C. Applying MDA and UML in the development of a healthcare system. In: Jardim Nunes N, , Selic B, , Rodrigues da Silva A, Toval Alvarez A, editors. UML satellite activities 2004, 3297. Heidelberg: LNCS, Springer; 2005. p. 203–18.

[20] Quaglini S, Stefanelli M, Lanzola G, Caporusso V, Panzarasa S. Flexible guideline-based patient careflow systems. Artif Intell Med 2001;22(1):65–80.

[21] Field MJ, Lohr KN, editors. Clinical practice guidelines: directions for a new program. Institute of Medicine, Washington, DC: National Academy Press; 1990.

[22] Latoszek-Berendsen A, Tange H, van den Herik HJ, Hasman A. From clinical practice guidelines to computer-interpretable guidelines. A literature overview. Methods Inf Med 2010;49(6):550–70.

[23] Mulyar N, van der Aalst WM, Peleg M. A pattern-based analysis of clinical computer-interpretable guideline modeling languages. J Am Med Inform Assoc 2007;14(6):781–7.

[24] Panzarasa S, Maddè S, Quaglini S, Pistarini C, Stefanelli M. Evidence-based careflow management systems: the case of post-stroke rehabilitation. J Biomed Inform 2002;35(2):123–39.

[25] Petri CA, Reisig W. Petri net. Scholarpedia 2008;3(4):6477.

[26] Jensen K. Coloured petri nets. Springer Verlag; 1997.

[27] ter Hofstede AH, van der Aalst WM. YAWL: yet another workflow language. Inform Syst 2005;30(4):245–75.

[28] van der Aalst WM, ter Hofstede AH, Kiepus-zewsky B, Barros AP. Workflow patterns. Distrib Parallel Dat 2003;14(1):5–51.

[29] Workflow patterns home page. <http://www.workflowpatterns.com>.

[30] van der Aalst WM, Aldred L, Dumas M, ter Hofstede AH. Design and implementation of the YAWL system. In: Proceedings of the 16th intelligence conference on advanced information systems engineering (CAiSE 04). Riga, Latvia; June 2004.

[31] Leonardi G, Panzarasa S, Quaglini S, Stefanelli M, Van der Aalst WM. Interacting agents through a web-based health serviceflow management system. J Biomed Inform 2007;40:486–99.

[32] Reichert M, Rinderle S, Dadam P. ADEPT workflow management system. In: van der Aalst WMP, ter Hofstede AHM, Weske M, editors. Proceedings of international conference on business process management, BPM 2003, Eindhoven, The Netherlands, June 26–27, 2003. Lecture notes in computer science, vol. 2678. Springer; 2003. p. 370379.

[33] Adams M, ter Hofstede AH, Edmond D, van der Aalst WM. Implementing dynamic flexibility in workflows using worklets. BPM Center Report BPM-06-06; 2006. BPMcenter.org.

[34] van der Aalst WM, van Dongen BF, Herbst J, Maruster L, Schimm G, Weijters AJ. Workflow mining: a survey of issues and approaches. Data Knowl Eng 2003;47(2):237–67.

[35] Mans RS, Schonenberg MH, Leonardi G, Panzarasa S, Cavallini A, Quaglini S, van der Aalst WM. Process mining techniques: an application to stroke care. Stud Health Technol Inform 2008;136:573–8.

[36] Bellazzi R, Ferrazzi F, Sacchi L. Predictive data mining in clinical medicine: a focus on selected methods and applications. WIREs Data Min Knowl Disc 2011;1(5):416–30. doi: http://dx.doi.org/10.1002/widm.23

[37] Augusto JC. Temporal reasoning for decision support in medicine. Artif Intell Med 2005;33(1):1–24.

[38] Mitsa T. Temporal data mining. CRC Press; 2010.

[39] Stamkopoulos T, Diamantaras K, Maglaveras N, Strintzis M. ECG analysis using nonlinear PCA neural networks for ischemia detection. IEEE Trans Signal Process 1998;46(11):3058–67.

[40] Sternickel K. Automatic pattern recognition in ECG time series. Comput Methods Programs Biomed 2002;68(2):109–15.

[41] Chaovalitwongse WA, Prokopyev OA, Pardalos PM. Ann Oper Res 2006;148(1):227–50.

[42] Zhang H, Ho T, Lin M-S, Liang X. Feature extraction for time series classification using discriminating wavelet coefficients. In: Advances in neural networks—ISNN 2006. Berlin/Heidelberg: Springer; 2006. p. 1394–9.

[43] Chuah MC, Fu F. ECG anomaly detection via time series analysis. In: ISPA workshops; 2007. p. 123–35.

[44] Joshi A, Rajshekhar Chandran S, Phadke S, Jayaraman V, Kulkarni B. Arrhythmia classification using local hölder exponents and support vector machine. In: Pattern recognition and machine intelligence. Lecture notes in computer science, vol. 3776. Springer; 2005. p. 242–7.

[45] Asl BM, Setarehdan SK, Mohebbi M. Support vector machine-based arrhythmia classification using reduced features of heart rate variability signal. Artif Intell Med 2008;44(1):51–64.

[46] Shahar Y. A framework for knowledge-based temporal abstraction. Artif Intell 1997;90(1–2):79–133.

[47] Stacey M, McGregor C. Temporal abstraction in intelligent clinical data analysis: a survey. Arif Intell Med 2007;39(1):1–24.

[48] Siadaty MS, Knaus WA. Locating previously unknown patterns in data-mining results: a dual data- and knowledge-mining method. BMC Med Inform Decis Mak 2006;6:13.

[49] Silberschatz A, Tuzhilin A. What makes patterns interesting in knowledge discovery systems. IEEE Trans Knowl Data Eng 1996;8(6):970–4.

[50] Ohsaki M, Abe H, Tsumoto S, Yokoi H, Yamaguchi T. Evaluation of rule interestingness measures in medical knowledge discovery in databases. Artif Intell Med 2007;41(3):177–96.

[51] Bellazzi R, Magni P, De Nicolao G. Dynamic probabilistic networks for modelling and identifying dynamic systems: a MCMC approach. Intell Data Anal 1997;1:245–62.

[52] Hovorka R, Tudor RS, Southerden D, Meeking DR, Andreassen S, Hejlesen OK, Cavan DA. Dynamic updating in DIAS-NIDDM and DIAS causal probabilistic networks. IEEE Trans Biomed Eng 1999;46(2):158–68.

[53] Evers S, Lucas P. Constructing Bayesian networks for linear dynamic systems. In: Nicholson Ann, editor. Proceedings of the eighth UAI Bayesian modeling applications workshop (UAI-AW 2011), CEUR, Barcelona, Spain; 14th July, 2011, p. 26–33.

[54] Åström Karl J, Murray Richard M. Feedback systems: an introduction for scientists and engineers. Princeton University Press; 2008.

[55] <http://en.wikibooks.org/wiki/Systems-Theory>.

[56] Magni P, Bellazzi R, De Nicolao G. Bayesian Function learning using MCMC methods. IEEE Trans Pattern Anal Mach Intell 1998;20:1319–31.

[57] Sorenson HW. Kalman filtering: theory and application. IEEE 1985.

[58] Dagum P, Galper A. Time series prediction using Belief Networks models. Int J Human-Comput Stud 1995;42:617–32.

[59] Russel S, Norvig P. Artificial intelligence: a modern approach. Prentice Hall; 1995.

[60] Nodelman U, Shelton C, Koller D. Continuous time Bayesian networks. In: Darwiche Adnan, Friedman Nir, editors. Proceedings of the Eighteenth Conference Conference on Uncertainty in Artificial Intelligence, August 1–4, 2002, Alberta, Canada. San Francisco, CA: Morgan Kaufman; 2002. p. 378–87.

[61] Fan Y, Shelton CR. Learning continuous-time social network dynamics. In: Bilmes Jeff, Ng Andrew, editors. Proceedings of the Twenty-Fifth Conference Conference on Uncertainty in Artificial Intelligence, June 18–21, 2009, Montreal, QC, Canada. Corvallis, Oregon: AUAI Press; 2009. p. 161–8.

[62] Gatti E, Luciani D, Stella F. A continuous time Bayesian network model for cardiogenic heart failure. Flex Serv Manufact J 2011:1–20.

[63] Nodelman U, Koller D, Shelton CR. Expectation propagation for continuous time Bayesian networks. In: Bacchus Fahiem, Jaakkola Tommi, editors. Proceedings of the Twenty-First Conference Conference on Uncertainty in Artificial Intelligence, July 26–29, 2005, Edinburgh, Scotland. Arlington, Virginia: AUAI Press; 2005. p. 431–40.

[64] Stella F, Amer Y. Continuous time Bayesian network classifiers. J Biomed Inform 2012;45:1108–19.

[65] Fan Y, Xu J, Shelton CR. Importance sampling for continuous time Bayesian networks. J Mach Learn Res 2010;11:2115–40.

[66] El-Hay T, Friedman N, Kupferman R. Gibbs sampling in factorized continuous time Markov processes. In: McAllester David, Myllymaki Petri, editors. Proceedings of the Twenty-Fourth Conference Conference on Uncertainty in Artificial Intelligence, July 9–12, 2008, Helsinki, Finland. Corvallis, Oregon: AUAI Press; 2008. p. 169–78.

[67] Sacchi L, Larizza C, Combi C, Bellazzi R. Data mining with temporal abstractions: learning rules from time series. Data Mining Knowl Disc 2007;15(2):217–47.

[68] Verduijn M, Sacchi L, Peek N, Bellazzi R, de Jonge E, de Mol BA. Temporal abstraction for feature extraction: a comparative case study in prediction from intensive care monitoring data. Artif Intell Med 2007;41(1):1–12.

[69] Moskovitch R, Peek N, Shahar Y. Classification of ICU patients via temporal abstraction and temporal patterns mining. In: IDAMAP09. Verona; 2009.

[70] Bellazzi R, Larizza C, Magni P, Montani S, Stefanelli M. Intelligent analysis of clinical time series: an application in the diabetes mellitus domain. Artif Intell Med 2000;20(1):37–57.

[71] Silva A, Cortez P, Santos MF, Gomes L, Neves J. Rating organ failure via adverse events using data mining in the intensive care unit. Artif Intell Med 2008;43(3):179–93.

[72] Bellazzi R, Abu-Hanna A. Data mining technologies for blood glucose and diabetes management. J Diabetes Sci Technol 2009;3(3):603–12.

[73] Seyfang A, Paesold M, Votruba P, Miksch S. Improving the execution of clinical guidelines and temporal data abstraction high-frequency domains. Stud Health Technol Inform 2008;139:263–72.

[74] Bellazzi R, Larizza C, Magni P, Bellazzi R. Temporal data mining for the quality assessment of hemodialysis services. Artif Intell Med 2005;34(1):25–39.

[75] Bellazzi R, Zupan B. Predictive data mining in clinical medicine. Current issues and guidelines. Int J Med Inform 2008;77(2):81–97.

[76] P. Chapman, J. Clinton, R. Kerber, T. Khabaza, T. Reinartz, C. Shearer, R. Wirth. CRISP-DM 1.0: Step-by-step data mining guide: The CRISP-DM Consortium, 2000.

[77] Witten IH, Frank E. Data mining: practical machine learning tools and techniques with Java implementations. San Francisco, Calif: Morgan Kaufmann; 1999.

[78] Friedman CP, Wyatt JC. Evaluation methods in biomedical informatics. New York: Springer; 2006.

[79] Kaplan B, Harris-Salamone KD. Health IT success and failure: recommendations from literature and an AMIA workshop. J Am Med Inform Assoc 2009;16(3):291–9.

[80] Beynon-Davies P. Information systems failure: the case of the London ambulance service's computer aided despatch project. Eur J Inf Syst 1995;4:171–84.

[81] Kaplan B, Shaw N. Future directions in evaluation research: people, organizational, and social issues. Methods Inf Med 2004;43(3–4):215–31.

[82] Bloxham A. £13 Billion NHS computer system failures affecting patient care. Telegraph; August 10, 2008. <http://www.telegraph.co.uk/news/uknews/2535099/13-bn-NHScomputer-system-failures-affecting-patient-care.html> [accessed 27.12.12].

[83] Aarts J, Berg M. Same system, different outcomes. Methods Inf Med 2006;45:53–61.

[84] Han Y, Carcillo J, Venkataraman S, et al. Unexpected increased mortality after implementation of a commercially sold computerized physician order entry system. Pediatrics 2005;116(6):1506–12.

[85] Silverstein S. Contemporary issues in medical informatics: good health IT, bad health IT, and common examples of healthcare IT difficulties. <http://www.ischool.drexel.edu/faculty/ssilverstein/cases> [accessed 27.12.12].

[86] Aarts J, Callen J, Coiera E, Westbrook J. Information technology in health care: socio-technical approaches. Int J Med Inform 2010;79(6):389–90.

[87] Coiera E, Aarts J, Kulikowski C. The dangerous decade. J Am Med Inform Assoc 2012;19(1):2–5.

Biomedical Informatics Methods for Personalized Medicine and Participatory Health

Fernando Martin-Sanchez[a], Guillermo Lopez-Campos[a], and Kathleen Gray[b]

[a]Health and Biomedical Informatics Centre, Melbourne Medical School, Faculty of Medicine, Dentistry & Health Sciences, The University of Melbourne, Melbourne, VIC, Australia
[b]Health and Biomedical Informatics Centre, Melbourne Medical School, Faculty of Medicine, Dentistry & Health Sciences and Department of Computing and Information Systems, The University of Melbourne, Melbourne, VIC, Australia

Contemporary medicine faces major challenges, among which are the increasing incidence of chronic diseases, rise of unhealthy life habits (e.g., sedentary lifestyle, fast food, alcohol, tobacco), escalating costs of medical technology, aging of the population in the developed world and spread of infectious diseases ensuing from climate change. All these factors call into question the sustainability of healthcare systems. There is clear need for a far-reaching transformation from the current approach in healing diseases toward a stronger focus on prevention.

To advance disease prevention, the scientific and medical community has been working on two solutions, so far quite independently.

On one hand, advances in analytical technologies in the biomedical laboratory have enabled a greater potential for analysis of patient molecular information and deciphering the molecular basis of disease. This work stream has advanced the concept of personalized medicine, which has proved successful in various ways, such as the availability of earlier diagnostic methods, more personalized therapies, more efficient clinical trials, and improved disease classification systems, among others.

On the other hand, advances in technologies associated with the social web (e.g., mobile devices and smartphones, games and sensors, used in conjunction with social networking sites, blogging and video-sharing tools) are giving rise to a wave of innovation in which patients and consumers take more responsibility for the maintenance of their own health and demand a greater role in the processes of clinical decision-making. This trend is based on the availability of technological tools that let patients collect data about their health, manage this information, share it with colleagues or clinicians, and even conduct analyses to gain knowledge that could help them to improve their health. This area is known as *participatory health*. Some successful experiences in this area report that they contribute to more preventive approaches through improved risk profiling, better models of disease prediction, and redirection of healthcare costs.

Both trends are based on an intensive use of information and therefore pose major challenges for biomedical informatics. In this chapter, we review the main data sources and methods for their use in the fields of personalized medicine and participatory health.

Both trends are likely to overlap in the near future. To study, cure, and ultimately prevent diseases that are a result of complex interactions between genetic and environmental factors, we need to have access to a multitude of biomedical data. Until recently, this capability has been limited to major research centers and hospitals, which are able to maintain sophisticated data collection and data processing equipment. However, now individuals are able to access technologies that can measure their personal genetic, environmental, and physiological profiles. Many do not hesitate to share this information with the community. Although there are still many unknowns in terms of the clinical value of these data, medicine should not miss this opportunity and should use this information for care and research to the fullest extent possible.

11.1 INTRODUCTION TO PERSONALIZED MEDICINE

Personalized medicine can be defined as an emerging practice in medicine that uses an individual's genetic profile to guide decision-making about the prevention, diagnosis, and treatment of disease. Knowledge of a patient's genetic profile can help doctors select the proper medication or therapy and administer it using the proper dose or regimen. Personalized medicine is being advanced through data from the Human Genome Project (Glossary of genetic terms, National Human Genome Research Institute, National Institutes of Health). Personalized medicine will facilitate the advent of a more precise approach in which preventive, diagnostic, and therapeutic solutions will be tailored to groups of individuals taking into account their molecular fingerprint (genome) [1], phenotype—the term used for the entirety of an individual's scientifically observable characteristics, such as morphology, biochemical and physiological properties—(phenome) and environmental exposure (exposome).

Although in recent years there has been some discussion on whether it is more appropriate to use the term "individualized" or "stratified" medicine to refer to this concept, it is clear that regardless of the term used, biomedical informatics has a key role to play in its exploration and application. Biomedical informatics creates new knowledge about the tools and methods required for the storage, integration, analysis, and visualization of a plethora of data with the aim of improving current diagnostic, prognostic, and therapeutic methods by adjusting them precisely to each individual patient based on her or his unique characteristics.

The aim of this chapter is to provide an overview of some of the currently available methods and tools discovered in biomedical informatics that can enable the delivery of more individualized care. Brief descriptions of current initiatives and resources associated with these different areas are arranged under two main subheadings—data storage and data analysis—illustrating just some of the biomedical informatics approaches that are enabling current applications and the development of personalized medicine.

As stated previously, personalized medicine requires the integrated use of genomic, phenotypic, and environmental information for its development. In medicine, the phenotype can be described in terms of the physiopathological parameters affecting an individual. These characteristics are determined by the interplay between specific genetic background and environment. Therefore, the equation "Genome * Exposome = Phenome" is at the core of our understanding of personalized medicine.

Throughout this chapter, we first review the basic management of genomic, phenotypic, and environmental data for personalized medicine; this includes everything from generation, collection, and data storage to their validation, annotation, and standardization, as well as issues related to searching, accessing, and retrieving such information. Then, following the same scheme, we review aspects of the integrated analysis of these data (genomic, phenotypic, and environmental) as well as their visualization and interpretation for future use in personalized medicine.

11.2 DATA SOURCES FOR PERSONALIZED MEDICINE

In the last two decades, we have witnessed advances in molecular biology and biotechnology that have revolutionized biomedical research. One of the most important advances has resulted from the availability of sophisticated laboratory equipment that is capable of generating unprecedented amounts of data from different experimental sources ranging from nucleic acid sequences to massive analyses of protein profiles. The vast amount of molecular data of potential interest for personalized medicine has overwhelmed the scientific community, and as a result new resources have been developed to facilitate the storage of these data and to provide public access to these datasets.

The fact that numerous inherited disorders exist has been known for a long time, but several hurdles have prevented us from understanding the underlying molecular causes of those disorders. The development of the Human Genome Project propelled advances in the methods used in molecular biology and bioinformatics technology, setting the basis for the development of a new way of practicing medicine where individual aspects encoded in each individual's genome could be factored into clinical decision processes. Advances in deoxyribonucleic acid (DNA) analysis technology, DNA microarrays, and next-generation sequencing technologies have further enabled massive genotyping by means of the analysis of SNPs (single nucleotide polymorphisms), exome (regions of DNA that code for proteins) sequencing, and whole genome sequencing at an affordable cost and in a short time. These processes are turning the idea of personalized medicine into a reality.

We note that although formally gene expression, proteomic data, and metabolomic data should be considered as part of the phenotype of a particular cell (i.e., how a particular genotype is expressed in response to an exposure), for the purpose of this chapter the main types of molecular data will be grouped under the "Genome" term of the "Genome * Exposome = Phenome" equation (i.e., how the entirety of a person's hereditary information is expressed).

Microarray data represent a good example of these new sources of data with potential application in the medical field. Originally microarrays were intended for clinical applications related to genotyping. An example was the development of a microarray for the detection of antiviral resistance mutations on HIV [2,3]. Methods for gene expression data analysis were then developed and microarrays were used heavily to generate expression profiles associated with various pathological conditions and identify gene expression signatures of clinical interest [4,5]. As these studies became more popular, the amount of generated data grew. This led to the development of specific repositories for these data such as the European Bioinformatics Institute's (EBI) ArrayExpress, the National Center for Biotechnology Information's (NCBI) Gene Expression Omnibus (GEO), and the United States Food and Drug Administration's (FDA) ArrayTrack. In an effort to improve the reproducibility of the analyses, a set of standards was developed to represent the resulting data and enable annotations to be included with the samples (e.g., clinical details and parameters). Lately, microarrays have been extensively used again in the area of genotyping. Many research studies using SNP microarrays have attempted to identify or link certain common genetic variants with common diseases. These technologies are used increasingly and valued widely.

With recent advances in next-generation DNA sequencing technologies, new data repositories associated with these technologies have emerged. Notable in this context is the laudable and significant work of the 1000 Genomes Project (www.1000genomes.org), which aims to sequence the genomes of more than 1000 people of different races and genetic backgrounds and freely provide the data for clinical research.

Having access to molecular sequence data is one of the most remarkable achievements in the development of personalized medicine. However, to explain observed phenotypes and hence understand the intricate processes involved in disease development, it is necessary to combine molecular information with environmental data, such as diet, exposure to infectious or chemical agents, drugs, and medications. Traditionally, these data have been captured by different means such as environmental monitoring with sensors or life habits surveys, and in some cases this information has been included in patients' clinical records. Nevertheless, environmental data capture is an evolving area and interest in it is rising, thanks to the availability of new portable devices and citizens' growing willingness to use such devices and share their personal environmental exposure data for biomedical research.

Clinical records have always been a valuable resource for research in biomedical sciences. With the advent of these new technologies and the huge amounts of information generated at the molecular level, clinical records must be adapted. In future, they will need to mesh clinical data with these new data types and feed data into cohort and population studies, thus providing valuable information regarding the phenotype and the most detailed description of patients' characteristics. Recent years have witnessed an expansion in the use and application of electronic health records (EHRs). These systems have simplified access to relevant clinical data required for combination with molecular data in order to achieve the goals of personalized medicine.

11.2.1 Retrieving and Using Phenotypic Data

The clinical record has been considered a gold mine for phenotypic annotation of patients' samples. But whereas in traditional experiments, it was feasible to use manual methods for extraction and interpretation of clinical data, advances in experimental technologies for gathering molecular data have created a new high-throughput approach that has outpaced our capability to transform them into accurate and complete medically actionable data.

The growth in the implementation and use of EHRs promises to reduce the effort required to extract clinical data, providing high-throughput phenotyping methods that can be coordinated with their molecular counterparts. Nevertheless, this promise comes with significant challenges for biomedical informatics. On one hand, the use of EHRs opens a new opportunity for data capture and exchange between research and clinical practice, linking genomic analyses with the data contained within the EHR. On the other hand, the application of molecular and genomic data in clinical practice requires including them as essential data elements within the EHR. It is still a challenge to design EHRs that can function as the bridge between clinical care and research in personalized medicine.

11.2.1.1 *Data Retrieval in EHRs*

Clinical records are an essential element in health care and from a research perspective they represent a high-quality information source. The trend to develop and deploy EHRs widely in the health sector has facilitated access to massive and valuable information sources for personalized medicine through processes based on large-scale, automated text mining.

Accessing the data within EHRs is faced with many hurdles. Although huge efforts have been devoted to implementing standardized terminologies and codes to describe these data, in many cases they are applied only for billing purposes or laboratory results reporting. Most of the phenotypic data in an EHR are stored as free text, often available only in narrative form. Thus the EHR contains much implicit information that clinicians readily comprehend but that is not encoded for systematic retrieval. There are other limitations faced in the extraction and interpretation of phenotypic data stored in EHRs in terms of their granularity, completeness, and accuracy, or rather the lack of these—factors that are due to the complexity of the clinical environment where the data are captured. For these reasons, accessing and extracting data from EHRs is a challenging area of biomedical informatics where many different approaches have been developed.

Natural Language Processing (NLP) systems are automated approaches that aim to understand natural (human) language. NLP systems can be used to extract unstructured information contained within narrative sections of the EHRs. Generally this extracted information is transformed into a structured format such as a controlled vocabulary or an ontology that will have further

Table 11.1 Description of the different tasks for NLP systems identified by Nadkarni et al. (2011).

Low-Level NLP Tasks

1. *Sentence boundary detection*. At this step the text is divided into sentences to be further processed
2. *Tokenization*. It is the process where the sentences are divided into individual tokens, usually words
3. *Part-of-Speech (POS) tagging*. The previously identified tokens are assigned to a grammatical category
4. *Morphological decomposition*. Identification of compound words which are abundant in medical vocabulary and decompose them to their root
5. *Shallow parsing*. Consists in the identification of phrases made of syntactic units such as noun phrases where a noun and modifiers (e.g., adjectives) are together

High-Level NLP Tasks

1. *Spelling and grammatical error identification*. This is an important aspect in the analysis of EHRs because they are prone to have these kind of errors
2. *Name Entity Recognition (NER)*. At this step the phrases identified by the shallow parsing step or the words are categorized and often mapped to terms in controlled vocabularies or concepts in ontologies such as SNOMED-CT, NCI-Thesaurus, or ICD codes
3. *Word Sense Disambiguation (WSD)*. Identifies the correct "meaning" of a word in its particular context
4. *Negation and uncertainty identification*. This task is focused in context of the extracted items and tries to infer whether the entity is present or absent, and measure the uncertainty of such inference
5. *Relationship extraction*
6. *Temporal relationships*. In the narrative context of the EHR there are some temporal relationships and this step is focused on identifying or inferring those relationships

different uses. Data extraction is a multi-step process [6] (Table 11.1), where different tasks and parameters can be adjusted.

A multitude of NLP systems have been developed and used in biomedical informatics [7,8] (Table 11.2) for many years, and their different algorithms are typically based on the use of hand-written rule-based tools and heuristic iterative approaches, machine learning methods, and combinations of these strategies.

The use of rule-based methods can be successful, but these approaches are time consuming, require manual effort, and are generally difficult to scale,

Table 11.2 Example of NLP (Natural Language Processing) tools used to extract information from the EHRs (electronic health records).

NLP Program
HITEX[a]
MedLEE[b]
cTAKES[c]
MPLUS[d]
MEDSYNDITAKE[e]
BioTeKS[f]
ACCCA[g]
MetaMap[h]
ODIE[i]
SymText[j]
SPIN[k]

[a]*Zeng QT, Goryachev S, Weiss S, Sordo M, Murphy SN, Lazarus R. Extracting principal diagnosis, co-morbidity and smoking status for asthma research: evaluation of a Natural Language Processing system. BMC Med Inform Decis Mak. 2006 Jul 26;6:30.* [b]*Friedman C. Towards a comprehensive medical language processing system: methods and issues. Proc AMIA Annu Fall Symp. 1997:595–9.* [c]*Savova GK, Masanz JJ, Ogren PV, Zheng J, Sohn S, Kipper-Schuler KC, Chute CG. Mayo clinical Text Analysis and Knowledge Extraction System (cTAKES): architecture, component evaluation and applications. J Am Med Inform Assoc. 2010 Sep-Oct;17(5):507–13.* [d]*Christensen L, Haug P, Fiszman M. MPLUS: A Probabilistic Medical Language Understanding System. Proceedings of the Workshop on Natural Language Processing in the Biomedical Domain. 2002:29–36. BioNLP 2002.* [e]*Hahn U, Romacker M, Schulz S. Creating knowledge repositories from biomedical reports: the MEDSYNDIKATE text mining system. Pac Symp Biocomput. 2002:338–49.* [f]*Mack R. Mukherjea S, Soffer A, Uramoto N, Brown E, Coden A. Cooper J, Inokuchi A, Iyer B, Mass Y, Matsozawa H, SubramaniamLV. Text analytics for life science using the unstructured information management architecture. IBM Syst J. 2004; 43:490–515.* [g]*Kang N, Afzal Z, Singh B, van Mulligen EM, Kors JA. Using an ensemble system to improve concept extraction from clinical records. J Biomed Inform. 2012 Jun;45(3):423–8. doi: 10.1016/j.jbi.2011.12.009. Epub 2012 Jan 3.* [h]*Aronson AR. Effective mapping of biomedical text to the UMLS Metathesaurus: the MetaMap program. Proc AMIA Symp. 2001:17–21.* [i]*https://bmir-gforge.stanford.edu/gf/project/odie/ Accessed November 2012.* [j]*Haug PJ, Koehler S, Lau LM, Wang P, Rocha R, Huff SM. Experience with a mixed semantic/syntactic parser. Proc Annu Symp Comput Appl Med Care. 1995:284–8.* [k]*Liu K, Mitchell kJ, Chapman WW, Crowley RS. Automating tissue bank annotation from pathology reports—comparison to a gold standard expert annotation set. AMIA Annu Symp Proc 2005:460–4.*

so they can be used for simple queries only. The alternative approach—machine learning methods—uses statistical approaches and algorithms that allow the software to infer rules based on the analysis of annotated training datasets. These analyses are then used to make predictions about the studied dataset, which then can be applied to new datasets of the same type. Chapter 6 provides more details about the these types of NLP techniques.

The eMERGE (Electronic Medical Records and Genomics) network is a multi-center project funded by the United States National Human Genome

Research Institute (NHGRI) for the purpose of developing and testing methods that combine information from EHRs with DNA biobanks to foster high-throughput genetic research [9]. In the first phase of the project, the goal was to develop algorithms associated with the retrieval of data corresponding to 14 different phenotypes. For this purpose, methods based on either NLP or structured data were developed and used successfully across participating centers to extract the target information. In this research, NLP-based methodologies performed better than extraction from structured data, identifying more cases with the desired phenotypes because they could analyze data that were available only as free text. Therefore, NLP has been shown to be a key tool for the retrieval of data associated with phenotypes of interest [10]. For more discussion on the leveraging of EHRs for translational research, see Chapter 12.

11.2.1.2 *Uses of EHR Data in Personalized Medicine*

The development of personalized medicine is tightly linked with advances in translational research. In this setting, the EHR is a potential data source for research. It can also be a valuable resource for research in related areas such as pharmacogenomics or pharmacovigilance.

The effect of different drugs on different patients is affected by each patient's genetic variants on those genes related to the metabolism of the drug, which affect drug pharmacodynamics and pharmacokinetics. Pharmacogenomics represents a paradigmatic area of personalized medicine, wherein the patient's genetic information is associated with the different possible responses to drugs. There are drugs currently available that include pharmacogenomics data in their labeling [11] and that require a patient to have a genetic test before the treating clinician proceeds with drug selection, prescription, or dosing. In these cases, it is extremely important to be able to integrate the patient's genetic data into the clinical record in order to combine both types of information. Examples of these relationships between commonly used drugs and genetic background are warfarin, for which there is a well known relationship between their effects and the different single nucleotide variants (SNVs) in the genes CYP2C9 and VKORC [12], as well as clopidogrel and SNVs in the gene CYP2C19 [13].

In practice, the use of this information requires that the practitioner is able to access information about the relationship between a certain drug and the genetic background of the patient, the availability of genetic tests to elicit genetic information of interest for the prescription of the drug and existing dosing guidelines. The Pharmacogenomics Knowledge Base (PharmGKB) is a publicly available online resource containing a variety of curated pharmacogenomics information [14] (Figure 11.1). PharmGKB stores information related with genomic SNV annotation including references to the literature, clinical annotation, and interpretation of data on the basis of the genotype. Information about important genes from a pharmacogenomics perspective, or VIP (Very Important Pharmacogenes), is also provided. Finally, this resource offers information about pathways involved in drug metabolism. All of this information is oriented to application, divided into "Clinical Pharmacogenomics information" (Clinical PGx) or "Pharmacogenomics Research" (PGx Research), with details presented through tabbed web browsing.

Within the Clinical PGx tab, it is possible to find information related to dosing guidelines, including excerpts from the guidelines and access to dosing algorithms and literature references, drug labels extracted from the US Food and Drug Administration, clinical annotations where each genetic variant is associated with a level of evidence supporting its clinical relevance, and finally some of the available tests for measuring the previously reported variants.

As a consequence of the extension in the use of pharmacogenomics in clinical practice combined with the increasing amount of available information, there is demand for the development of more sophisticated clinical decision support systems (CDSS). In this context, these systems have been referred to as Personalized Decision Support Systems (PDSS) [15,16]. These CDSSs

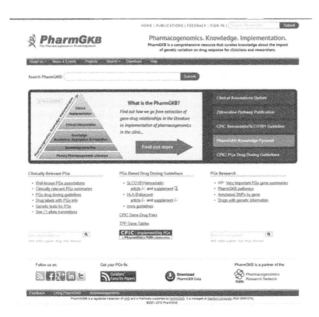

■ **FIGURE 11.1** PharmGKB Screenshots. PharmGKB is a curated database containing information relating to genes and drugs in pharmacogenomics.

are designed so that they can guide clinicians' decisions about the prescription and dosing of certain drugs when patient genetic data are available and the drug has pharmacogenomic dosing guidelines. An important success factor in the implementation of these CDSSs is that information is correctly represented and available in the system [17].

Interestingly, the first CDSS to support the prescription of drugs based on genetic analysis and SNVs was designed in the infectious diseases domain, for the management of HIV infected patients [18,19]. In this system, the genetic information used consisted of patterns of drug-resistant mutations detected in the viral populations infecting patients. The system used that information to support the selection of a drug regimen and provided an explanation supporting that choice. More recently, the advances carried out by pharmacogenomics combined with the inclusion of structured genetic information within an EHR have led to the development of what is generally considered "personalized medicine oriented" CDSS. Examples of these types of systems have been developed for psychiatric medication [20], warfarin and clopidogrel [21,22]. In all these systems, computational models of information associated with different SNPs and their effect in drug metabolism are used to support the dosing adjustment recommendations.

In recent years, there has been an increase in the number of biobanks (repositories of biological samples) where the samples can be matched up with the EHRs of the donors. In this scenario, the analysis of samples stored in the biobank can be correlated with features of clinical phenotypic data. This degree of data linking enables the use of the samples for multiple purposes in research and can drive new research in personalized medicine.

The existence of repositories with biological samples combined with clinical information facilitates the development of studies where sampling is carried out based on the use of certain clinical parameters of interest. This approach is especially relevant for the design of association studies. In this case, the phenotypic information can be mined to identify those biobank samples associated specifically with the phenotype of interest, helping to reduce the confounding variables in the experiment. Alternatively, the information contained in an EHR can be used to enrich the information of an already ongoing study or to expand the scope of studies by adding new samples with the required phenotypes. Both of these approaches have been defined as EHR-driven genomic research for phenotyping selection or phenotypic augmentation [23]. Examples of these kinds of approaches are the previously cited eMERGE Network, the Vanderbilt University Biobank BioVU, and the Danish National Biobank.

Another important role of biomedical informatics regarding the use of EHR as a valuable data source lies in the ethical and legal challenges posed by the use of this information. These challenges include developing reliable and robust methods for sample and data anonymization and the opposite, namely re-identification in cases where clinically important information may be discovered incidentally during research processes.

11.2.2 **Retrieving and Using Environmental Data**

The role played by the environment in the complex balance between health and diseases states is well known. The concept of an "exposome" was recently coined as an analogy to the genome: it highlights the need to obtain more data about an individual's environmental exposure [24]. More recently the "exposome" concept has been divided into three categories of exposures: internal, specific external, and general external [25]. The *internal exposures* refer to the internal environment of an organism and include aspects such as metabolites, hormones, etc. The *specific external exposures* refer to elements such as infectious agents, radiation, and other exposures to different pollutants. Finally, the *general external factors* refer to other aspects such as socio-economic and cultural aspects. This situation can be even more complex because it is known that some environmental factors may cause irreversible changes in the DNA sequences (e.g., ionizing radiation). Furthermore, thanks to recent advances in epigenomic studies, more subtle methods of reversible genome modification have been identified. Epigenomic changes work by altering genomic information as a response to environmental changes. For the purpose of this section, we will refer only to the second class of exposures, specifically external, keeping the elements involved in the internal exposures or the elements associated with epigenomics for the section on the genomic (molecular) data.

Ironically, environmental data surround us but accessing these data is an extremely challenging task, especially from a personalized medicine perspective where exposures to various environmental factors must be captured individually for each person. This departs from the traditional population-based approach, consisting of surveys measuring the effects of various environmental factors on groups of people. The development of this scientific area of enquiry, and of a more comprehensive process for collecting "personalized environmental" data, are closely connected with the development of participatory medicine. In participatory medicine, patients are starting to measure and manage many aspects of their exposure to risks that are related to environmental factors (as discussed further in Section 11.4 of this chapter).

Management of environmental factors associated with diseases and disease risk traditionally has been addressed by the disciplines of public health and epidemiology. Considering the phenotype as a combination of the genotype and the effect of the environment poses a new challenge for biomedical informatics: the need to develop sound methods to gather and manage personal environmental information. This could be vital in the development of personalized medicine.

Some important sources of data related to environmental factors of interest for personalized medicine are those where different toxic elements (such as small molecules or even drugs) are studied using a molecular perspective. Toxicogenomics was defined as the use of "-omics" technologies in toxicology more concretely, starting with microarrays [26]. Biomedical informatics has had a strong influence in the development of toxicogenomics and contributed to the creation of databases and analytical tools. As a result, there are several data resources associated with toxicogenomics and other chemical compounds, including drugs, which include relevant information that may be useful for personalized medicine (Table 11.3).

An important bridge between toxicogenomics and personalized medicine is the use of ontologies and controlled vocabularies. The Gene Ontology (GO) is an example of an ontology that plays a bridging role. An example of a controlled vocabulary is MEDIC (MErged DIsease voCabulary) [27] a fusion of OMIM (Online Mendelian Inheritance in Man), MeSH (Medical Subject Headings) "Diseases" branch, and the Comparative Toxicogenomic Database (CTD). The use of MEDIC has enabled the generation of more than 2.5 million disease-associated relationships in CTD.

It is possible to access some types of environmental exposure information through the clinical record, such as smoking or alcohol drinking habits, but more commonly these data are gathered either in population surveys or for specific purposes (for example measuring food intake in people on specific diets or medication regimens).

As a consequence of this fragmentation in sources of information there is a clear need for the development of data harmonization strategies to enable the use of multiple distributed data sources. To alleviate this problem, the PhenX (Consensus Measures for Phenotypes and Exposures) project has identified a set of important consensus measures [28]. The aim of the PhenX project (www.phenx.org), funded by the NHGRI and developed by RTI International, is to develop and provide a series of recommended measures to be used in large-scale genomic studies, such as genome-wide association studies (GWAS), that integrate epidemiological and genomic research. The proposed measures are built around 21 research domains covering aspects such as: alcohol, tobacco, and other substances, environmental exposures, physical activity, and physical fitness; social environment; nutrition and dietary supplements. For each

Table 11.3   Resources of interest for toxicogenomics with information that might be of interest for personalized medicine.

Name	Description
CEBS (Chemical Effects in Biological Systems)	Public resource with curated data about toxicogenomics http://www.niehs.nih.gov/research/resources/databases/cebs/index.cfm
LTKB (Liver Toxicity Knowledge Base)	US FDA system with data knowledge and data mining tools to analyze drug-induced liver injury. Benchmark dataset contains information related to 287 prescription drugs http://www.fda.gov/ScienceResearch/BioinformaticsTools/LiverToxicityKnowledgeBase/default.htm
CTD (Comparative Toxicogenomic Database)	A manually curated database containing information about gene products and environmental chemical substances and their linkage with diseases http://ctdbase.org/
ChemProt	Database related to systems pharmacology based on chemical-protein resources and disease-associated protein-protein interactions http://www.cbs.dtudk/services/ChemProt/
PubChem	Set of databases (PubChem Compound, PubChem Substance, and PubChem BioAssay) http://pubchem.ncbi.nlm.nih.gov/
ChEBI (Chemical Entities of Biological Interest)	Database containing data from other resources (such as KEGG Compound or ChEMBL). It contains information about the molecules and it is cross-referenced to other resources containing molecular information such as pathways, gene expression results, or proteins www.ebi.ac.uk/chebi/
Drugbank	Combines more than 150 fields related to drug and target data (such as sequence, structure, and pathway) for more than 6500 elements associated with more than 4000 proteins http://www.drugbank.ca/
ChEMBL	EBI Database with bioactive small molecules (around 500,000) containing information on molecular properties and bioactivities such as pharmacology and ADMET data. It offers a query system based on the compounds, the targets or the assays. It contains data from PubChem. **e** http://www.ebi.ac.uk/chembl/

of these domains, the project identifies and catalogues 15 different measures and detailed protocols associated with each of those measures. The catalogue containing these recommended elements is freely accessible and allows users to browse and query the system via a web interface called "PhenX Toolkit" (http://www.phenxtoolkit.org/) (Figure 11.2).

PhenX RISING (Real-world Implementation, SharING) is an effort to incorporate those measures defined in the PhenX project into existing population-based genomic studies. To ensure compatibility of PhenX measures with other relevant biomedical informatics standards, there are ongoing collaborations with LOINC (Logical Observation Identifiers Names and Codes) [29] and other projects [30].

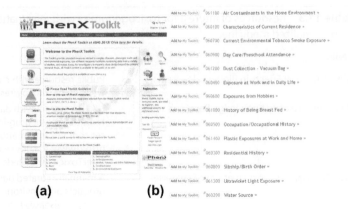

(a) **(b)**

■ **FIGURE 11.2** Screenshots of PhenX. (a) Screenshot of the main interface of PhenX toolkit. (b) Detail of the environmental exposures.

An alternative view on the harmonization of information is offered by the Data Schema and Harmonization Platform for Epidemiological Research (DataSHaPER—http://www.datashaper.org) [31]. This approach is based on a flexible harmonization scheme and supports retrospective data analysis, whereas the more stringent approach based on the use of PhenX enhances the analysis of studies using elements from this catalogue [32].

11.2.3 **Retrieving and Using Genetic Data**

Probably the best known and developed aspect of personalized medicine consists of the use of genomic and molecular information. Following the structure of this discussion of personalized medicine around the equation, "Genome * Exposome = Phenome," this section discusses the major information resources and methods to share not only genetic information but also molecular information from individuals more globally.

As previously mentioned, changes in available technologies in biological research have had a huge impact on the ways that experiments are conducted and data are managed. The development of "-omics" approaches at every possible level (genomics, transcriptomics, proteomics, metabolomics, etc.) has created unprecedented amounts of data that are of interest for medicine whether for clinical practice or for biomedical research. The latest disruptive technology is massively parallel sequencing (MPS) also known as next-generation sequencing (NGS). These techniques threaten to deliver a deluge of data for potentially routine use in clinical medicine. As a consequence of advances in these methods there is a huge number of genetic and molecular data resources freely available over the Internet (Table 11.4).

Table 11.4 Examples of Internet resources related with molecular data of interest for personalized medicine.

Resource	Type of Data Stored
	These are the three major DNA databases, where all the DNA sequences are stored.
Genbank	http://www.ncbi.nlm.nih.gov/genbank/
ENA	http://www.ebi.ac.uk/ena/
DDBJ	http://www.ddbj.nig.ac.jp/
ENSEMBL	Genome Browser with highly annotated data. http://www.ensembl.org/index.html
UCSC GenomeBrowser	Genome Browser with highly annotated data. http://genome.ucsc.edu/
Entrez Gene	Integrates information related genes including the reference sequences, variations, phenotypes… http://www.ncbi.nlm.nih.gov/gene
GeneCards/GeneTests	Database with information about known and predicted human genes. http://www.genecards.org/
HUGO/HGNC	Human Genome Organization gene nomenclature committee provides unique names and symbols for human loci and includes links to related genomic, proteomic or phenotypic information. http://www.genenames.org/
dbSNP	Database containing information about short genetic variations. http://www.ncbi.nlm.nih.gov/projects/SNP/
ClinVar	Still in development, this database intends to capture and aggregate information about sequence variation and its relationship with human health. http://www.ncbi.nlm.nih.gov/clinvar/
dbVar	Contains information about large genomic variants. http://www.ncbi.nlm.nih.gov/dbvar/
HGMD	Humane Gene Mutation database provides information about mutations found in humans. http://www.hgmd.cf.ac.uk/
LOVD	Leiden Open Variation Database is genecentric and provides information about DNA variations. http://www.lovd.nl/2.0/
DGV	Database of Genomic Variants is a curated catalogue of structural genomic variants. http://projects.tcag.ca/variation/
MitoMap	Genome database with genetic variants in mitochondrial DNA http://www.mitomap.org
1000Genomes	Resource with information about human genome variation. http://www.1000genomes.org
Kegg	Kyoto Encyclopaedia of Gens and Genomes. Resource built up with different databases for understanding high-level functions of biological systems. KEGG contains different databases and entry points covering pathways (KEGG Pathway), genomes (KEGG Genomes), diseases (KEGG Disease), drugs (KEGG Drug) among others. More recently has developed KEGG Medicus as a health-related information resource linking several of its different data-oriented modules. http://www.genome.jp/kegg/
Reactome	Open source, open access, and manually curated pathway database. It is highly cross-referenced. http://www.reactome.org/
mirBase	Database containing information about microRNA sequences and annotation. http://www.mirbase.org/
ArrayExpress	Database of functional genomics experiments. http://www.ebi.ac.uk/arrayexpress/

(Continued)

Table 11.4 Examples of Internet resources related with molecular data of interest for personalized medicine (Continued).

Resource	Type of Data Stored
Gene Expression Atlas	Subset of curated and re-annotated data extracted from ArrayExpress. http://www.ebi.ac.uk/gxa/
GEO	Gene Expression Omnibus. Public functional genomics repository. http://www.ncbi.nlm.nih.gov/geo/
Genetic Testing Registry	Central repository for the voluntary submission of genetic test information. http://www.ncbi.nlm.nih.gov/gtr/
Orphanet	Portal for rare diseases and orphan drugs. http://www.orpha.net/consor/cgi-bin/index.php
EDDNAL	European Directory of DNA Diagnostic Laboratories. http://www.eddnal.com/
OMIM	Online Mendelian Inheritance in Man. It is a comprehensive repository of human genes and phenotypes about all known Mendelian disorders. http://www.omim.org/
ClinicalTrials	Database of publicly and privately supported clinical studies of human participants conducted around the world. http://clinicaltrials.gov/
dbGAP	Database of Genotypes and Phenotypes. It is an archive of studies that have investigated the interaction of genotype and phenotype. It offers controlled access. http://www.ncbi.nlm.nih.gov/gap.
EGA	European Genome-Phenome Archive. Repository of genetic studies linked with phenotypes. It offers controlled access. https://www.ebi.ac.uk/ega/
UniProt	Comprehensive high-quality protein sequence and function information resource. http://www.uniprot.org/
Prosite	Resource containing documentation entries describing protein domains, families, and functional sites as well as the patterns and profiles used to identify them. http://prosite.expasy.org/
InterPro	Resource for the functional analysis of proteins classifying them into families and predicting domains and important sites. http://www.ebi.ac.uk/interpro/
PDB	Protein Data Bank. Biological macromolecular resource contains the structure of different molecules as well as tools to visualize the structures. http://www.rcsb.org/pdb/home/home.do
Brenda	Comprehensive and high-quality curated database with information about enzymes. http://www.brenda-enzymes.info/
HOMER	Human Organ-specific Molecular Electronic Repository. Contains information about organ-specific molecules associated with disease-organ and disease-gene relationships. http://discern.uits.iu.edu:8340/Homer/index.html
HMDB	Human Metabolome database. Database containing information about human metabolites and small molecules, contains chemical, clinical, and biochemical data. http://www.hmdb.ca/

A revolution in biomedical informatics is coming not just because of the use of new types of data, but also because of the vast amount and diversity of data that must be stored, shared, and analyzed.

11.2.3.1 *Data Sharing and Molecular Information*

Accompanying the explosion of data in "-omics" technologies is the need to share all these data. Great efforts have been devoted to the development of data sharing standards at different levels and for different technologies. Many of these methods were initially developed by bioinformaticians for their use in research, but as the "-omics" technologies found their way in medicine these standards have been introduced into clinical information systems also. As a result, organizations such as the US Food and Drug Administration and various health information system vendors have increased their involvement in standards development and adoption.

The standards for data sharing in "-omics" can be grouped into two major categories: (1) experiment description and (2) experiment execution [33]. Experiment description standards have been developed for the different "-omics" and represent a major achievement for data sharing. The paradigmatic example is the MIAME (Minimum Information About a Microarray Experiment) standard. These standards can be subdivided into standards for:

- *Reporting*. These standards cover all the "minimum information" required to describe an experiment. The MIBBI (Minimal Information about Biological and Biomedical Investigations) project [34] has made an effort to promote the elaboration and later use of these reporting standards for biological and biomedical investigations. The use of these standards has been endorsed by many publications (such as *The Lancet*, *Nature*, *Science*, and *Cell*) thus requiring their use. A list of these initiatives can be found at the website of MIBBI (http://mibbi. sourceforge.net/), which notes their relevance and their possible impact in clinics and personalized medicine. Some of those standards include the previously cited MIAME (related with microarray experiments), MISFISHIE (for In Situ Hybridization and Immunohistochemistry Experiments), and the more recent MINSEQE (for high-throughput Sequencing Experiments).
- *Data exchange and modeling*. These standards have been developed to facilitate interoperability and exchange of data and often have been jointly produced with data modeling standards. In many cases, these systems are based on XML solutions. Examples are MAGE-ML/ MAGE-OM (Mark-up language developed for microarray experiment data exchange and object model) or the SBML (Systems Biology Mark-up Language). The development of the standards based on XML has faced some challenges by experimentalists. For this reason, an alternative tabulated format called MAGE-TAB was initially developed for microarray experiments to interact with MAGE-ML. This MAGE-TAB format was the seed for the further extension to other

environments of the more general ISA-TAB format (where ISA refers to Investigation/Study/Assay). The aim of the ISA-TAB format is *"to facilitate standards-compliant collection, curation, management and reuse of datasets in an increasingly diverse set of life science domains"* [35], and it provides a general framework for data collection and exchange through linking data and metadata. The ISA-TAB flexibility has been used to develop a customized version of the standard for nanotechnology called ISA-TAB Nano. A description of the ISA-TAB format and tools can be found at (http://isacommons.org). Another very important experiment description standard for personalized medicine and complementary to the ISA-TAB format is the Study Data Tabulation Model (SDTM). This format, created by the CDISC (Clinical Data Interchange Standards Consortium, http://www.cdisc.org), is very similar to the ISA-TAB format, overlapping in many aspects. It provides a structured framework and format to submit both clinical and non-clinical toxicological data to the authorities. From the clinical perspective, several efforts have been made to incorporate the "-omics" information into the different standards available such as HL7-GTR (Health Level 7 Genetic Testing Report), which at the time of this writing was not approved and distributed for testing.

■ *Terminology.* The development of standards for the "-omics" aspects of personalized medicine has created common ground for clinical and research perspectives as "-omics" results were included in clinical standards. Probably one of the most successful and well-known examples of these "-omics" standards is the Gene Ontology (GO). The use of these standards has facilitated interaction between different "-omics" linking them and enabling their adoption by personalized medicine. An example of an interesting ontology in personalized medicine is the Human Phenome Ontology. The increasing number of terminologies and ontologies developed in recent years has highlighted the need for repositories. The EBI Ontology Lookup Service (http://www.ebi.ac.uk/ontology-lookup) together with NCBO web portal (http://bioportal.bioontology.org) are important resources that provide access to the most relevant ontologies developed in the field of "-omics."

Experiment execution standards cover the definition of reference materials and the associated metadata. The development and adoption of massive parallel sequencing is a clear example of the need for these standards. There is currently a range of proposals for the development of these reference materials to be used in clinical settings to calibrate equipment and analytical pipelines. An example of these initiatives is a standard recently proposed by the US Centers for Disease Control and Prevention [36].

11.2.3.2 *Data Sharing and Privacy Concerns in a Genomic Era*

The development of new tests and methods based on genomic information, particularly those involving DNA sequencing, represents a new and important challenge for data sharing between clinical and research environments. As previously stated in this chapter, there is an increasing demand from research for access to clinically annotated samples. Previously, privacy issues in data sharing of clinical information for research have been resolved using anonymization methods, where any information enabling patient identification is removed. However, the new data that are shared for research related to personalized medicine are genomic data; two key characteristics of genetic data make privacy preservation in data sharing especially complex. Genetic data by their nature provide a way to identify unique patients or sample donors, and they also provide information about future susceptibility to certain diseases (either in patients themselves or in their families). In this context, biomedical informatics must develop new solutions for ethically, legally, and socially acceptable genomic data sharing [37].

GWAS studies are an example of the complexity of some privacy concerns. In the early development of these studies, screening for SNPs was carried out in different populations; in this situation the privacy of the individual participants relied on aggregation of the data. In 2006, the US National Institutes of Health began offering aggregated data through the Database of Genotypes and Phenotypes (dbGAP, http://www.ncbi.nlm.nih.gov/gap), where the individualized study data were kept private and under controlled access. However, advances in genomic knowledge and informatics methods have shown that it is theoretically possible to determine whether the DNA of a certain individual is within the pool of data of a GWAS study [38]. This has changed previous conceptions of privacy issues related to sharing of genomic data and prompted some modifications in the dbGAP data access policy. The present policy requires controlled access to all contents in a database containing genomic and other identifying information. Similarly, the policy in the European database EGA (European Genome-Phenotype Archive, http://www.ebi.ac.uk/ega) offers only controlled access to its contents.

Some biomedical informatics solutions have been suggested. One example is an encryption system developed to protect the transmission of genomic sequences between the sequencing laboratories and the hospitals [39]. The proposed system is based on a two-way encryption method that uses some of the genetic data of the sample for decrypting purposes.

An alternative and opposite model of data sharing in this context is used in the 1000 Genomes Project (http://www.1000genomes.org/) and the Personal

Genomes Project (PGP, http://www.personalgenomes.org/) where genomic information is made available freely and publicly for research. In the 1000 Genomes Project, researchers have collected over 1000 human genomes from volunteers in 14 different populations at the time of this writing and aim to double these numbers, to provide a deep view of human genetic variation that may lead to understanding better the genetic contribution to different diseases [1]. In the PGP, genetic information is obtained through genotyping analyses services such as those offered by companies like 23andMe or complete genome sequencing. In addition, PGP brings together other data like phenotypic data associated with health records and even the clinical interpretation of genetics variants associated with each sample. For that purpose, PGP uses the GET-Evidence system (Genome-Environment-Trait Evidence) [40] that presents and processes genomic information and automatically prioritizes variants for their interpretation by a peer production model.

11.3 DATA ANALYSIS FOR PERSONALIZED MEDICINE

This section covers the methods used on integrated analyses of the different data types aiming to provide some insight into the solution of the "Genome * Exposome = Phenome" equation.

11.3.1 Data Mining

New technologies are transforming biomedical science and clinical medicine due to the vast amounts of information produced. This is prompting a paradigm shift from hypothesis-driven to data-driven approaches to knowledge discovery. The exploitation of these complex and diverse datasets requires the use of data mining techniques and methods (see Chapter 7).

11.3.1.1 From "-omics" to "-WAS"

In recent years, one of the most commonly used methods for the advance of personalized medicine has been known as wide association studies. Originally developed for genomics as GWAS (Genome Wide Association Studies) the aim of these methods was to identify those SNVs associated with a particular phenotypical characteristic of interest (for example, having a particular disease or having a susceptibility to it). Although initially designed and developed for genomics data, as happened with "-omics" technologies (which were extended to create other areas of specialization such as proteomics, metabolomics, etc.), the "-WAS" approaches have been applied in other domains. Some of them are gene expression based: (eGWAS), epigenomics (EpWAS), environmental (EnWAS), or phenome (PheWAS). Note that in the literature both epigenomic and environmental "WAS" approaches may be termed EWAS; to prevent confusion, in this chapter the terms EpWAS and EnWAS are used for epigenomic and environmental WAS, respectively.

11.3.1.1.1 Genome-Wide Association Studies—GWAS

These studies try to associate susceptibility to certain diseases with the natural genetic variation occurring within the genomes of a given population. The underlying idea is that susceptibility to common diseases should be linked with common alleles across the populations [41]. In these studies, hundreds of thousands to millions of different genetic variants, SNPs, and copy number variations (CNVs) are analyzed simultaneously. Although these approaches have been able to identify susceptibility loci for different traits [42], in many cases these associations have shown only a small increase in the risk factor or the utility for risk assessment.

The development of these studies requires the use of data mining and machine learning approaches to analyze the relationships between the thousands of SNVs and the phenotypic characteristic measured (e.g., disease susceptibility). In many cases, these studies have relied on the application of parametric approaches such as logistic regression. These methods have been widely used for GWAS analyses, but are sometimes based on simplifications that do not consider possible dominance effects; their power is limited when dealing with high-order non-linear interactions that may happen in complex diseases [43]. As an alternative, the use of Bayesian methods allows the inclusion of more complex interaction effects and takes into account previous biological knowledge [44].

The limitations of the parametric approaches have led to the use of other methods borrowed from data mining and machine learning, acknowledging that the use of these techniques makes fewer assumptions about the models. A range of different methods have been used. Tree-based methods (e.g., random forest [RF]) and non-parametric machine learning methods (e.g., multi-dimensional reduction [MDR]) have been extensively applied in this domain [45]. Other techniques like neural networks have also been used in these studies [46].

Another useful approach for the analysis of GWAS studies consists of using attribute selection methods to reduce the complexity of high-order combinations possible among the hundreds of thousands of SNVs analyzed in GWAS studies. The filter-based methods select those high-quality SNVs that are going to be used as input for the machine learning algorithms. Some examples of software using these approaches are ReliefF [47] or TuRF [48]. The use of these methods implies discarding some elements that might be relevant for the analysis. Alternatively, and to overcome the risk of discarding important variants, wrapper algorithms have been included.

The use of available knowledge such as GO annotation or biochemical pathways represents an important trend in the analysis of "-omics" data and has also been used in GWAS to provide biological insight into results and guiding associations [49]. However, an important limitation of the current analyses using these approaches is the quality of the data sources used for the inferences. It is therefore strongly recommended to make use of only the highest quality curated resources, to avoid misleading interpretations.

The visualization methods used for representing the results obtained in GWAS studies are usually based on Manhattan plots, where p-values of each association test are represented against the chromosomal position of the analyzed SNV.

11.3.1.1.2 Gene Expression-Based Gene Wide Association Studies—eGWAS

In the last 15 years, gene expression studies have generated large amounts of data that have been made publicly available through different databases, including GEO or ArrayExpress. The concept of gene expression-based wide association studies appeared in 2012 and refers to an alternative meta-analysis method for the analysis of gene expression data using analytical approaches borrowed from GWAS. This method combines, in a single study, methods developed for analysis of gene expression and SNVs. Thus, the eGWAS method exploits the large amounts of gene expression data available in public databases and combines them into a single analysis that aims to identify genes and calculate the likelihood of finding the same differentially expressed gene repeated in a large number of case-associated samples. The researchers who originated this method successfully applied it in the analysis of Type 2 Diabetes to identify new genes and contribute to a better understanding of this pathology [50].

11.3.1.1.3 Epigenome Wide Association Studies—EpWAS

Epigenomics is the "-omics" approach to studying of the chemical modifications of DNA that play an important role in the regulation of gene activity and expression. Epigenomic regulation is a highly dynamic process that interfaces genomic regulation with environmental factors such as diet and other environmental exposures. These modifications, which can be inherited, do not alter the genomic sequence but are very important elements in the generation of the final phenotypes and are essential for many developmental stages. Modification of epigenomic patterns may result in different clinical phenotypes; the influence of these regulation methods has been studied in psychiatric disorders, obesity, and cancer. As with other "-omics" approaches, the evolution of molecular techniques in recent years has allowed the development of large-scale initiatives for the study of these processes and has generated huge amounts of data that have been collected and made available through different databases, such as the recently developed NCBI Epigenomics database (http://www.ncbi.nlm.nih.gov/epigenomics). An increasing number of computational methods for predictive modeling, using different machine learning techniques such as artificial neural networks or support vector machines, have been developed in recent times to analyze these new sets of epigenetic data.

In GWAS studies, whole genome analyses are carried out to identify the influence of SNVs on phenotypic traits. Similarly, to study the influence of epigenomic variations, large-scale approaches called EpWAS (epigenome-wide association studies) [51] have been designed. EpWAS and GWAS share many of their analytical methods, but the interpretation of EpWAS is more complex—the epigenetic modification can be either the cause or the consequence of the analyzed phenotypic trait. Another important factor in EpWAS is the dynamic nature of epigenomic data, which enables longitudinal analyses and may exploit linkages with EHR data. An example of this is the use of Guthrie cards (neonatal blood cards used for the screening of metabolic diseases) and the comparison of epigenomic profiles between subjects at birth and 3 years later [52].

11.3.1.1.4 Metabolome-Wide Association Studies—MWAS

Metabolomics encompasses the massive characterization of the metabolites present in a sample at a given time. The metabolome offers a window into the phenotype of the cells as well as an interface between the physiological and environmental factors such as diet or the microbiome (the set of different microbial species interacting with a human body on different body sites). The existence of metabolome data and GWAS methods set the stage for the development of metabolome-wide association studies in 2008 [53,54]. Initially Nuclear Magnetic Resonance (NMR) spectra from more than 4000 urine samples were analyzed, using diet and blood pressure as phenotypic traits, with the goal of identifying the different biomarkers involved.

Associated with the development of these studies is an alternative that is truly the combination of GWAS and the use of metabolomics information, called mGWAS [55]. In this approach, a combination of a traditional GWAS study with over 500,000 SNPs and a panel of 163 metabolites as final traits was analyzed, including the use of gene and pathways annotation data.

11.3.1.1.5 Phenome-Wide Association Studies—PheWAS

Phenome-wide association study, or PheWAS [56], is another recent "-WAS" approach derived from GWAS and is based on the use of rich data available in the EHR. PheWAS studies could be considered as a "transposition" of GWAS.

In GWAS analyses, a single phenotype is studied to identify those genomic variants associated with it whereas in PheWAS analyses, the aim is to identify the phenotypic traits associated with a given genotype (Figure 11.3). PheWAS analyses complement GWAS analyses and provide new insights about the biological mechanisms associated with diseases.

The original article describing this methodology as a proof of concept used only five SNPs with previously known association with different diseases and ICD-9 code derived data as the phenotypic source for around 6000 patients. However, the potential of the PheWAS approach is to use hundreds or thousands of SNVs for the analyses. The original algorithm divided individuals in a case-control manner for each phenotype and then used a chi-square test to calculate the p-value and odds ratio for each allele.

More recently, a PheWAS approach has been used by the NHGRI-supported PAGE (Population Architecture using Genetics and Epidemiology) Network [57]. An important aspect addressed by this work was the need to adjust for multiple testing errors associated with the complexity of these tests.

The visualization of PheWAS analysis results represents a challenge because the Manhattan plots used for representation of GWAS are too simple for these studies where several phenotypical traits and genotypes are analyzed simultaneously. PheWas-View is a tool designed to visualize the complex relationships and pleiotropy observed in PheWAS studies [58].

11.3.1.1.6 **Environmental-Wide Association Studies—EnWAS**

"WAS" studies have inspired the use of analytical techniques to find relationships among different factors and certain phenotypic traits. In environmental-wide association studies (EnWAS), the variables analyzed are environmental exposures to different agents [59]. In the original work

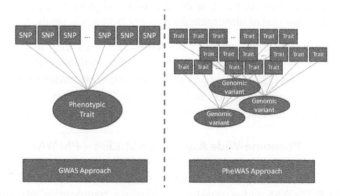

■ **FIGURE 11.3** Schematic representation of the GWAS and the PheWAS approaches.

where the concept of EnWAS was established, researchers analyzed the influence of a set of 266 environmental factors in the development of Type 2 Diabetes. In this study, the environmental factors were "equivalent" to the SNVs used in GWAS analyses on different patient cohorts and representation of the results was done using a modified Manhattan plot graph.

11.3.2 Using Massive Parallel Sequencing Data in Personalized Medicine

The development of massive parallel sequencing (MPS) techniques is also called next-generation sequencing (NGS). The decrease in the cost of sequencing is extending the use of these methods. It is expected that MPS will become more frequent in the near future, bringing new challenges for biomedical informatics in the analysis, interpretation, and management of data generated by these methods.

There are different uses of MPS methods covering areas such as genome sequencing, gene expression analysis or epigenetics analyses. Most of the current clinical approaches are focused on the use of whole exome sequencing (WES) and whole genome sequencing (WGS). WES limits the sequencing process to DNA regions that code for proteins, considering that disease-associated SNVs are more likely to be found in those regions (around 85% of human disease-causing mutations) [60]. The aim of this method is to identify those variants previously associated with a disease or identify novel variants that might be causative. For this purpose, different methods and algorithms have been developed and are discussed further in this section.

As the costs of WGS fall spectacularly, the use of this methodology is increasing in importance since it provides insight about the whole genomic content of a sample. WGS has been successfully applied in clinics in several cases [61]. The biomedical informatics challenges associated with the application of these technologies are amplified compared to those found in WES, since the search space for the identification of different genomic variants is much larger and it is necessary to identify a possible causative variant among the several million SNVs and thousands of CNVs that can be usually found in a human genome. To increase the complexity of this situation, the results obtained by the Personal Genomes Project showed that there are thousands of non-synonymous changes within the genome of an individual and that there are a few tens of heterozygous deleterious variants with the potential of causing a Mendelian disease. Therefore one of the tasks for biomedical informatics is to incorporate all of this knowledge into analytical pipelines for decision support in clinical medicine.

It is also possible to apply MPS methods for functional genomics and use data from these methods for personalized medicine. The use of MPS technologies for the analysis of the transcriptome is commonly referred to as RNA-Seq. There is open debate on whether MPS-based approaches will mean the end of microarray-based transcriptomic analyses or when this will happen. This debate has some significance for biomedical informatics, since current microarray-based gene expression experiments require a data sharing policy based on the MIAME standard. RNA-Seq approaches are equivalent to a WES experiment and therefore the privacy concerns must be taken into consideration.

11.3.2.1 *MPS Data Analysis*

The large amounts of data generated by MPS-based methods demand multistage (Figure 11.4) approaches to transform sequence reads generated from sequencers into information that may be used in clinical applications.

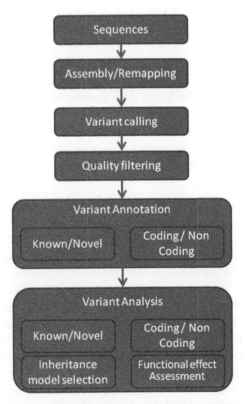

■ **FIGURE 11.4** Example of the steps required for the clinical interpretation of a MPS analysis. Although there is a variety of tools available at each of these steps in some cases these tools are constrained to certain MPS technologies.

The first step in dealing with MPS data is the assembly and quality control process. There are two major categories of MPS assemblers depending on the problem and whether the genome is being generated *de novo* or is being re-sequenced. The latter is usually the case in most personalized medicine applications where a human genome reference sequence is available for the mapping process. Currently these two approaches use different algorithms. Most *de novo* assemblers use De Bruijn graphs methods, whereas remapping methods commonly use hash-based algorithms or the Burrows-Wheeler transform. Burrows-Wheeler transform-based methods are faster but less sensitive than hash-based ones for genomic insertions or deletions ("indels"). "Classic" alignment methods (e.g., BLAST or BLAT) are too slow for these analyses, although in some pipelines these methods are still used for refining purposes [62]. Another important aspect to consider in the selection of a particular assembly algorithm is the purpose of the analysis; genome sequencing requires colinear alignments, whereas RNA analyses require methods that take into account RNA structure (introns and exons). Table 11.4 earlier in this chapter shows some examples of assembly software and tools. The selection of tools and parameters used at this step may have a strong influence on further steps in the analysis.

Once assembly of sequence reads has been carried out, the next step is variant calling. The objective of this step is to identify the different genomic variants found in the assembled genome. This step is strongly influenced by the parameters used in the assembly process. For example, a too-stringent alignment will not allow any mismatches during the mapping process and will prevent the detection of any variants with respect to the reference genome used. Current methodologies for variant calling are based on probabilistic methods and require sufficient coverage. One of the challenges found at this step is the discrimination between sequencing errors, the SNVs, and especially on those heterozygous SNVs where the SNV will appear only in a fraction of the reads.

In personalized medicine applications, this is usually the most important step because it is here that the different genomic variants can be identified and therefore associated with a particular disease or susceptibility. This is a challenging process and there are several algorithms available, such as GATK (Genome Analysis Tool Kit) [63]. However, the use of different algorithms may detect different variations as well as provide misleading results due to detection of false positives and false negatives. There are multiple causes for these types of artifacts, some of them associated with the MPS platform used or with problems in previous steps in the analyses.

Once the sequence is available, the next step is to assess the effects of the variants identified. In many cases, this assessment is carried out by analyzing the position where the variant is mapped and its characteristics. For example, if the variability is located in a protein-coding gene and causes a non-synonymous change in the protein sequence, then it may have clinical consequences. Equally, if the variant disrupts a splicing site then clinical effects may ensue. For this assessment, several methods and algorithms have been developed to evaluate the impact of SNVs in proteins providing an *in silico* prediction of their effect and functional consequences. An example of one such program is PolyPhen2 [64].

Running these types of analyses can be very time consuming and therefore can limit their potential application in some scenarios (e.g., detecting newborns affected with rare diseases). Researchers recently described a pipeline that makes it possible to perform these types of analyses in 50 h using a symptom- and sign-assisted genome analysis (SSAGA) tool that maps clinical characteristics of 591 genetic diseases to their phenotypes and genes known to cause those symptoms. The use of this system was shown to help prioritize clinical information for interpreting sequencing results because it was able to focus the sequence analyses on only those regions associated with clinical findings [65].

11.4 INTRODUCTION TO PARTICIPATORY HEALTH

"Gimme my damn data!," "The patient will see you now...," "Let patients help," "Nothing about me without me!." These are some of the slogans coined by patient advocates including Dave de Bronkart, Regina Holliday, Hugo Campos, Salvatore Iaconesi, and Marian Sandmaier. All of them are demanding actions to make patients more empowered, informed, and involved in decision making, prevention, and learning. This movement has attracted the attention of not only consumer associations and patients, but also of the scientific and clinical communities and even governments. In recent years, conferences like Medicine 2.0, Health 2.0, mHealth Summit, Quantified Self, Medicine X, and TEDMED have been swamped with bookings from thousands of people interested in this new area, which may be referred to as Personal Health Informatics, Consumer Health Informatics, Participatory Health, or Participatory Medicine. A Society for Participatory Medicine was established and began publishing its own journal in 2009 (http://participatorymedicine.org).

The concept of participatory medicine has its roots in social philosophy. The ideal of participatory medicine has been expressed as cooperation between mature patients and committed, responsive physicians [66]. Participatory medicine is proposed as an alternative to *"traditional interest in only the physical manifestation of symptoms and scientific ideology, not the patients' ideology*" [67]. Patient participation in health care may encompass performing clinical or daily living skills in ambulatory settings, as well as being active in decision making from admission to discharge in in-patient settings; however, it cannot be assumed that either patients or clinicians universally accept it as an approach to care [68].

Early references to practical applications of participatory medicine predate the popularization of the Internet, for example:

> *"Health systems agencies frequently have a citizen participation structure, and in some instances there is a requirement for 50 percent consumer participation in planning processes and administrative decisions. ...Some planners I have dealt with are beginning to believe that good medicine requires participatory medicine"* [69].

However, the widespread implementation of participatory medicine was problematic with the technology of the time. At present, two main elements can be identified as the drivers of this trend in health care. Firstly, the digital revolution in other domains (including banking, insurance, leisure, and government) has outpaced the incorporation of digital systems in the health sector, for many possible reasons (the complexity of health-related data, volume of data, privacy concerns, or lack of demand). For some time this fact did not greatly affect health care at the level of health service providers or research centers, but things are changing now that the digital revolution has turned medicine into an arena for widespread patient and citizen participation.

Secondly, convergence is occurring between mature and affordable technologies such as wearable sensors, DNA sequencing, the personal health record, mobile devices, games, the Internet of things, and Web 2.0 platforms—especially social networks. This is making it possible for anyone to collect, store, manage, exchange, and even analyze their own health information. This convergence is also predicted to bring consumer-oriented changes in health service dynamics, such as *"the patient will see you now"* [70].

In this section, we review the latest developments in this area, from the perspective of informatics. We identify new ways to collect and store personal health data first, and then provide some examples of trends in the use of these data, from exchange to analysis.

11.5 DATA COLLECTION FOR PARTICIPATORY HEALTH

11.5.1 Personal Health Records

Both the US Surgeon General (through the 2010 "My Family Health Portrait" initiative) and the UK National Health Service (through the 2012 "Power of Information" strategy for public health and adult social care) have started to emphasize patient-centric healthcare records. In Australia, the Commonwealth Government is in the process of rolling-out a Personally Controlled Electronic Health Record (PCEHR) enabling all citizens to have and control access to their health information.

At the same time, consumers are beginning to maintain their own clinical records independently of national health systems. One example of a web-based tool for this purpose is HealthVault (www.healthvault.com); a directory of dozens more is maintained by the American Health Information Management Association at myPHR (www.myphr.com). The PHR has the potential to transform health care, changing the doctor-patient encounter and empowering individuals to take a more proactive approach toward their health [71]. This poses challenges relating to continuity of health records for individuals who may have multiple health professionals during the course of their treatment [72]. For optimal safety and quality of care, these systems must be able to link with hospital and primary care information systems, at the patient's discretion, in order to provide data for clinical decision support and monitoring of clinical care.

11.5.2 Personal Diagnostic Testing

"Test at home, treat online." This is the motto of one of the new services (Quick Check Health http://quickcheckhealth.com) planning to offer over-the-counter home diagnostic tests for common illnesses such as urinary tract infection, strep throat, flu, cholesterol, Lyme disease, sexually transmitted diseases, yeast infections, and others. If a test were positive, the user could launch an online clinical consultation. A clinician then would review the case and, if appropriate, a prescription would be sent to the consumer's pharmacy. Such services are still under development and will need regulatory approval to proceed but have been shown to be technologically and economically feasible.

11.5.3 Personal Medical Images Management

An easy way to share, store, and manage results of medical images exams is now available to patients using services such as XRFiles (www.xrfiles. com) and MediCle (https://medicle.radiologyservicesonline.com). In these examples, X-rays, CT scans, ultrasounds, mammograms, and other diagnostic quality medical images can be managed online through a private log-in identification process. Patients can then send images securely and in full fidelity, for instance to a clinician to seek a second opinion, or to an educational or research project as donor data. These services may integrate with a personal health record (PHR) and allow patients the option to share their medical images, in the context of their medical history, with any clinician or researcher.

11.5.4 **Personal Sensing and Monitoring**

One current technology trend that is helping to mainstream participatory medicine is the so-called "Internet of things"—pervasive, location-sensitive, mobile, wearable, wireless devices linked to social media services [73]. These include everything from physical and physiological tracking devices, to easy-to-use software that records one's data, analyzes them, interprets them graphically, and allows one to share and compare them with others [74]. This is expected to enable more reliable self-monitoring and more self-management of health care, including mental health care, more often than not home based rather than hospital based.

The Quantified Self (www.quantifiedself.com) is a movement with the motto "*self knowledge through numbers*" that aims to support citizens who are using different technologies to collect data on aspects of their daily life (e.g., food intake), physiology (e.g., blood oxygen levels), and other factors (e.g., mood) with the belief that gathering and analyzing those data can help them improve their lives [75] (see Figure 11.5).

Such self-monitoring and self-sensing, which combines wearable sensors (EEG, ECG, video, etc.) and wearable computing, is also known as "life logging," "self-tracking," "auto-analytics," "body hacking," and "self-quantifying." The term "quantified self" was proposed by Wired Magazine editors Gary Wolf and Kevin Kelly in 2007 as "*a collaboration of users and*

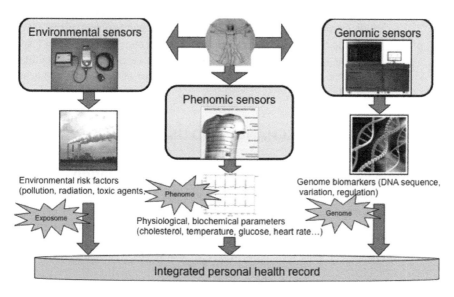

■ **FIGURE 11.5** Sensors collecting personal genetic, environmental, and phenotypical information and storage in the personal Health Record.

tool makers who share an interest in self knowledge through self-tracking." Membership of this group is doubling every year with more than 16,000 members and 100 meet-up groups across the world in 2013.

11.5.5 **Personal Genome Services**

Advances in DNA sequencing technology now make possible the collection of information on the genomic sequence of an individual in a short time (days) and at low cost (hundreds of dollars) [76]. This has facilitated the birth of a new industry that is known as personal, DTC ("Direct to Consumer"), or DIY ("Do It Yourself") genomics. For a few years now, companies such as 23andMe, Navigenics, and others have offered services of personal DNA sequencing and analysis directly to the consumer [77]. Typically these services can be arranged online. Anyone can hire the service, receive a kit, send a sample of their DNA and within a few weeks access their results on the Internet, in a secure environment, along with their DNA sequence features and a page that informs them about various aspects related to personal genetic information (for instance, ancestors, risk or susceptibility to a panel of diseases, reactions to various drugs). Although most of these services are based on the analysis of a more or less wide panel (about 1 million) of SNPs (single nucleotide polymorphisms), they also offer exome analysis (areas of the genome which code for proteins) or even complete genome analysis for higher prices. The number of people who know their genomic information is growing exponentially, with web tools such as Interpretome [78] becoming available to help patients interpret these data. It is anticipated that in the coming years this information may become a standard part of the patient electronic health record. It therefore may be taken into account as a matter of course when making decisions about health care and may be routinely exchanged over communication networks as part of health data and health record sharing.

11.6 **DATA EXCHANGE AND USE IN PARTICIPATORY HEALTH**

11.6.1 **Patients Accessing Health Information**

The popularization of the World Wide Web supported growing interest in participatory medicine through providing access to information in new ways and by different people, and new forms of shared information [79]. The explosion of curated health information freely and openly available on the Internet [80] has been far in excess of other fields of knowledge [81].

The accompanying problem of massive amounts of freely and openly available health information that is not evidence based has given rise to a suite of quality management standards and tools. Examples are the HONcode (www.hon.ch) and its Worldwide online Reliable Advice to Patients and Individuals (WRAPIN) knowledge base, which allows lay people to compare the content of any health information they find online with an authoritative source on the same topic.

These consumer health information standards and tools include visualization resources, for instance the easily recognizable HONcode logo that may be displayed on participating health information websites. Another good example is the growing interest in the use of the "Blue Button." This symbol has been used since 2010 to indicate that a health information system is compliant with the functionality of making data available for patients. The Veteran Administration started using this symbol and now several organizations (including Health Level 7) are developing tools that allow patients to view and download their personal health information. Blue Button was developed by the Department of Veterans Affairs and gave veterans and their families access to their health records. The first version was limited to text. Recently, a design challenge supported by the US ONCHIT (Office of the National Coordinator for Health IT) has reimagined the patient health record (http://healthdesignchallenge.com/).

The development of the social web has facilitated medical knowledge management for patients and consumers. Resources like Webicina (http://www.webicina.com/) provide free, curated medical social media resources for over 80 medical topics in more than 17 languages.

The rapid expansion of social web health information resources includes a wide range of directory services. One example is Medline Plus (http://www.nlm.nih.gov/medlineplus), which in turn lists links to other directories, primarily for the United States health system. Another example is the first edition of the "European Directory of Health Apps" launched in 2012 (http://www.patient-view.com/uploads/6/5/7/9/6579846/pv_appdirectory_final_web_300812.pdf). This resource contains facts about 200 smartphone health apps capable of helping patients self-manage their medical conditions. The Directory does not represent the first occasion that such information has been gathered together on a large number of medical conditions—the key difference about this Directory is that the health apps it lists have all been recommended by patient groups and empowered consumers, then categorized and indexed in several ways (including by local language), to make it easy for readers to find details.

Isabel Symptoms Checker (from symptoms to diagnosis) gives patients access to a highly sophisticated medical diagnosis tool that can take a pattern of symptoms in everyday language and instantly compute, from a vast database of 6000 diseases, the most likely ones. It is based on the same system that doctors and nurses rely on [82] around the world to help with diagnosis (see Figure 11.6).

11.6.2 **Patients Reading Doctor's Notes**

A recent report [83] on the first results of the OpenNotes project raises another interesting aspect of participatory health. In 2010, more than 100 primary care doctors from three diverse medical institutions across the United States began sharing their medical notes online with their patients. Each site was part of a 12-month study to explore how sharing doctors' notes may affect health care.

The OpenNotes study started a movement to make it easy for patients to read notes written about their care, and to bring more transparency to medical records. It is an initiative that invites patients to review the notes written about them by their doctors, nurses, or other clinicians during or after an appointment. By engaging directly with this information, patients may be able to question and analyze the information in these records, understand more about their medical conditions, spot and correct misinformation in their records, and ultimately make their treatment more efficient and effective [84].

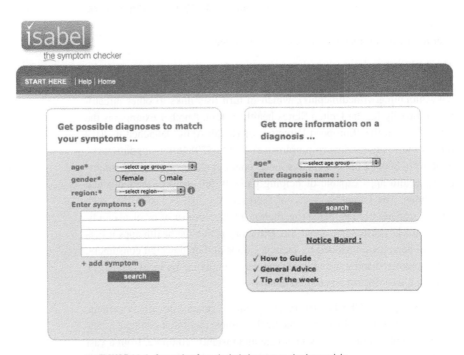

■ **FIGURE 11.6** Screenshot from the Isabel symptom checker module.

Patients can benefit because they have the chance to read and discuss notes with their doctor or family member, helping them take more control of their health and health care. Healthcare professionals can build better relationships with their patients and take better care of them when they share their visit notes. Opening up visit notes to patients may make care more efficient, improve communication, and most importantly may help patients become more actively involved with their health and health care.

11.6.3 Patients Sharing Decision Making

Shared decision making refers to those processes in which patients choose between the different treatment options available, based on their needs and preferences. Information systems are an essential support in this process, enabling patients to ask questions, explore options, and decide on a treatment for a particular health condition, in collaboration with their clinical professional [85].

In the last few years, a number of projects have developed shared decision-making support systems, such as one for dental restoration [86]. The Ottawa Personal Decision Guide (http://decisionaid.ohri.ca) is a tool designed for anyone making health-related decisions. It was collaboratively developed by patients and clinicians in a hospital setting, with a focus on "tough" decisions, in other words where there are many options, where the outcomes are uncertain, or where different people may value the benefits and risks differently. It can help people assess their decision-making needs, plan next steps, and track their progress in decision making. Another version, the Ottawa Family Decision Guide, is aimed at relatives and caregivers involved in healthcare decisions. Finally, an application called iShould works in connection with Facebook. iShould helps people make and share decisions with their friends.

11.6.4 Patients Reporting Outcomes

It is recognized that patients' experience of care is a major metric of quality and there has been an enormous interest in the development and application of questionnaires, interviews, and rating scales that measure states of health and illness from the patient's perspective. Patient-reported outcome measures (PROMs) provide a means of gaining an insight into the way patients perceive their health and the impact that treatments or adjustments to lifestyle have on their quality of life. These instruments can be completed by a patient or individual about themselves, or by others on their behalf [87–94].

Bibliographic databases and systematic reviews of PROMs relevant to specific disease and population (demographic) groups can provide guidance regarding the selection of appropriate instruments for use in clinical trials, clinical practice, and population surveys, links to related websites (organizations, research groups, and journals). PROMIS (see Table 11.5) is an information system specifically designed for handling patient-reported outcomes.

11.6.5 Patients Sharing Health Information on Social Media and Crowdsourced Clinical Trials

The emergence of Web 2.0 and social media has supported public collaboration around healthcare concerns. Through the use of tools such as wikis, social networks, blogs, virtual worlds, a worldview sometimes described as Health 2.0 or Medicine 2.0 has developed, characterized by communal exchanges and comparison of personal experiences [95]. The use of these tools has fostered wider and faster citizen responses in public health crisis situations, such as epidemics and natural disasters. It has also generated more vocal and visible advocacy groups for particular health interests or causes, such as tissue donors or rare disease sufferers.

Participatory medicine will come to mean that many patients are willing and able to selectively share their health data, including genetic and metabolic data, in real time. Such activities are enabling crowdsourcing of data for clinical trials and preventive health research, thus shortening the continuum between bench and bedside [96].

PatientsLikeMe, Genomera, CureTogether, and CancerCommons represent good examples of this trend, often referred to as: "*clinical research with the patients, not on the patients*":

- 23andMe (www.23andme.com) offers personal genomics services, but it also collects data for research. It recently published an article [97] describing two new genetic associations in Parkinson's Disease.
- PatientsLikeMe (www.patientslikeme.com) currently groups more than 175,000 patients and more than 1000 conditions. Self-reported data from 600 patients on the use of lithium for Amyotrophic Lateral Sclerosis (ALS) were reported in 2011 [98].
- CureTogether (www.curetogether.com) offers access to millions of ratings comparing the real-world performance of treatments across more than 600 health conditions.
- CancerCommons (www.cancercommons.org) was founded in 2011 by an Internet commerce expert and cancer sufferer, to link cancer patients, clinicians, and biomedical scientists in "rapid learning communities," with the goal that patients are treated in accord with the

Table 11.5 Examples of Internet resources related to participatory health.

Functionality	Resource	URL
Personal genome services	23andMe	https://www.23andme.com/
	Navigenics (now Life Technologies)	http://www.navigenics.com/
	DecodeMe	http://www.decodeme.com/
	Knome	http://www.knome.com
Personal diagnostic testing	QuickCheck	http://quickcheckhealth.com/
Personal medical image management	MediCle	https://medicle.radiologyservicesonline.com/
	XRFiles	http://www.xrfiles.com/
Personal sensing and monitoring	Quantified Self	http://quantifiedself.com/
		http://quantified-self.meetup.com/
		http://quantifiedself.com/guide/
Personal health records	AHIMA PHR	http://www.myphr.com/
	Microsoft HealthVault	http://www.microsoft.com/en-gb/healthvault/default.aspx
	Australian PCEHR	http://www.nehta.gov.au/ehealth-implementation/what-is-a-pcehr
Patient reading doctor's notes	Open Notes project	http://www.myopennotes.org/
Patient sharing health information on social media and crowsourced clinical trials	CureTogether (now part of 23andMe)	http://curetogether.com/
	Patients like me	http://www.patientslikeme.com/
	Genomera	http://genomera.com/
	DIY Genomics	http://diygenomics.org/
Patient reporting outcomes	PROMIS (NIH)	http://www.nihpromis.org/
	PROM (NHS)	http://phi.uhce.ox.ac.uk/
Patient accessing health information	Webicina	http://www.webicina.com/
	European Directory of Health Apps (2012–2013)	http://g3ict.org/download/p/fileId_955/productId_265
	Isabel HealthCare	http://www.isabelhealthcare.com/home/default
Shared decision making	RightCare (NHS)	http://www.rightcare.nhs.uk/index.php/shared-decision-making/
	Ottawa Personal Decision Guide	http://decisionaid.ohri.ca/decguide.html

latest knowledge on therapies, and to continually update that knowledge based on each patient's response. At this site, patients, clinicians and researchers can all report their observations and outcomes. New data are analyzed by collaborative, interinstitutional teams in relation to current knowledge and hypotheses about cancer.

11.7 **CONCLUSIONS AND FUTURE DIRECTIONS**

11.7.1 **Similarities and Differences Between Personalized Medicine and Participatory Health**

So far, personalized medicine and participatory health have followed quite independent paths. However, they do share a number of aspects. These include the need for systems approaches to tackle the complexity of the many interactions across different levels, along with the required integration of multiple sources of data. Additionally, personalized medicine and participatory health share their dependence on advances in analytical technologies and their requirement for platforms and tools able to provide the storage and computational capacity to mine and compare billions of bits of data ("big data") [99].

Despite this, these trends still present some differences. Personalized medicine more than participatory health is clinician focused, deals with molecular data,and puts a major emphasis on reactive medicine (curing disease). In contrast, participatory health is mainly patient centered, focuses on environmental risk factors, and puts more emphasis on preventive medicine.

11.7.2 **Convergence Between Personalized Medicine and Participatory Health**

The advantage of managing and sharing vast amounts of data across networks was clearly demonstrated in a recent longitudinal study [100]. In this study, one of the researchers monitored his molecular data for 14 months. Over 3 billion data points were collected on his genome, gene expression, proteins and antibodies, and metabolites during this period. In the course of the investigation, he was able to detect two viral infections, one of which triggered Type 2 Diabetes that responded to medication and changes in diet and physical activity. This study illustrates the clinical utility of an integrated approach to collecting and interpreting all the molecular information of a patient and of generating personalized -omics profiles. This data explosion (from the genome to the transcriptome, proteome, and metabolome as well as immunological data) will require enormous capacity both in computing power and in the capability of the networks that connect laboratories, clinical centers, and the patient's home.

This work represents a good example of the convergence between the two areas developed in this chapter, personalized medicine and participatory health. Specifically, this work supports the trend known as self-quantification—in this case, the tracking of the molecular information of an individual by that individual. Personal "omics" sits at the intersection between participatory health and personalized medicine. It is expected that these advances will lead to a greater ability to develop a more responsive preventative medicine where diseases can be detected before even the first symptoms appear.

11.7.3 **Advantages and Disadvantages of Personalized Medicine and Participatory Health**

Various forums have noted several positive aspects associated with personalized medicine and participatory health. Among these are increased motivation of individuals, a deeper understanding of their health, wider possibilities for self-improvement, broader risk profiling, more timely and targeted preventive measures. Additional benefits are expressed in terms of reducing pressures on the tertiary level of health services (generally, the most expensive) by allowing more of the care provision to occur in secondary, primary, and even home-based care, also being described as ambient-assisted living (www.aal-europe.eu).

Among the suggested disadvantages, there are still unknowns around concepts such as privacy, security, education, cyberchondria (hypochondria exacerbated by consulting too much or inappropriate online information), regulation and accreditation of changed practices, the changing role of the clinician, increased infrastructure needs, the therapeutic gap between clinical advice and patient adherence, and the ethical foundations of biomedical research in this new era. Most of these uncertainties have direct connections with information processing. Therefore, biomedical informatics is well positioned to address concerns, overcome barriers, and enable improvements in people's health. However, the emergence of more sophisticated technologies will not by itself guarantee participatory health for all. Getting the educational and economic settings right for global participation by consumers and clinicians alike is a challenge that may not be within the scope of biomedical informatics to resolve.

11.7.4 **Key Directions for Biomedical Informatics in Personalized Medicine and Participatory Health**

Personalized medicine and participatory health are intertwined technology-based innovations that are changing biomedical research, clinical practice, and patient and consumer expectations of health care, all at the same time. They represent innovations in thinking about the potential of data processing and information management to generate and apply new knowledge in medicine. Key characteristics of these trends are big data, public access, -omics approaches, and preventive medicine.

Biomedical informatics has made an important contribution to these the innovations, devising new methods and tools that have supported and extended personalized medicine and participatory health, particularly taking advantage of large-scale distributed computing, new web technologies, and smart sensors. Biomedical informatics nevertheless faces further challenges as computational technologies, social movements, and scientific discoveries that range from the microbiome to the biome continue to erode old paradigms of biomedical research and health care.

The future of research and service provision in health will continue to demand biomedical informatics specialists with very sophisticated repertoires of solutions to problems that may be ethical, statistical, or biological. To achieve all that personalized medicine and participatory health may make possible will also require a greater level of biomedical informatics knowledge and skill in the future than is present today, in everyone who is involved including citizens and patients, clinicians and health service administrators, researchers, and research managers.

REFERENCES

[1] Clarke L, Zheng-Bradley X, Smith R, Kulesha E, Xiao C, Toneva I, et al. The 1000 Genomes Project: data management and community access. Nature Methods 2012;9(5):459–62. Epub 2012/05/01.

[2] Kozal MJ, Shah N, Shen N, Yang R, Fucini R, Merigan TC, et al. Extensive polymorphisms observed in HIV-1 clade B protease gene using high-density oligonucleotide arrays. Nat Med 1996;2(7):753–9. Epub 1996/07/01.

[3] Vahey M, Nau ME, Barrick S, Cooley JD, Sawyer R, Sleeker AA, et al. Performance of the Affymetrix GeneChip HIV PRT 440 platform for antiretroviral drug resistance genotyping of human immunodeficiency virus type 1 clades and viral isolates with length polymorphisms. J Clin Microbiol 1999;37(8):2533–7. Epub 1999/07/16.

[4] Sorlie T, Perou CM, Tibshirani R, Aas T, Geisler S, Johnsen H, et al. Gene expression patterns of breast carcinomas distinguish tumor subclasses with clinical implications. Proc Natl Acad Sci USA 2001;98(19):10869–74. Epub 2001/09/13.

[5] van de Vijver MJ, He YD, van't Veer LJ, Dai H, Hart AA, Voskuil DW, et al. A gene-expression signature as a predictor of survival in breast cancer. New Engl J Med 2002;347(25):1999–2009. Epub 2002/12/20.

[6] Nadkarni PM, Ohno-Machado L, Chapman WW. Natural language processing: an introduction. J Am Med Inform Assoc 2011;18(5):544–51. Epub 2011/08/19.

[7] Meystre SM, Savova GK, Kipper-Schuler KC, Hurdle JF. Extracting information from textual documents in the electronic health record: a review of recent research. Yearb Med Inform 2008:128–44. Epub 2008/07/30.

[8] Hripcsak G, Albers DJ. Next-generation phenotyping of electronic health records. J Am Med Inform Assoc 2013;20(1):117–21. Epub 2012/09/08.

[9] McCarty CA, Chisholm RL, Chute CG, Kullo IJ, Jarvik GP, Larson EB, et al. The eMERGE Network: a consortium of biorepositories linked to electronic medical records data for conducting genomic studies. BMC Med Genom 2011;4:13. Epub 2011/01/29.

[10] Kho AN, Pacheco JA, Peissig PL, Rasmussen L, Newton KM, Weston N, et al. Electronic medical records for genetic research: results of the eMERGE consortium. Sci Transl Med 2011;3(79):79re1. Epub 2011/04/22.

[11] Frueh FW, Amur S, Mummaneni P, Epstein RS, Aubert RE, DeLuca TM, et al. Pharmacogenomic biomarker information in drug labels approved by the United States food and drug administration: prevalence of related drug use. Pharmacotherapy 2008;28(8):992–8. Epub 2008/07/29.

[12] Johnson EG, Horne BD, Carlquist JF, Anderson JL. Genotype-based dosing algorithms for warfarin therapy: data review and recommendations. Mol Diagn Ther 2011;15(5):255–64. Epub 2011/11/04.

[13] Mega JL, Close SL, Wiviott SD, Shen L, Hockett RD, Brandt JT, et al. Cytochrome p-450 polymorphisms and response to clopidogrel. New Engl J Med 2009;360(4):354–62. Epub 2008/12/25.

[14] Thorn CF, Klein TE, Altman RB. Pharmacogenomics and bioinformatics: PharmGKB. Pharmacogenomics 2010;11(4):501–5. Epub 2010/03/31.

[15] Kouris I, Tsirmpas C, Mougiakakou SG, Iliopoulou D, Koutsouris D. E-Health towards ecumenical framework for personalized medicine via Decision Support System. In: Conference proceedings: annual international conference of the IEEE engineering in medicine and biology society; 2010. p. 2881–5. Epub 2010/11/26.

[16] Leong TY. Toward patient-centered, personalized and personal decision support and knowledge management: a survey. Yearb Med Inform 2012;7(1):104–12. Epub 2012/08/15.

[17] Overby CL, Tarczy-Hornoch P, Hoath JI, Kalet IJ, Veenstra DL. Feasibility of incorporating genomic knowledge into electronic medical records for pharmacogenomic clinical decision support. BMC Bioinform 2010;11(Suppl.9):S10. Epub 2012/11/10.

[18] Pazzani MJ, See D, Schroeder E, Tilles J. Application of an expert system in the management of HIV-infected patients. J Acquir Immune Defic Syndr Hum Retrovirol 1997;15(5):356–62. Epub 1997/08/15.

[19] Tural C, Ruiz L, Holtzer C, Schapiro J, Viciana P, Gonzalez J, et al. Clinical utility of HIV-1 genotyping and expert advice: the Havana trial. AIDS (London, England) 2002;16(2):209–18. Epub 2002/01/25.

[20] Pestian J, Spencer M, Matykiewicz P, Zhang K, Vinks AA, Glauser T. Personalizing drug selection using advanced clinical decision support. Biomed Inform Insights 2009;2:19–29. Epub 2009/11/10.

[21] Deshmukh VG, Hoffman MA, Arnoldi C, Bray BE, Mitchell JA. Efficiency of CYP2C9 genetic test representation for automated pharmacogenetic decision support. Methods Inf Med 2009;48(3):282–90. Epub 2009/04/24.

[22] Pulley JM, Denny JC, Peterson JF, Bernard GR, Vnencak-Jones CL, Ramirez AH, et al. Operational implementation of prospective genotyping for personalized medicine: the design of the Vanderbilt PREDICT project. Clin Pharmacol Therapeut 2012;92(1):87–95. Epub 2012/05/17.

[23] Kohane IS. Using electronic health records to drive discovery in disease genomics. Nat Rev Genet 2011;12(6):417–28. Epub 2011/05/19.

[24] Wild CP. Complementing the genome with an "exposome": the outstanding challenge of environmental exposure measurement in molecular epidemiology. Cancer Epidemiol Biomarkers Prev 2005;14(8):1847–50. Cosponsored by the American Society of Preventive Oncology. Epub 2005/08/17.

[25] Wild CP. The exposome: from concept to utility. Int J Epidemiol 2012;41(1):24–32. Epub 2012/02/03.

[26] Nuwaysir EF, Bittner M, Trent J, Barrett JC, Afshari CA. Microarrays and toxicology: the advent of toxicogenomics. Mol Carcinogenesis 1999;24(3):153–9. Epub 1999/04/16.

[27] Davis AP, Wiegers TC, Rosenstein MC, Mattingly CJ. MEDIC: a practical disease vocabulary used at the Comparative Toxicogenomics Database. Database: J Biol Databases Curation 2012;2012:bar065. Epub 2012/03/22.

[28] Stover PJ, Harlan WR, Hammond JA, Hendershot T, Hamilton CM. PhenX: a toolkit for interdisciplinary genetics research. Curr Opin Lipidol 2010;21(2):136–40. Epub 2010/02/16.

[29] Vreeman DJ, McDonald CJ, Huff SM. Representing patient assessments in LOINC(R). AMIA Annu Sympos Proc 2010;2010:832–6. Epub 2011/02/25.

[30] Hamilton CM, Strader LC, Pratt JG, Maiese D, Hendershot T, Kwok RK, et al. The PhenX Toolkit: get the most from your measures. Am J Epidemiol 2011;174(3): 253–60. Epub 2011/07/14.

[31] Fortier I, Burton PR, Robson PJ, Ferretti V, Little J, L'Heureux F, et al. Quality, quantity and harmony: the DataSHaPER approach to integrating data across bioclinical studies. Int J Epidemiol 2010;39(5):1383–93. Epub 2010/09/04.

[32] Fortier I, Doiron D, Burton P, Raina P. Invited commentary: consolidating data harmonization – how to obtain quality and applicability? Am J Epidemiol 2011;174(3):261–4. author reply 5–6, Epub 2011/07/14.

[33] Chervitz SA, Deutsch EW, Field D, Parkinson H, Quackenbush J, Rocca-Serra P, et al. Data standards for Omics data: the basis of data sharing and reuse. Methods Mol Biol (Clifton, NJ) 2011;719:31–69. Epub 2011/03/04.

[34] Taylor CF, Field D, Sansone SA, Aerts J, Apweiler R, Ashburner M, et al. Promoting coherent minimum reporting guidelines for biological and biomedical investigations: the MIBBI project. Nat Biotechnol 2008;26(8):889–96. Epub 2008/08/09.

[35] Sansone SA, Rocca-Serra P, Brandizi M, Brazma A, Field D, Fostel J, et al. The first RSBI (ISA-TAB) workshop: can a simple format work for complex studies? Omics: J Integr Biol 2008;12(2):143–9. Epub 2008/05/02.

[36] Gargis AS, Kalman L, Berry MW, Bick DP, Dimmock DP, Hambuch T, et al. Assuring the quality of next-generation sequencing in clinical laboratory practice. Nat Biotechnol 2012;30(11):1033–6. Epub 2012/11/10.

[37] Bohannon J. Genealogy databases enable naming of anonymous DNA donors. Science 2013;339(6117):262. Epub 2013/01/18.

[38] Homer N, Szelinger S, Redman M, Duggan D, Tembe W, Muehling J, et al. Resolving individuals contributing trace amounts of DNA to highly complex mixtures using high-density SNP genotyping microarrays. PLoS Genet 2008;4(8):e1000167. Epub 2008/09/05.

[39] Cassa CA, Miller RA, Mandl KD. A novel, privacy-preserving cryptographic approach for sharing sequencing data. J Am Med Inform Assoc 2013;20(1):69–76. Epub 2012/11/06.

[40] Ball MP, Thakuria JV, Zaranek AW, Clegg T, Rosenbaum AM, Wu X, et al. A public resource facilitating clinical use of genomes. Proc Natl Acad Sci USA 2012;109(30):11920–7. Epub 2012/07/17.

[41] Reich DE, Lander ES. On the allelic spectrum of human disease. Trends Genet 2001;17(9):502–10. Epub 2001/08/30.

[42] Manolio TA, Collins FS, Cox NJ, Goldstein DB, Hindorff LA, Hunter DJ, et al. Finding the missing heritability of complex diseases. Nature 2009;461(7265): 747–53. Epub 2009/10/09.

[43] Moore JH, Williams SM. New strategies for identifying gene-gene interactions in hypertension. Ann Med 2002;34(2):88–95. Epub 2002/07/11.

[44] Aschard H, Lutz S, Maus B, Duell EJ, Fingerlin TE, Chatterjee N, et al. Challenges and opportunities in genome-wide environmental interaction (GWEI) studies. Human Genet 2012;131(10):1591–613. Epub 2012/07/05.

[45] Moore JH. Detecting, characterizing, and interpreting nonlinear gene-gene interactions using multifactor dimensionality reduction. Adv Genet 2010;72:101–16. Epub 2010/10/30.

[46] Gunther F, Wawro N, Bammann K. Neural networks for modeling gene-gene interactions in association studies. BMC Genet 2009;10:87. Epub 2009/12/25.

[47] Robnik-Sikonja M, Cukjati D, Kononenko I. Comprehensible evaluation of prognostic factors and prediction of wound healing. Artif Intell Med 2003;29(1–2):25–38. Epub 2003/09/06.

[48] Greene CS, Penrod NM, Kiralis J, Moore JH. Spatially uniform relieff (SURF) for computationally-efficient filtering of gene-gene interactions. BioData Mining 2009;2(1):5. Epub 2009/09/24.

[49] Baranzini SE, Galwey NW, Wang J, Khankhanian P, Lindberg R, Pelletier D, et al. Pathway and network-based analysis of genome-wide association studies in multiple sclerosis. Human Mol Genet 2009;18(11):2078–90. Epub 2009/03/17.

[50] Kodama K, Horikoshi M, Toda K, Yamada S, Hara K, Irie J, et al. Expression-based genome-wide association study links the receptor CD44 in adipose tissue with type 2 diabetes. Proc Natl Acad Sci USA 2012;109(18):7049–54. Epub 2012/04/14.

[51] Rakyan VK, Down TA, Balding DJ, Beck S. Epigenome-wide association studies for common human diseases. Nat Rev Genet 2011;12(8):529–41. Epub 2011/07/13.

[52] Beyan H, Down TA, Ramagopalan SV, Uvebrant K, Nilsson A, Holland ML, et al. Guthrie card methylomics identifies temporally stable epialleles that are present at birth in humans. Genome Res 2012;22(11):2138–45. Epub 2012/08/25.

[53] Holmes E, Loo RL, Stamler J, Bictash M, Yap IK, Chan Q, et al. Human metabolic phenotype diversity and its association with diet and blood pressure. Nature 2008;453(7193):396–400. Epub 2008/04/22.

[54] Nicholson JK, Holmes E, Elliott P. The metabolome-wide association study: a new look at human disease risk factors. J Proteome Res 2008;7(9):3637–8. Epub 2008/08/19.

[55] Gieger C, Geistlinger L, Altmaier E, Hrabe de Angelis M, Kronenberg F, Meitinger T, et al. Genetics meets metabolomics: a genome-wide association study of metabolite profiles in human serum. PLoS Genet 2008;4(11):e1000282. Epub 2008/12/02.

[56] Denny JC, Ritchie MD, Basford MA, Pulley JM, Bastarache L, Brown-Gentry K, et al. PheWAS: demonstrating the feasibility of a phenome-wide scan to discover gene-disease associations. Bioinformatics (Oxford, England) 2010;26(9):1205–10. Epub 2010/03/26.

[57] Pendergrass SA, Brown-Gentry K, Dudek SM, Torstenson ES, Ambite JL, Avery CL, et al. The use of phenome-wide association studies (PheWAS) for exploration of novel genotype-phenotype relationships and pleiotropy discovery. Genet Epidemiol 2011;35(5):410–22. Epub 2011/05/20.

[58] Pendergrass SA, Dudek SM, Crawford DC, Ritchie MD. Visually integrating and exploring high throughput Phenome-Wide Association Study (PheWAS) results using PheWAS-View. BioData Mining 2012;5(1):5. Epub 2012/06/12.

[59] Patel CJ, Bhattacharya J, Butte AJ. An Environment-Wide Association Study (EWAS) on type 2 diabetes mellitus. PloS One 2010;5(5):e10746. Epub 2010/05/28.

[60] Choi M, Scholl UI, Ji W, Liu T, Tikhonova IR, Zumbo P, et al. Genetic diagnosis by whole exome capture and massively parallel DNA sequencing. Proc Natl Acad Sci USA 2009;106(45):19096–101. Epub 2009/10/29.

[61] Bainbridge MN, Wiszniewski W, Murdock DR, Friedman J, Gonzaga-Jauregui C, Newsham I, et al. Whole-genome sequencing for optimized patient management. Sci Transl Med 2011;3(87):87re3. Epub 2011/06/17.

[62] Stein LD. An introduction to the informatics of "next-generation" sequencing. In: Baxevanis Andreas D et al. Current protocols in bioinformatics; 2011 [chapter 11]: Unit 11 1. Epub 2011/12/14.

[63] McKenna A, Hanna M, Banks E, Sivachenko A, Cibulskis K, Kernytsky A, et al. The Genome Analysis Toolkit: a MapReduce framework for analyzing next-generation DNA sequencing data. Genome Res 2010;20(9):1297–303. Epub 2010/07/21.

[64] Adzhubei IA, Schmidt S, Peshkin L, Ramensky VE, Gerasimova A, Bork P, et al. A method and server for predicting damaging missense mutations. Nat Methods 2010;7(4):248–9. Epub 2010/04/01.

[65] Saunders CJ, Miller NA, Soden SE, Dinwiddie DL, Noll A, Alnadi NA, et al. Rapid whole-genome sequencing for genetic disease diagnosis in neonatal intensive care units. Sci Transl Med 2012;4(154):154ra135. Epub 2012/10/03.

[66] Fuchs C. Knowledge and society from the perspective of the unified theory of information (UTI) approach. In: Petitjean M, editor. Proceedings of FIS2005: third conference on the foundations of information science, Paris, 4–7 July 2005. Molecular Diversity Preservation International (MDPI), Basel, Switzerland, <http://www.mdpi.org/fis2005/F.24.paper.pdf> [accessed 20.12.12].

[67] Geist P, Dreyer J. The demise of dialogue: a critique of medical encounter ideology. West J Commun 1993;57(2):233–46.

[68] Cahill J. Patient participation – a review of the literature. J Clin Nursing 1998; 7:119–28.

[69] Gawthrop L, Waldo D. Civis, civitas, and civilitas: a new focus for the year 2000. Public Administration Review 1984, 44 March 101–111.

[70] Kruger J. The patient will see you now. J Participatory Med 2011:3. <http://www.jopm.org/perspective/narratives/2011/12/28/the-patient-will-see-you-now/> [accessed 03.05.12].

[71] Wagholikar A, Fung M, Nelson C. Improving self-care of patients with chronic disease using online personal health record. Austr Med J 2012;5(9):517–21. <http://dx.doi.org/10.4066/AMJ.2012.1358>.

[72] Santos C, Pedrosa T, Costa C, Oliveira JL. Concepts for a personal health record. Stud Health Technol Inform 2012;180:636–40.

[73] Swan M. Emerging patient-driven health care models: an examination of health social networks, consumer personalized medicine and quantified self-tracking. Int J Environ Res Public Health 2009;6(2):492–525.

[74] Dyson E. Why participatory medicine? J Participatory Med 2009;1(1):e1. <http://www.jopm.org/opinion/editorials/2009/10/21/why-participatory-medicine/> [accessed 03.05.12].

[75] Smarr L. Quantifying your body: a how-to guide from a systems biology perspective. Biotechnol J 2012;7(8):980–91.

[76] Schneider GF, Dekker C. DNA sequencing with nanopores. Nat Biotechnol 2012;30(4):326–8.

[77] Weaver M, Pollin TI. Direct-to-consumer genetic testing: what are we talking about? J Genet Couns 2012.

[78] Karczewski KJ, Tirrell RP, Cordero P, Tatonetti NP, Dudley JT, Salari K, et al. Interpretome: a freely available, modular, and secure personal genome interpretation engine. Pac Sympos Biocomput 2012:339–50.

[79] Stead W. Positioning the library at the epicentre of the networked biomedical enterprise. Bull Med Libr Assoc 1998;86(1):26–30.

[80] Fox S, Jones S. The social life of health information. Pew Internet Am Life Project 2009. <http://www.pewinternet.org/~/media/files/reports/2009/piphealth2009.pdf> [accessed 03.05.12].

[81] Laakso M, Bjork B-C. Anatomy of open access publishing: a study of longitudinal development and internal structure. BMC Med 2012;10(124):9.

[82] Vardell E, Moore M. Isabel, a clinical decision support system. Med Ref Serv Quart 2011;30(2):158–66.

[83] Delbanco T, Walker J, Darer JD, Elmore JG, Feldman HJ, Leveille SG, et al. Open notes: doctors and patients signing on. Ann Intern Med 2010;153(2):121–5.

[84] Vicdan Handan, Dholakia Nikhilesh. Medicine 2.0 and beyond: from information seeking to knowledge creation in virtual health communities (29 March 2012). Belk Russell W, Llamas Rosa, editors. The Routledge companion to digital consumption. New York and London: Routledge; 2012. Available at SSRN: <http://ssrn.com/abstract=2030844> [accessed 20.12.12].

[85] Braddock CH. The emerging importance and relevance of shared decision making to clinical practice. Med Decis Making 2010;30(Suppl. 1):5S–7S.

[86] Park S, Lee S, Kim M, Kim H. Shared decision support system on dental restoration. Expert Syst Appl 2012;39(14):11775–81.

[87] Cohen RM, Greenberg JM, Ishak WW. Incorporating multidimensional patient-reported outcomes of symptom severity, functioning, and quality of life in the individual burden of illness index for depression to measure treatment impact and recovery in MDD. JAMA Psych 2013;2:1–8.

[88] Sugrue R, Macgregor G, Sugrue M, Curran S, Murphy L. An evaluation of patient reported outcomes following breast reconstruction utilizing Breast Q. Breast 2013.

[89] Bhumbra R. Experts point out pitfalls of using patient reported outcomes to guide NHS care. BMJ 2012(345):e8133.

[90] Paz SH, Spritzer KL, Morales LS, Hays RD. Evaluation of the Patient-Reported Outcomes Information System (PROMIS()) Spanish-language physical functioning items. Qual Life Res 2012. [Epub ahead of print] PubMed PMID: 23124505.

[91] Cascade E, Marr P, Winslow M, Burgess A, Nixon M. Conducting research on the Internet: medical record data integration with patient-reported outcomes. J Med Internet Res 2012;14(5):e137.

[92] Ahmed S, Berzon RA, Revicki DA, Lenderking WR, Moinpour CM, Basch E, et al. International Society for Quality of Life Research. The use of patient-reported outcomes (PRO) within comparative effectiveness research: implications for clinical practice and health care policy. Med Care 2012;50(12):1060–70.

[93] Ohno-Machado L. Informatics 2.0: implications of social media, mobile health, and patient-reported outcomes for healthcare and individual privacy. J Am Med Inform Assoc 2012;19(5):683.

[94] Hinds PS, Nuss SL, Ruccione KS, Withycombe JS, Jacobs S, Deluca H, et al. PROMIS pediatric measures in pediatric oncology: valid and clinically feasible indicators of patient-reported outcomes. Pediatr Blood Cancer 2013;60(3):402–8.

[95] Swan M. Scaling crowdsourced health studies: the emergence of a new form of contract research organization. Personal Med 2012;9(2):223–34.

[96] Silber D. Medicine 2.0: the stakes of participatory medicine. Presse Med 2009; 38(10):1456–62. [in French].

[97] Do CB, Tung JY, Dorfman E, Kiefer AK, Drabant EM, Francke U, et al. Web-based genome-wide association study identifies two novel loci and a substantial genetic component for Parkinson's disease. PLoS Genet 2011;7(6).

[98] Wicks P, Vaughan T, Massagli M, Heywood J. Accelerated clinical discovery using self-reported patient data collected online and a patient-matching algorithm. Nat Biotechnol 2011;29:411–4.

[99] Hood L, Friend S. Predictive, personalized, preventive, participatory (P4) cancer medicine. Nat Rev Clin Oncol 2011;8:184–7.

[100] Chen R, Mias GI, Li-Pook-Than J, Jiang L, Lam HY, Chen R, et al. Personal omics profiling reveals dynamic molecular and medical phenotypes. Cell 2012;148(6): 1293–307.

Linking Genomic and Clinical Data for Discovery and Personalized Care

Joshua C. Denny[a] and Hua Xu[b]

[a]*Department of Biomedical Informatics and Medicine, Vanderbilt University, Nashville, TN, USA*
[b]*School of Biomedical Informatics, University of Texas Health Science Center at Houston, Houston, TX, USA*

CHAPTER OUTLINE

12.1 INTRODUCTION

Electronic Health Record (EHR) adoption in the United States and worldwide has been increasing significantly over the past few decades. Once primarily found only in select academic and tertiary care medical centers, EHRs are now being widely installed throughout academic medical centers, community hospitals, and in small outpatient clinics, spurred in part by major national investments in health care information technology and increased reimbursement in the United States via "Meaningful Use" legislation [1]. EHRs may not only improve clinical care [2–4] and reduce cost [5], they also create a very real opportunity to enable clinical and translational research. Volumes of clinical data, which once could only be mined through time-consuming and costly manual chart reviews, can now be processed using electronic means.

Coupling EHR data with DNA biobanks may foster a new generation of genomic research that may greatly accelerate existing models for genomic discovery. The typical model of DNA research has used purpose-collected cohorts or clinical trial populations. Enrolling and testing patients in these models is expensive and time consuming. Accrual of rare events (e.g., rare drug adverse reactions, rare exposures, or rare diseases) requires very large sample sizes. Furthermore, given the high cost of many health care tests (e.g., magnetic resonance imaging), the cost of such testing can be prohibitive to perform on large cohorts, whereas this testing may occur frequently within large clinical settings. EHR data provide a longitudinal resource for research, which is produced as a byproduct of routine health care. However, since EHR data are primarily captured to support clinical care, EHRs are not an ideal research environment. EHR data are captured in busy clinical settings, often governed by reimbursement rules and time-pressured encounters, and require processing in order to be translated into meaningful "phenotypes" amenable for genomic study. This chapter explores methods and techniques for mining EHR data to perform genetic association tests, and describes some of the necessary steps to deploy genetics to support personalized medicine.

12.2 REPURPOSING EHRs FOR CLINICAL AND TRANSLATIONAL RESEARCH

12.2.1 Creating Research-Enabled EHRs

EHRs are designed to optimize patient care and administrative functions. As such, they facilitate rapid access of patient data on a per-patient basis, and are designed to provide a complete capture of necessary information to support clinical care and billing. Querying across all patients for a given diagnosis, lab result, or textual keyword can be a non-trivial task within existing EHR systems. Furthermore, while a clinical EHR may be well suited for many chart review tasks (e.g., allowing full view of the electronic record on a per-patient basis), it still may be non-optimal for many other tasks. For example, did the patient have influenza in, for example, 2004? Such data may often not be recorded in problem lists, and can be restricted (depending on institutional culture) to chronic problems and acute ones with lasting impact (e.g., myocardial infarction). Moreover, review of billing codes (to correlate with other clinical data) may not be easily retrieved by a provider viewing a patient's record in the EHR. Or, does the patient have drug-induced liver injury? Such a question often requires finding the elevated liver tests and all the medication that were prescribed around that time. An EHR is typically adept at rapid retrieval of the patient's current medications, and can easily let one find the liver function tests, but combining the two with temporal relationships requires manual synthesis of the data.

Thus, to make EHR data more research-accessible, clinical data are often extracted from the operational system and reformatted into research data repositories, typically employing relational databases. One model is the creation of enterprise data warehouses (EDWs), which typically are relational database stores of EHR data. Taken outside of the clinical workflow, complicated search queries can be run against these systems across large patients without fear of slowing down the clinical systems. However, EDWs may not always represent a full collection of EHR data. For example, some EDWs store only structured EHR data, such as laboratory results and billing codes, eschewing clinical documentation (see Section 12.3 below). A number of research data warehouse systems have been developed. Examples created in academic medical centers include the Informatics for Integrating Biology and the Bedside (i2b2) [6], the Utah Population Database [7], Marshfield Clinic's Personalized Medicine Research Program [8], and Vanderbilt's Synthetic Derivative [9], among many others. The i2b2 system provides a graphical user interface and has been installed in many sites across the United States and world [10]. Additionally, commercial EHR venders have also developed research repositories that are attached to their EHRs. For example, Epic users can add Clarity, an EDW module, to ease mining of their clinical data by placing EHR data into a SQL-based relational database. Epic is also developing a business intelligence package, called Cogito, which provides EDW-like functionality with integrated analytics. Another useful addition to EHRs for clinical research has been the Research Electronic Data Capture (REDCap) system, which as of this writing has 529 institutional partners worldwide [11]. REDCap provides secure, web-based software for custom data capture form design and usage, along with surveys and data processing tools.

12.2.2 **EHR-Associated Biobanks**

More recently, researchers have been linking EHR data with biological databanks, or "biobanks." The most popular of these currently have been the collection of germline DNA, although other sources, such as plasma, urine, and pathology specimens, could be recorded as well. DNA can be collected from purpose-collected samples, such as through a consented study that isolates DNA from either blood samples or buccal swabs. For instance, buccal swabs have been used by the pharmacy benefits manager Medco to test patients for genetic variants related to certain drugs of interest, as well as to establish the Kaiser Permanente North California biobank, which has as its target the collection of 500,000 participants [12]. An alternate method that can be used by hospitals and clinics is isolation of DNA from samples that are either left over from routine blood testing (e.g., from an ordered laboratory test) or from a separate sample collected at the sample time as other routine testing. Such methods have been deployed by sites within the Electronic Medical Records and Genomics (eMERGE) Network [13] and in the Million Veterans Project [14].

The Personalized Medicine Research Population (PMRP) project of the Marshfield Clinic (Marshfield, WI) [15] was one of the earliest examples of EHR-linked DNA biobanks. The PMRP project selected 20,000 individuals who receive care in the geographic region of the Marshfield Clinic. These patients have been consented, surveyed, and have given permission to the investigators for re-contact in the future if additional information is needed. Similar EHR-linked biobanks exist at other eMERGE Network sites—Northwestern University (Chicago, IL), Geisinger Health System (Geisinger, PA), Mount Sinai School of Medicine (New York, NY), Cincinnati's Children's Hospital, the Mayo Clinic. Other hospitals, such as Aurora Health Care (Milwaukee, WI), have also established DNA biobanks. Each of these uses an opt-in approach, whereby patients consent to be part of the DNA biobank. Many of these sites include both EHR data and purpose-collected data (such as patient surveys) as part of the phenotype data [8,16]. Some of these biobanks have been designed as a repository for non-DNA biologic specimens as well.

An alternative "opt out" approach is used by Vanderbilt University's BioVU, which associates DNA with de-identified EHR data [9]. In the BioVU model, patients can opt out of the DNA biobank during completion of a standard "Consent to Treatment" form administered during check-in for routine clinic appointments. A majority of patients (>85%) do not opt out [9]. Patients that do not complete the consent to treatment form are excluded from BioVU. To ensure that no one knows with certainty if a subject's DNA is in BioVU, an additional small percentage of patients are randomly excluded. DNA for the remaining patients is extracted from blood that is scheduled to be discarded after clinical testing is done. Partners HealthCare employs a similar model linking de-identified EHR data with leftover blood from routine clinical testing for the Crimson biobank.

The BioVU model requires that the DNA and associated EHR data are de-identified to ensure that the model complies with the policies of non-human subjects research. The de-identified EHR is called the Synthetic Derivative. This process has been described in detail previously [9]. The full text of the EHR undergoes a process of de-identification with software programs that remove the 18 Health Insurance Portability and Accountability Act (HIPAA) Safe Harbor identifiers from all clinical documentation in the medical record. Multiple reviews by both the local institutional review board and the federal Office for Human Research Protections have affirmed BioVU's status as non-human subjects research according to 45 Code of Federal Regulations 46 [9]. EHR data are linked to DNA through a common identifier generated from a one-way hash of the medical record number. Using a hashed medical record number as an identifier allows for the Synthetic Derivative to be continually updated and still associated with the DNA samples while also preventing back-linkage to the medical record number.

12.3 PHENOTYPING ALGORITHMS: FINDING MEANINGFUL POPULATIONS OF PATIENTS FROM EHR DATA

12.3.1 Classes of Data Available in EHRs

EHRs contain heterogeneous types of data, as they are designed primarily to support clinical care, billing, and, increasingly, other functions such as quality monitoring and reporting. Thus, the types of data and their storage are optimized to support these missions. There are different ways to categorize EHR data (e.g., based on care settings such as inpatient vs. outpatient) or content of the data (e.g., labs vs. medications). As the focus here is to introduce the methods for processing EHR data, we divide EHR data into two broader categories based on their formats: structured vs. unstructured data. Structured data often include billing codes, laboratory results, and some types of medication data, available in most systems as structured "name-value pair" data. Unstructured data include narrative or semi-narrative text formats, such as clinical documentation, pathology and radiology results, and some test results (such as echocardiograms). Phenotyping algorithms are logical combinations of multiple types of data (e.g., billing codes, laboratory results, and medication data) that are designed to achieve high accuracy when identifying cases and controls from the EHR.

12.3.1.1 *Structured Data*

Demographics: Demographic data, such as age/date of birth, gender, and race/ethnicity, are key covariates for most clinical and genetic studies and are fairly ubiquitously available as structured data in EHRs. However, these variables are not always reliably recorded, and may be encoded in a variety of different formats and have different allowable values. Early experiences within the eMERGE Network with the creation of data dictionaries for cross-institution studies found that initial data dictionary variable names and allowable values for demographics differed significantly between phenotypes and sites [17]. Improved use of available standard terminology systems such as caDSR (Cancer Data Standards Registry and Repository) and SNOMED CT (Systematized Nomenclature of Medicine, Clinical Terms) has improved the portability and similarity of eMERGE dictionary [17]. Additionally, genetic testing has shown that the EHR sex is correctly recorded [9].

Since alleles can vary greatly between different ancestral populations, accurate knowledge of genetic ancestry information, as recorded by race/ethnicity variables, is essential to allow for proper control of population stratification when performing association studies. Race/ethnicity as recorded within an EHR may be entered through a variety of sources, typically entered by administrative staff via structured data collection tools, which may differ from that of self-determination. Moreover, this field can often be left blank or completed with nonspecific values such as "Unknown" or "Other." Patients without EHR-defined race/ethnicity information ranges between 9% and 23% of subjects [18,19]. A Veterans Administration (VA) hospital system study noted that >95% of all EHR-derived race/ethnicity agreed with self-reported race/ethnicity using nearly 1 million records [20]. Moreover, research comparing genetic ancestry to that entered in the EHR found that genetic ancestry agreed well with genetic determinations [21]. Thus, despite concerns over EHR-derived ancestral information, such information, when present, appears similar to self-report and genetic ancestry information. (It is important to note that if a sufficiently large number of ancestry informative markers [e.g., single nucleotide polymorphisms, or SNPs] are tested, genetic ancestry can be calculated [22] or population stratification can be adjusted for through principal components analysis [23]. Genetic ancestry is superior to self-report race/ethnicity information, since many people are a composite of multiple ancestries.)

Billing codes: The International Classification of Diseases (ICD) and Current Procedural Terminology (CPT) are two typical types of codes for billing purposes in EHR. ICD is maintained by the World Health Organization (WHO) and contains codes of diseases, signs, symptoms, and procedures. While the majority of the world uses ICD version 10 (ICD-10), the United States (as of 2013) uses ICD version 9-CM (ICD9-CM, with clinical modification) within clinical environments (public health reporting, such as associated with death certification, does use ICD10); the current Center for Medicare and Medicaid Services guidelines mandate a transition in clinical settings to ICD-10-CM in the United States by October 1, 2014. Because of their widespread use as required components for billing, and due to their ubiquity within EHR systems, billing codes are frequently used for research purposes [24–29]. Prior research has demonstrated that use of a single ICD code alone to indicate a given diagnosis can have poor sensitivity and/or specificity [30,31]. Despite this, they remain an important part of more complex phenotype algorithms that achieve high performance [18,19,32].

ICD-9 and ICD-10 codes follow a hierarchy defined by numerical codes (ICD-9-CM) or alphanumerical codes (ICD-10). ICD-9 Disease or Symptom codes consist of a three-digit number (termed a "category") followed, in most cases, by one or two additional specifying digits. For example, the three-digit code "250" specifies diabetes mellitus and further digits are added to specify the type of diabetes, whether the diabetes is controlled or not, and certain diabetic complications, such as "Type 1 diabetes, not stated as uncontrolled" (250.01). ICD-9 procedure codes are two-digit codes, followed by two digits following the decimal; e.g., 10.21 "Biopsy of conjunctiva." Among Disease and Symptom codes, there are 18 chapters, such as Infectious and parasitic diseases (001-139), neoplasms (140-239), etc. (ICD-10 has 19 chapters, splitting the ICD-9 chapter "Diseases of the sense organs" into separate chapters for "Diseases of the eye and adnexa" and "Diseases of the ear and mastoid process.") Chapters are divided into sections (e.g., "Diseases of other endocrine glands," ICD-9 codes 249-259) that contain a number of three-digit codes (i.e., categories).

Since ICD-9 (and ICD-10) can contain greater granularity than what may be desired when performing research (e.g., you want all the Type 2 diabetes patients), groupings of codes are often used. While convenient to use the ICD-9 hierarchical relationships, these are often non-ideal for research purposes. The ICD-9 250 category includes all Type 1 and Type 2 diabetes, but each Type 1 and Type 2 also has digits to specify controlled vs. uncontrolled diabetes, and whether it has the complications of neuropathy, ophthalmic disease, renal disease, circulatory disease, or other complications. Similarly, codes for tuberculosis are found in ICD-9 categories 010-018, 137, and several V codes. Thus, clinical groupings have been published that group the ICD-9 codes into more useful groupings for research. One published grouping is the Clinical Classifications Software (CCS) created as part of the Health care Cost and Utilization Project from the Agency for Health care Research and Quality [33]. CCS is available for download with association software from http://www. hcup-us.ahrq.gov/toolssoftware/ccs/ccs.jsp. CCS groups the >14,000 ICD-9 diagnosis codes into >700 hierarchical codes. Another is the classification made for use in genomic analysis, the phenome-wide association study (PheWAS) code groups [34]. The original PheWAS code grouping grouped the Disease and Symptom codes into 776 diseases; current versions [35] contain about 1500 disease codes that are arranged hierarchically. A unique feature of the PheWAS code groupings is that they contain a corresponding "control group" for each case grouping; these control groups exclude related diseases from being a potential control when doing a case-control analysis (e.g., a patient with ischemic heart disease cannot serve as a control for acute myocardial infarction). The PheWAS groupings are also available for download at http://knowledgemap.mc.vanderbilt.edu/research/content/phewas. Table 12.1 gives example groupings for both CCS and the PheWAS hierarchy.

CPT codes are created and maintained by the American Medical Association. Providers use CPT codes to bill for clinical services, and represent everything from the type and complexity of a patient visit (which correspond to different reimbursement rates) to orderable tests, procedures, and surgeries. Typically, CPTs are paired with ICD diagnosis codes, the latter providing the reason (e.g., a disease or symptom) for a clinical encounter or procedure. This satisfies the requirements of insurers, who require certain allowable diagnoses and symptoms to pay for a given procedure. For example, insurance companies

Table 12.1 ICD-9 code groupings in the Clinical Classifications Software and using PheWAS codes. The ICD-9 descriptions have been shortened to more easily fit in a table while still preserving their meaning.

ICD-9		Clinical Classifications Software		PheWAS	
Code(s)	Description	Code	Description	Code	Description
10.*-18.*	Various tuberculosis codes and sites of infection				
137.*	Late effects of respiratory or unspecified tuberculosis	1.1.1	Tuberculosis	10	Tuberculosis
V12.01	Personal history of tuberculosis				
250.00	Diabetes mellitus type II, not uncontrolled, no complication	3.2	Diabetes mellitus without complication	250.2	Type 2 diabetes
250.01	Diabetes mellitus Type I, not uncontrolled, no complication	3.2	Diabetes mellitus without complication	250.1	Type 1 diabetes
250.40	Diabetes mellitus Type II, not uncontrolled, with renal manifestations	3.3.2	Diabetes with renal manifestations	250.22	Type 2 diabetes with renal manifestations
250.41	Diabetes mellitus Type I, not uncontrolled, with renal manifestations	3.3.2	Diabetes with renal manifestations	250.12	Type 1 diabetes with renal manifestations

will pay for a brain magnetic resonance imaging (MRI) scan that is ordered for a number of complaints (such as known cancers or symptoms such as headache), but not for unrelated symptoms such as chest pain.

When using billing codes to establish a particular diagnosis using EHR data, procedure codes (i.e., CPT or ICD procedure codes) tend to have high specificity but low sensitivity, while ICD diagnosis codes have comparatively lower specificity but higher sensitivity. Many physicians, for instance, may use a diabetes ICD code to test a patient for diabetes, because the physician clinically suspects the diagnosis, before a confirmatory test has been performed. A procedure code is typically only billed when the procedure has actually been performed; however, it is just a marker for a disease, and many procedures may be nonspecific for a given diagnosis. For instance, to establish the diagnosis of coronary artery disease, one could look for a CPT code for "coronary artery bypass surgery" or "percutaneous coronary angioplasty," or for one of several ICD-9 codes. If the CPT code is present, there is a high probability that the patient has corresponding diagnosis of coronary disease (indicating high specificity). However, many patients without these CPT codes also have coronary disease (indicating lower sensitivity), but either has not received these interventions or received them at a different hospital. Prior studies have shown that CPT codes are highly accurate to predict the occurrence of a given procedure [36]; however, if the procedure was performed at another hospital, recall may be low. Thus, in health systems linked to a comprehensive regional Health Information Exchange or in which insurance information is available for individuals (e.g., a health maintenance organization [HMO]), a query of CPT codes could result in both high precision and recall for performed procedures.

Laboratory and vital signs: Vital signs and most laboratory tests are stored in structured formats. In addition, these data are often repeated many times in the record and are often numerical with well-defined normal ranges, which aid in computation. Since vital signs and laboratory values play important roles in the diagnosis and monitoring of disease progression and treatment response, they play a useful role in identifying population of interest from the EHR. Often, they are stored as name-value pair data in the EHR or EDW systems, and often these fields can be encoded using standard terminologies. The Logical Observation Identifiers Names and Codes (LOINC®) vocabulary was originally created to provide a common encoding for these data. LOINC is a Consolidated Health Informatics standard for representation of laboratory and test names and is part of Health Language 7 (HL7) [37,38]. Despite the growing use of LOINC, many (perhaps most) hospital lab systems often use local terminologies to encode laboratory results internally. Since laboratory systems or testing companies may change over time, translation efforts are needed.

Both internal mappings and external translation are greatly facilitated by mapping to standard vocabularies, such as LOINC. Important aspects for laboratory data are recording the units and reference ranges, which may both change over time. Weights and heights were also recorded by different systems using different field names and stored internally with different units (e.g., kilograms, grams, or pounds for weight; centimeters, meters, inches, or feet for height).

Structured Medication Data: With the increased use of computerized provider order entry (CPOE) systems and medication administration record systems for the inpatient setting, and *electronic* prescribing (e-prescribing) tools in the outpatient setting, medication records in the EHR are becoming increasingly available as structured entries. Prescriptions can be mapped to local vocabularies but are also often mapped to controlled vocabularies such as RxNorm or proprietary vocabularies, such as First Databank. Many hospital systems also have installed automated barcode medication administration records, which capture inpatient medication records [39]. The combination of electronic inpatient records and outpatient e-prescribing systems can allow construction of accurate drug exposures, especially for more recent medication histories. However, most outpatient records still have a number of non-structured medication records through either handwritten prescriptions or other communications with pharmacies, such as faxed refill requests or telephoned prescriptions. Such medication data is often found in clinical documentation.

12.3.1.2 *Unstructured Data*

Provider documentation: Clinical documentation represents perhaps the richest and most diverse source of phenotype information. Provider documentation is required for nearly all billing of tests and clinical visits, and is frequently found in EHR systems. To be useful for phenotyping efforts, clinical documentation must be in the form of electronically available text that can be used for subsequent manual review or automated text processing programs. Although a number of users have created structured documentation tools, clinical notes are still typically created in unstructured, free-text formats [40]. Historically, providers dictated notes for transcription services, which involved a human typing the note for them. More often today, notes are created via semi-automated computer-based documentation (CBD) systems. These notes typically produce narrative-text documents that are amenable to free-text searching and text-processing techniques (see below). Sometimes, important documents may only be available as hand-written documents. Unavailability may result from clinics that are slow adopters, have very high patient volumes, or have specific workflows not well accommodated by the EHR system [41].

Documentation from reports and tests: Radiology, pathology, and some test and procedure results are often in the form of narrative reports. Many of these contain a mixture of structured and unstructured results, which may or may not be separately recorded in the EHR. Examples include an electro-cardiogram report, which typically has structured interval durations, heart rates, and overall categorization (e.g., "normal" or "abnormal"), as well as a narrative-text "impression" representing the cardiologist's interpretation of the result (e.g., "consider anterolateral myocardial ischemia") [42].

Unstructured Medication Data: Outpatient medication records are often recorded via narrative-text entries within clinical documentation, patient problem lists, or communications with patients through telephone calls or patient portals. Many EHR systems have incorporated outpatient e-prescribing systems, which create structured medical records during generation of new prescriptions and refills. However, within many EHR systems, e-prescribing tools are optional, not yet widely adopted, or have only been used within recent history. Thus, accurate construction of a patient's medication exposure history often requires information embedded in clinical narratives. When searching for specific phenotypes, focused free-text searching for a specific set of medications can be efficient and effective [18]. This approach requires the researcher to generate the list of brand names, generics, combination medications, and abbreviations that would be used, but has the advantage that it can be easily accomplished using keyword searching methods. The downside is that this approach requires re-engineering for each medication or set of medications to be searched, and does not allow for the retrieval of other medication data, such as dose, frequency, and duration.

12.3.2 **EHR Data Extraction and Normalization**

As described in the previous section, EHRs contain heterogeneous types of clinical data that are collected for purposes other than research. Before an electronic phenotyping algorithm can be executed, clinical data have to be processed and normalized to standard representations. Natural language processing (NLP) technologies, which can extract structured information from free text, are becoming an essential tool for many EHR data-extraction tasks. NLP has been successfully applied to the medical domain to identify detailed clinical information from narrative clinical documents. As clinical findings are often represented by different standards (e.g., terminologies), ontology-based approaches have been developed to map concepts in different clinical terminologies and to normalize them to standard representations for precise and consistent semantic interoperation across multiple care providers and health care enterprises.

12.3.2.1 *NLP to Extract Structured Information from Clinical Text*

For detailed NLP methods in the biomedical domain, please refer to Chapter 6. In this section, the focus is to briefly introduce clinical NLP systems and their use in extracting phenotypic information from clinical text. A number of studies have shown that coded data (e.g., ICD-9) alone were not sufficient or accurate enough for identifying disease cohorts [43–45]. Information extracted from clinical narratives by NLP systems is often complementary to structured data. For example, Penz et al. found that ICD-9 and CPT codes identified less than 11% of the cases in a study of detecting adverse events related to central venous catheters, while NLP methods achieved a sensitivity of 0.72 and a specificity of 0.80 [46]. Moreover, Li et al. compared the results of ICD-9 encoded diagnoses and NLP-processed discharge summaries for clinical trial eligibility queries [30]. They concluded that NLP-processed notes provide more valuable data sources for clinical trial pre-screening because they provide past medical histories as well as more specific details about diseases that are generally unavailable as ICD-9 coded data.

Over the last three decades, many clinical NLP systems have been developed. Most of them are information extraction systems and can be used to extract phenotypic information from clinical text. Based on the purposes of NLP systems, they can be divided into three categories: general-purpose, entity-specific, and task-specific systems. General-purpose clinical text processing systems, which often take significant amount of time and effort to develop, are able to recognize broad types of clinical findings (e.g., disease, drug, procedure, etc.). Widely used general-purpose clinical NLP systems include MedLEE (Medical Language Extraction and Encoding System) [47], cTAKES (clinical Text Analysis and Knowledge Extraction System) [48], MetaMap [49], and KnowledgeMap [50], all of which have been applied to EHR phenotyping tasks. Entity-specific systems only recognize certain types of clinical entities. For example, a number of systems have been developed to recognize medications and their signature information (e.g., dose, route, and frequency) in clinical text in the 2009 i2b2 NLP challenge [51]. Task-specific ones refer to systems that aim at extracting very specific concepts from clinical text. For example, Garvin et al. developed a regular expression-based system to extract ejection fraction rate in echocardiograms from seven VA medical centers [52]. How to determine which NLP tool(s) to use is a practical question for end-users that is dependent on the specific phenotyping task. An efficient strategy would be to combine general-purpose systems with user-specified rules to achieve high performance on specific phenotyping tasks. For example, Xu et al. developed a customized preprocessor and integrated it with the general-purpose MedLEE system to accurately extract breast cancer-specific information from pathology reports [53]. Similarly, a generic medication extraction engine (called MedEx) were combined with specific rules to effectively calculate warfarin weekly dose, which was used to replicate a genetic association using EHR data [54].

12.3.2.2 **Ontology-Based Methods for Clinical Data Normalization**

Structured clinical data (either originally recorded in EHRs or extracted by NLP systems from clinical documents) can be represented by different controlled vocabularies. For example, in EHR databases, disease names can be coded as ICD-9 codes or SNOMED-CT codes, and drug names can be coded as National Drug Data File (NDDF) Plus by First Databank or National Drug Code (NDC) by US FDA (Food and Drug Administration). To achieve efficient and accurate phenotyping, it is critical to map similar concepts across different clinical vocabularies. Fortunately, the National Library of Medicine has developed (in 1986) and maintains a comprehensive biomedical thesaurus, the Unified Medical Language System (UMLS) [55]. The UMLS is a compendium of over 100 controlled vocabularies in the biomedical domain, including terminologies such as ICD-9, CPT, and SNOMED-CT. It can serve as an interlingua of biomedical vocabularies by providing a mapping structure among these vocabularies and allowing one to translate among the various terminologies. The UMLS is concept oriented—different terms with the same meaning (such as "hypertension" or "high blood pressure") will be assigned to the same Concept Unique Identifier (CUI). A subset of UMLS, called RxNorm, provides normalized names for clinical drugs and links its names to many of the drug vocabularies commonly used in pharmacy management and drug interaction software, such as First Databank and Micromedex. Many clinical NLP systems use the UMLS or UMLS components as the terminology to encode clinical findings to increase the interoperability of heterogeneous clinical data.

To increase semantic interoperability, more detailed clinical models have been developed to represent clinical events and observations. The Clinical Element Model (CEM) developed at the Intermountain Healthcare is a typical example, which provides a single normalized logical structure for a data element. For example, a "Systolic Blood Pressure" measure can be represented as (Key="Systolic Blood Pressure" and data="120 mm hg") in the CEM model [56,57]. CEMs are written in the Constraint Definition Language (CDL) that can be compiled into objects such as XML Schema Definitions (XSDs) or Semantic Web Resource Description Framework (RDF) to make them computable. In addition, CEM is compatible with other efforts for standardizing clinical information, such as the HL7 Detailed Clinical Model (DCM), which aims at developing an information model of a discrete set of precise clinical knowledge that can be used in a variety of contexts. Currently, many efforts have been devoted to build a standards-based infrastructure for secondary use EHR data. A prominent example is the consortium of secondary use of EHR data in the Strategic Health IT Advanced Research Projects (SHARPn) program funded by Office of the National Coordinator for Health

Information Technology (ONC) [58]. The SHARPn team is developing open source services and software for normalizing disparate EHR data, both structured and narrative, to support biomedical research. As mentioned above, another important informatics framework for repurposing of EHR data for biomedical research is the i2b2 software developed by the Informatics for Integrating Biology and the Bedside, a National Center for Biomedical Computing based at Partners Healthcare System. The i2b2 framework is in use at more than half of the national CTSA (Clinical and Transitional Science Award) institutions for managing clinical data for research purposes [10].

12.3.3 Building an Electronic Phenotype Algorithm

Phenotype algorithms begin with selection of the phenotype of interest, along with identification of key clinical elements that define that phenotype, usually in discussion with clinical experts. Phenotype algorithms often consist of combinations of billing codes, laboratory and test results, medication exposures, and natural language processing applied to unstructured text data combined with either Boolean operators (e.g., AND, OR, NOT) [18,59] or machine learning methods [60,61]. For laboratory data, certain thresholds are often used (serum potassium between 3.5 and 5 mEq/ dL, for instance, if one wanted to ensure normal potassium values). For billing data, requiring more than one code for a given diagnosis is also often helpful. A study on rheumatoid arthritis (RA) found that requiring 3 ICD-9 codes for RA increased the positive predictive value from 33% to 57% [62]. When finding cases of Crohn's disease (which can be difficult to distinguish clinically from ulcerative colitis) for a genetic study, Ritchie et al. required that more Crohn's disease codes than ulcerative colitis codes [18].

Medication records serve an important role in accurate phenotype characterization. They can be used to increase the precision of case identification, and to help ensure that patients believed to be controls do not actually have the disease. Medications received by a patient serve as confirmation that the treating physician believed the disease was present to a sufficient degree that they prescribed a treating medication. It is particularly helpful to find presence or absence of medications highly specific or sensitive for the disease. For instance, a patient with diabetes will receive either oral or injectable hypoglycemic agents; these medications are both highly sensitive and specific for treating diabetes, and can also be used to help differentiate Type 1 diabetes (treated almost exclusively with insulin) from Type 2 diabetes (which is typically a disease of insulin resistance and thus can be treated with a combination of oral and injectable hypoglycemic agents).

Control algorithms are of similar importance to case algorithms [18]. EHRs are opportunistic with regard to the collection of data based on contacts with the health care systems and diseases one has. The English poet William Cowper said, "absence of proof is not proof of absence," and the same is certainly true of the EHR. Thus, for common diseases, such as diabetes or hypertension, one typically needs to include queries for key elements to ensure that cases are not found commonly in controls. This may be unnecessary for very rare diseases; in these cases, exclusions of individuals with the specific diagnoses may be sufficient.

12.3.4 **Iterative Algorithm Development and Evaluation**

When evaluating phenotype algorithms, the most important consideration is often the positive predictive value (PPV), or precision, of the algorithm. Precision is defined as the ratio of true positives (TP) for an algorithm to the all positives (that is, $TP + $ false positives [FP]) identified by the algorithm ($PPV = TP/(TP + FP)$). Recall (or sensitivity) is the ratio of TP identified and all positives identified in a gold standard review (that is, $TP + $ false negatives [FN], or $Recall = TP/[TP + FN]$). Typically the gold standard is established by chart review via physicians [18,62] or trained chart abstractors using a standardized review instrument [63]. Since algorithms typically include a number of components, they often take a number of iterations to achieve high performance. The typical model is to set a pre-specified target of accuracy, typically a PPV of 90–95%, and then to iteratively review cases and controls returned by the algorithm with reviewers (see Figure 12.1). The PPV target is based some on the rareness of the phenotype. A high PPV will be the target for common phenotypes such as diabetes, heart disease; for rare phenotypes, such as drug adverse events like Stevens Johnson Syndrome, one may manually review all potential cases in order to not miss true cases. However, since the comprehensive review of a large set of records is often infeasible, especially for rare phenotypes, true recall measurements can be hard (or expensive) to achieve, and PPV becomes the more important metric [64].

Since record review of large patient charts can lead to disagreements, calculation of inter-rater agreement is important to ensure accuracy of the gold standard. Common measures of inter-rater agreement are percentage agreement

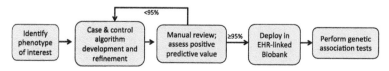

■ **FIGURE 12.1** Iterative phenotype development.

and Cohen's Kappa. The F1-measure, the harmonic mean of recall and precision (calculated as $F1 = 2 \times \text{Recall} \times \text{Precision}/[\text{Recall} + \text{Precision}]$), can also be used for inter-rater agreement, and provides an estimate very similar to Kappa [65].

12.3.5 PheKB: An Online Catalog of Phenotyping Algorithms

As described above, the creation of phenotype algorithms with high positive predictive value requires significant time and effort. In the eMERGE network, these algorithms typically take 6–12 months to develop through a process of design at an individual site, deployment and validation at external sites, and iterative redesign. Prior work has shown that these algorithms are transportable to multiple sites and EHR systems with good performance [35,59,62,63]. The Phenotype Knowledgebase (PheKB, http://phekb.org) is a website designed to aid in creation, validation, and sharing of phenotype algorithms (see Figure 12.2). PheKB's fundamental utility is as a repository for phenotype algorithms. Users can read, upload, search, and provide feedback on the phenotype algorithms, and upload a variety of documents and metadata regarding these phenotypes. Typically that includes a phenotype algorithm file and a data dictionary. Files of any common type (e.g., Microsoft Word,

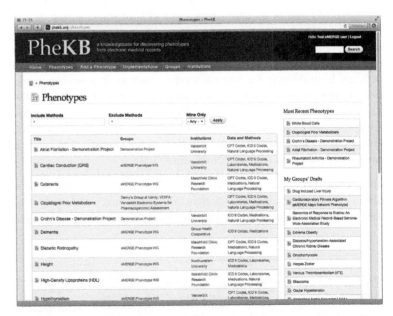

■ **FIGURE 12.2** PheKB is a resource for phenotype algorithm development—can also be used in the process of phenotype development.

PDF) can be uploaded and associated with the phenotype record. Algorithms can be published and shared publicly, or restricted to a particular "group" of users that can collectively develop or edit the algorithm. Users can comment and ask questions on phenotypes, receive email notification when updates are made, and create "implementation" records, which capture site-specific validation of a phenotype algorithm along with notes on any adaptations made. In eMERGE, phenotype algorithms on PheKB are validated at the creating site as well as at least 1–2 other institutions. PheKB is currently searchable by metadata fields (e.g., institution, author, keyword, or type of content used).

12.4 TYPES OF GENETIC ASSOCIATION STUDIES

12.4.1 Genetic Associations with Diseases and Traits

Candidate gene-variant studies and, more recently, genome-wide association studies (GWAS) have been the mainstay of genetic analysis over the last decade. GWAS typically investigate 500,000 SNPs or more. The more recent advent of next-generation sequencing technologies has increased the power of genetic analysis. Association studies with diseases or traits have been the primary focus of most genetic studies to date. For instance, most association studies cataloged in the NHGRI GWAS Catalog [66] or performed within EHR systems to date have focused on diseases and traits that can be defined as a binary or linear outcome in the medical record, such as cataracts [63], hypothyroidism [35], or Type 2 Diabetes [59].

A detailed example of a disease phenotype algorithm is provided in Figure 12.3, which shows an EHR algorithm developed to find primary

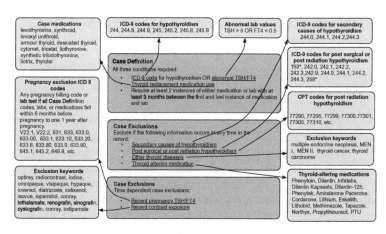

■ **FIGURE 12.3** Phenotype algorithm for primary hypothyroidism. This figure is reproduced with permission from [32]. The full algorithm is available on http://PheKB.org.

hypothyroidism (presumptive Hashimoto's thyroiditis) [35]. Of note, although the vast majority of cases of primary hypothyroidism should be Hashimoto's thyroiditis, primary hypothyroidism was selected as the target phenotype because physicians rarely check confirmatory autoantibodies or perform thyroid biopsies to firmly establish the diagnosis of Hashimoto's thyroiditis. As shown in the figure, the algorithm uses laboratory results, medication exposures, ICD and CPT codes, and some simple text queries of radiology reports and other clinical documentation. The algorithm was evaluated at five different sites (Group Health Cooperative, Marshfield Clinic, Mayo Clinic, Northwestern, and Vanderbilt), and the average positive predictive value was 92% (range by site, 82–98%). The algorithm was then deployed at each site to identify patients with existing GWAS data from other studies (e.g., patients genotyped for analysis of cardiac conduction, dementia, cataracts) as part of the eMERGE Network [13]. The GWAS noted a novel association with variants near *FOXE1*, a thyroid transcription factor, associated with hypothyroidism. This finding has since been validated by another GWAS, which also identified several other loci of interest [67].

12.4.2 Genetic Associations with Drug Response

Drug-response phenotypes include adverse drug events and therapeutic efficacy. Serum drug levels can also be the phenotype of interest for genetic associations studies, especially when the drug level has direct therapeutic indications (e.g., warfarin for anticoagulation, antibiotics, or antirejection medications in transplant patients). Performing genetic association studies on drug response can be especially challenging [68]. A key challenge is that the detection of a drug-response phenotype requires accurate identification of at least two "phenotypes"—the drug exposure and the outcome. In some cases, it requires resolving temporal sequences of more than two phenotypes. For instance, in studying cardiovascular events following initiation of clopidogrel, we required: (1) the patient to have a myocardial infarction or intracoronary stent, (2) treatment with clopidogrel, and (3) occurrence of a cardiovascular event while still taking clopidogrel [69]. Clopidogrel is typically given for 1–12 months following a myocardial infarction or stent, and patient adherence can be decreased by adverse reactions and high cost, especially before it became generic. Overall, only 44% (260/591) of the potential cases identified by electronic algorithms were judged true cases. Despite these challenges, pharmacogenetic associations studies have been successfully deployed in EHR data for warfarin steady-state dose and variants in *CYP2C9*, *VKORC1*, *CYP4F2*, and *CALU* [70], clopidogrel efficacy and variants in *CYP2C19* and *ABCB1* [69], and the antirejection drug tacrolimus and *CYP3A5* [71]. In addition, informatics tools such as MedEx [72], a medication information extraction system, have been applied to automatically extract drug dosing information for the warfarin pharmacogenetic study [54] (see Figures 12.2 and 12.3).

12.4.3 **Phenome-Wide Association Studies (PheWAS)**

Since EHRs contain broad collections of phenotypes limited only by their included patients and what the physician recorded, it permits the analysis of many different phenotypes against a particular genotype. A PheWAS is a type of "reverse genetics" approach that starts with a given genotype and asks with which phenotypes it may be associated. The PheWAS approach was first described using EHR data using five SNPs with known associations [34], but the same principle has also been applied to observational cohort methods [73]. As mentioned above, the initial EHR PheWAS method groups ICD-9-CM billing codes into related case groups and then also defines relevant control groups. Then, pairwise case-control analyses are performed for each phenotype using standard methods. Figure 12.4 presents a PheWAS for an HLA SNP, rs3135388, performed in BioVU with 6005 patients. This SNP is known to be associated with multiple sclerosis. The PheWAS also highlights associations with other autoimmune conditions, such as Type 1 diabetes and hypothyroidism. PheWAS analyses can also be performed with more dense EHR data, such as natural language processing data, though grouping is challenging [74] (see Figure 12.4).

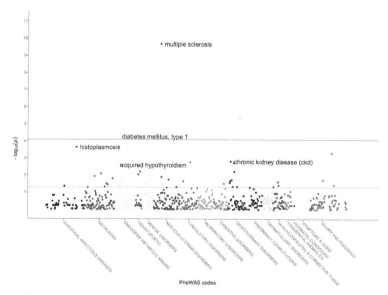

■ **FIGURE 12.4** A PheWAS plot for rs3135388 in HLA-DRA. This region has known associations with multiple sclerosis. The red line indicates statistical significance at Bonferroni correction. The blue line represents $p<0.05$. Figure reproduced from Denny JC. Chapter 13: Mining Electronic Health Records in the Genomics Era. PLoS Comput Biol 8(12): e1002823.

12.5 MOVING TO THE BEDSIDE: IMPLEMENTING GENETICS INTO THE EHR

12.5.1 Importance of Clinical Decision Support for Genetic Data

Genomic decision support can target both drug prescribing and other recommendations for care, both with a goal of "personalizing medicine." To date, most efforts have focused on pharmacogenomic support for the purpose of automated clinical decision support (CDS) advisors. However, geneticists routinely use genetic information in the clinical to personalize care for risk syndromes, such as screening for colon cancer in the setting of Lynch syndrome or breast cancer in patients with *BRCA1/2* mutations. In the future, CDS advisors may guide such care. Here, we focus primarily on CDS for prescribing.

CDS advisors to support prescribing have been shown in many contexts to improve the accuracy of prescriptions generated [75]. While no formal studies of CDS in the genomic context have been performed to date, it is expected that CDS will be equally if not more important for genomic data as for traditional risk factors such as poor renal function or drug-drug interactions. The key factors making genomic decision support essential to effective physician recognition of genomic factors during prescribing include:

1. Lack of physician knowledge regarding genomic variants influencing each medication, which vary by drug (e.g., clopidogrel is influenced by *CYP2C19* variants [76]; warfarin influenced by *CYP2C9*, *VKORC1*, *CYP4F2*, *CALU*, and others [70]) and can vary between drugs within a particular drug classes as well (simvastatin is influenced by *SLCO1B1* but this may not influence risk of toxicity from other statins [77]).

2. Nomenclature of variants does not itself provide interpretation of their meaningfulness (e.g., *CYP2C19*2* is a hypofunctioning variant; *CYP2C19*17* is a hyperfunctioning variant).

3. The number of variants discovered and our understanding of their importance is ever-expanding. Moreover, increased availability of high-density genotyping methods and next-generation sequencing has greatly increased the number of new variants discovered, and will likely continue to do so for at least the near future. Thus, one may expect pharmacogenomic-based decision support to change at a greater rate than traditional decision support rules. As one example, between 2010 and 2012, the pharmacogenomic advisor for clopidogrel at Vanderbilt (see below) included four major changes based on indications, genotype, and alternative medications recommended as more knowledge became available.

4. Clinical decision support for genomic variants may involve complex dose calculations. For instance, warfarin dose is adjusted using genomic variants through a linear regression equation. It would be challenging (and potentially errorprone) to ask providers to implement outside of the context of an EHR.

12.5.2 Determining Clinical Utility of Genetic Variants

Determining genetic variants with potential implications for clinical care is the first step of genomic medicine. However, it is not a trivial task to identify clinically relevant variants (or actionable variants) from the rapidly expanding literature on the association between molecular variation patterns and clinical phenotypes. National and institutional initiatives have expended significant resources on the evaluation of assays and the assessment of the underlying evidence. Table 12.2 shows a list of databases that contain clinically relevant variants, which represents the major ongoing efforts in this area.

Table 12.2 Resources of clinically relevant genetic variants.

Name	Creator	URL	Comments
ClinVar	National Center for Biotechnology Information (NCBI)	http://www.ncbi.nlm.nih.gov/clinvar/	It provides up-do-date relationships among human variations and phenotypes along with supporting evidence
Evaluation of genomic applications in practice and prevention	Centers for Disease Control and Prevention (CDC)	http://www.cdc.gov/genomics/gtesting/EGAPP/recommend/	It contains six recommendations on the validity and utility of specific genetic tests, as of December 2012
Pharmacogenomic biomarkers in drug labels	US Food and Drug Administration (FDA)	http://www.fda.gov/drugs/sciencere-search/researchareas/pharmacogenetics/ucm083378.htm	It lists FDA-approved drugs with pharmacogenomic information in their drug labels
Very important pharmacogenes	PharmGKB	http://www.pharmgkb.org/search/annotatedGene/	It provides annotated information about genes, variants, haplotypes, and splice variants of particular relevance for pharmacogenetics and pharmacogenomics
Clinical Pharmacogenetics Implementation Consortium (CPIC)	Pharmacogenomics Research Network	http://www.pharmgkb.org/page/cpic	Provides a list of the published guidelines for drug-genome interactions produced by CPIC

There are other databases containing broader genetic associations that may not be necessarily clinically relevant. One example of these is the National Human Genome Research Institutes Catalog of GWAS-associated SNPs at $p < 1 \times 10^{-5}$, which included 1467 publications and 8123 SNPs as of 12/21/12 [66]. Another example is the COSMIC database, which contains somatic mutations of cancers, but no evidence about clinical utility of these mutations [78]. Currently, most of such efforts are based on manual curation. Thus, automated or semi-automated approaches to identify clinically important variants, such as literature mining methods, would be highly desirable.

12.5.3 Genomic Data Collection, Storage, and Representation

An individual's genomic data such as "next generation" DNA sequencing could be at very large volume—hundreds of gigabytes to terabytes in their raw form, which exceeds the currently capacity of EHR systems in data storage, rapid availability, and transfer. As current knowledge about interpretation of sequence information as well as the clinical significance of molecular variants is constantly evolving, it is important to keep the raw genomic data for re-interpretation at a later date. However, common compression algorithms that are used for other high volume health care data such as digital images may not be appropriate for genomic data, as they reduce file size by removing single pixel level data. One approach to lossless data compression for genomic sequences is storage of the differences between an individual's genome sequence and a "Clinical Standard Reference Genome" [79]. The size of such differences in a roughly 3 billion nucleotide genome is estimated as 1–4 million, indicating a 100-fold reduction in data size.

Health care providers need to find relevant clinical data in the EHR in a timely fashion so that they can make decisions efficiently. A recent survey about genomic data in EHR systems showed that key stakeholders expected more structured and standardized documentation, organization, and display of genetic tests [80]. Therefore, creation of compact and user-friendly representations of molecular variations becomes an important practical question for integrating genomic data with EHRs. Informatics approaches to this problem have been implemented by St. Jude Children's Research Hospital [81] and Vanderbilt University [82]. One solution is to develop ontology-based approaches, such as the Clinical Bioinformatics Ontology (CBO), which can represent genetic test results by a compact code consisting of a few unique alphanumeric characters or a unique identifier in the vocabulary [83]. Software that can dynamically interpret and report genetic tests based on associated genomic knowledge bases is also being developed, such as the GeneInsight Suite [84]. There is also an established HL7 Clinical Genomics work group for creation of representation standards for genomic information [85].

12.5.4 Examples of Currently Available Genomic Decision Support

Historically, only a few uncommon medications were subject to genomic guidance. One example is thiopurines (e.g., azathioprine or mercaptopurine), which are given as immunosuppressants or chemotherapeutic agents, with thiopurine methyltransferase (TPMT) activity. Patients with reduced TPMT activity are at increased risk of potentially life-threatening bone marrow suppression with thiopurines [86]. About 10% of patients have intermediate gene activity, and 0.3% have extremely low or absent activity [87]; enzyme activity can also be predicted by genotype [86]. Thus, it is recommended by the FDA that providers check *TPMT* genotype before prescribing thiopurines [86]. In recent years, several institutions are deploying more widespread pharmacogenetic testing in clinical practice that can take advantage of cheaply available, multiplexed genotyping platforms to test for many genetic variants at the same time. In 2010, Vanderbilt began implementing the Pharmacogenomic Resource for Enhanced Decisions in Care and Treatment (PREDICT) [82]. The PREDICT program uses a multiplexed genotyping platform that contains 184 variants in 34 pharmacogenes to allow for multiple opportunities to provide genomic guidance now and in the future. The currently targeted medications are clopidogrel (the most commonly prescribed antiplatelet medication given following coronary stenting and myocardial infarctions), warfarin (the most commonly prescribed chronic anticoagulant), and simvastatin (one of the most commonly prescribed cholesterol lowering medications). Providers order genomic testing on patients as they are about to undergo cardiac catheterization (about 40% of which end up receiving clopidogrel), or based on a risk score calculation suggesting that the patient is at increased risk to receive one of three medications with pharmacogenetic guidance (clopidogrel, warfarin, or simvastatin). Genetic testing is performed within a Clinical Laboratory Improvement Amendment (CLIA) certified laboratory, and only results with high concordance and sufficient evidence are implemented into the EHR. Genotype results are placed within the EHR including both the actual genotype result (e.g., CYP2C19*2/*2) as well as a human-readable interpretation (e.g., "poor metabolizer, reduced antiplatelet effect"). CDS modules are provided for each of the implemented medications as well.

Genomic-based CDS are underway across other institutions as well. St. Jude Children's Research Hospital also uses a multiplexed genotyping platform to provide decision support for a number of medications [81]. They have modified their EHR to make genotype results quickly accessible and provide CDS for target medications as well. The Mayo clinic has studied the use of genotyping to assist in the use of anti-depressant medications, though this has focused on specific medications and genes instead of a broader, multiplexed approach [88]. The Scripps Institute has also implemented focused genotyping to guide clopidogrel therapy (personal communication).

12.6 SUMMARY

In this chapter, we summarized the role of EHR data in genetic discovery and implementation of genomic medicine, and the informatics methods that can be applied to translate EHR data into reliable phenotypic knowledge. Typically genomic and pharmacogenomic research has been performed with observational cohorts or clinical trials; use of EHR data for genetic studies is indeed a recent phenomena, as the first EHR-biobank genetic studies were performed in 2010 [18,34,89,90]. However, a growing body of evidence has supported the use of EHRs for genomic and pharmacogenomic research, as detailed herein. Use of EHR data for clinical and genomic research requires careful attention to informatics algorithms to achieve sufficient precision in case and control development. In some cases, EHR data may actually be superior to traditional research cohorts in that it allows an "unbiased" analysis of a wide variety of phenotypes in ways not possible with purposefully collected phenotypic information. Finally, EHRs are a necessary component for the realization of the vision of genomic medicine. The ever-increasing complexity of genomic medicine will rapidly exceed the capacity of physicians to stay abreast of and correctly implement at the point of care without seamless computerized decision support systems to manage large datasets of variants and adapt to rapidly changing guidelines.

12.7 SELECTED WEBSITES OF INTEREST

- NHGRI GWAS Catalog:
  http://www.genome.gov/gwastudies/
- Clinical Pharmacogenetics Implementation Consortium Guidelines:
  http://www.pharmgkb.org/page/cpic
- cTAKES (Clinical Text Analysis and Knowledge Extraction System):
  https://wiki.nci.nih.gov/pages/viewpage.action?pageId=65733244
- MetaMap:
  http://metamap.nlm.nih.gov

- Unified Medical Language System:
  http://www.nlm.nih.gov/research/umls/
- AHRQ's Clinical Classifications Software:
  http://www.hcup-us.ahrq.gov/toolssoftware/ccs/ccs.jsp
- PheWAS ICD9 code groupings and software:
  http://knowledgemap.mc.vanderbilt.edu/research/content/phewas
- Phenotype Knowledgebase (PheKB):
  http://phekb.org
- Electronic Medical Records and Genomics (eMERGE) Network:
  http://gwas.org
- Online Registry of Biomedical Informatics Tools (ORBIT) Project:
  http://orbit.nlm.nih.gov

REFERENCES

[1] Blumenthal D, Tavenner M. The 'Meaningful use' regulation for electronic health records. N Eng J Med 2010;363:501–4.

[2] Shojania KG, et al. The effects of on-screen point of care computer reminders on processes and outcomes of care. Cochrane Database Syst Rev CD001096 2009. http://dx.doi.org/10.1002/14651858.CD001096.pub2.

[3] Kuperman GJ et al. Medication-related clinical decision support in computerized provider order entry systems: a review. J Am Med Inform Assoc 2007;14:29–40.

[4] Kazley AS, Ozcan YA. Do hospitals with electronic medical records (EMRs) provide higher quality care?: an examination of three clinical conditions. Med Care Res Rev 2008;65:496–513.

[5] Kaushal R et al. Return on investment for a computerized physician order entry system. J Am Med Inform Assoc 2006;13:261–6.

[6] Murphy SN et al. Serving the enterprise and beyond with informatics for integrating biology and the bedside (i2b2). J Am Med Inform Assoc 2010;17:124–30.

[7] Hurdle JF et al. Identifying clinical/translational research cohorts: ascertainment via querying an integrated multi-source database. J Am Med Inform Assoc 2013;20:164–71.

[8] McCarty CA, Wilke RA, Giampietro PF, Wesbrook SD, Caldwell MD. Marshfield Clinic Personalized Medicine Research Project (PMRP): design, methods and recruitment for a large population-based biobank. Personalized Med 2005;2:49–79.

[9] Roden DM et al. Development of a large-scale de-identified DNA biobank to enable personalized medicine. Clin Pharmacol Ther 2008;84:362–9.

[10] i2b2: Informatics for Integrating Biology & the Bedside. <https://www.i2b2.org/work/i2b2_installations.html>.

[11] Harris PA et al. Research electronic data capture (RED Cap)—a metadata-driven methodology and workflow process for providing translational research informatics support. J Biomed Inform 2009;42:377–81.

[12] Kaiser Permanente, UCSF Scientists Complete NIH-Funded Genomics Project Involving 100,000 People. <http://www.dor.kaiser.org/external/news/press_releases/Kaiser_Permanente,_UCSF_Scientists_Complete_NIH-Funded_Genomics_Project_Involving_100,000_People/>.

[13] McCarty CA et al. The eMERGE Network: a consortium of biorepositories linked to electronic medical records data for conducting genomic studies. BMC Med Genomics 2011;4:13.

[14] Million Veteran Program (MVP). <http://www.research.va.gov/mvp/>.

[15] McCarty CA, Nair A, Austin DM, Giampietro PF. Informed consent and subject motivation to participate in a large, population-based genomics study: the Marshfield Clinic Personalized Medicine Research Project. Community Genet 2007;10:2–9.

[16] NUgene Project. <https://www.nugene.org/>.

[17] Pathak J et al. Mapping clinical phenotype data elements to standardized metadata repositories and controlled terminologies: the eMERGE Network experience. J Am Med Inform Assoc 2011;18:376–86.

[18] Ritchie MD et al. Robust replication of genotype-phenotype associations across multiple diseases in an electronic medical record. Am. J. Hum. Genet 2010;86:560–72.

[19] Liao KP et al. Electronic medical records for discovery research in rheumatoid arthritis. Arthritis Care Res (Hoboken) 2010;62:1120–7.

[20] Sohn M-W et al. Transition to the new race/ethnicity data collection standards in the Department of Veterans Affairs. Popul Health Metr 2006;4:7.

[21] Dumitrescu L et al. Assessing the accuracy of observer-reported ancestry in a biorepository linked to electronic medical records. Genet Med 2010;12:648–50.

[22] Pritchard JK, Stephens M, Donnelly P. Inference of population structure using multilocus genotype data. Genetics 2000;155:945–59.

[23] Price AL et al. Principal components analysis corrects for stratification in genome-wide association studies. Nat Genet 2006;38:904–9.

[24] Herzig SJ, Howell MD, Ngo LH, Marcantonio ER. Acid-suppressive medication use and the risk for hospital-acquired pneumonia. Jama 2009;301:2120–8.

[25] Klompas M et al. Automated identification of acute hepatitis B using electronic medical record data to facilitate public health surveillance. PLoS ONE 2008;3:e2626.

[26] Kiyota Y et al. Accuracy of Medicare claims-based diagnosis of acute myocardial infarction: estimating positive predictive value on the basis of review of hospital records. Am Heart J 2004;148:99–104.

[27] Dean BB et al. Use of electronic medical records for health outcomes research: a literature review. Med Care Res Rev 2009. <http://www.ncbi.nlm.nih.gov/entrez/query.fcgi?cmd=Retrieve&db=PubMed&dopt=Citation&list_uids=19279318>

[28] Elixhauser A, Steiner C, Harris DR, Coffey RM. Comorbidity measures for use with administrative data. Med Care 1998;36:8–27.

[29] Charlson ME, Pompei P, Ales KL, MacKenzie CR. A new method of classifying prognostic comorbidity in longitudinal studies: development and validation. J Chronic Diseases 1987;40:373–83.

[30] Li L, Chase HS, Patel CO, Friedman C, Weng C. Comparing ICD9-encoded diagnoses and NLP-processed discharge summaries for clinical trials pre-screening: a case study. In: Annual symposium proceedings/AMIA symposium; 2008. p. 404–8.

[31] Elkin PL et al. A randomized controlled trial of the accuracy of clinical record retrieval using SNOMED-RT as compared with ICD9-CM. Proceedings/annual symposium; 2001. p. 159–63.

[32] Conway M et al. Analyzing the heterogeneity and complexity of electronic health record oriented phenotyping algorithms. In: AMIA annual symposium proceedings; 2011. p. 274–83.

[33] Cowen ME et al. Casemix adjustment of managed care claims data using the clinical classification for health policy research method. Med Care 1998;36:1108–13.

[34] Denny JC et al. PheWAS: demonstrating the feasibility of a phenome-wide scan to discover gene-disease associations. Bioinformatics 2010;26:1205–10.

[35] Denny JC et al. Variants near FOXE1 are associated with hypothyroidism and other thyroid conditions: using electronic medical records for genome- and phenome-wide studies. Am J Hum Genet 2011;89:529–42.

[36] Denny JC et al. Extracting timing and status descriptors for colonoscopy testing from electronic medical records. J Am Med Inform Assoc 2010;17:383–8.

[37] Huff SM et al. Development of the logical observation identifier names and codes (LOINC) vocabulary. J Am Med Inform Assoc 1998;5:276–92.

[38] Logical Observation Identifiers Names and Codes. 2007. <http://www.regenstrief. org/medinformatics/loinc/>.

[39] Poon EG et al. Effect of bar-code technology on the safety of medication administration. N Engl J Med 2010;362:1698–707.

[40] Rosenbloom ST et al. Generating clinical notes for electronic health record systems. Appl Clin Inform 2010;1:232–43.

[41] Rosenbloom ST et al. Data from clinical notes: a perspective on the tension between structure and flexible documentation. J Am Med Inform Assoc 2011;18:181–6.

[42] Denny JC et al. Identifying UMLS concepts from ECG Impressions using KnowledgeMap. AMIA Annu Symp Proc 2005:196–200.

[43] Birman-Deych E et al. Accuracy of ICD-9-CM codes for identifying cardiovascular and stroke risk factors. Med Care 2005;43:480–5.

[44] Kern EFO et al. Failure of ICD-9-CM codes to identify patients with comorbid chronic kidney disease in diabetes. Health Serv Res 2006;41:564–80.

[45] Schmiedeskamp M, Harpe S, Polk R, Oinonen M, Pakyz A. Use of international classification of diseases, ninth revision, clinical modification codes and medication use data to identify nosocomial *Clostridium difficile* infection. Infect Control Hosp Epidemiol 2009;30:1070–6.

[46] Penz JFE, Wilcox AB, Hurdle JF. Automated identification of adverse events related to central venous catheters. J Biomed Inform 2007;40:174–82.

[47] Fan JW, Friedman C. Semantic classification of biomedical concepts using distributional similarity. J Am Med Inform Assoc 2007;14:467–77.

[48] Savova GK et al. Mayo clinical Text Analysis and Knowledge Extraction System (cTAKES): architecture, component evaluation and applications. J Am Med Inform Assoc 2010;17:507–13.

[49] Aronson AR. Effective mapping of biomedical text to the UMLS Metathesaurus: the MetaMap program. Proc AMIA Symp 2001:17–21.

[50] Denny JC, Smithers JD, Miller RA, Spickard A. 'Understanding' medical school curriculum content using KnowledgeMap. J Am Med Inform Assoc 2003;10:351–62.

[51] Uzuner Ö, Solti I, Cadag E. Extracting medication information from clinical text. J Am Med Inform Assoc 2010;17:514–8.

[52] Garvin JH et al. Automated extraction of ejection fraction for quality measurement using regular expressions in Unstructured Information Management Architecture (UIMA) for heart failure. J Am Med Inform Assoc 2012;19:859–66.

[53] Xu H, Anderson K, Grann VR, Friedman C. Facilitating cancer research using natural language processing of pathology reports. Medinfo 2004;11:565–72.

[54] Xu H et al. Facilitating pharmacogenetic studies using electronic health records and natural-language processing: a case study of warfarin. J Am Med Inform Assoc 2011;18:387–91.

[55] Humphreys BL, Lindberg DA, Schoolman HM, Barnett GO. The Unified Medical Language System: an informatics research collaboration. J Am Med Inform Assoc 1998;5:1–11.

[56] Coyle JF, Mori AR, Huff SM. Standards for detailed clinical models as the basis for medical data exchange and decision support. Int J Med Inform 2003;69:157–74.

[57] Huff SM, Rocha RA, Bray BE, Warner HR, Haug PJ. An event model of medical information representation. J Am Med Inform Assoc 1995;2:116–34.

[58] Rea S et al. Building a robust, scalable and standards-driven infrastructure for secondary use of EHR data: The SHARPn project. J Biomed Inform 2012;45:763–71.

[59] Kho AN et al. Use of diverse electronic medical record systems to identify genetic risk for type 2 diabetes within a genome-wide association study. J Am Med Inform Assoc 2012;19:212–8.

[60] Love TJ, Cai T, Karlson EW. Validation of psoriatic arthritis diagnoses in electronic medical records using natural language processing. Semin Arthritis Rheum 2011;40:413–20.

[61] Carroll RJ, Eyler AE, Denny JC. Naïve electronic health record phenotype identification for rheumatoid arthritis. In: AMIA annual symposium proceedings; 2011. p. 189–96.

[62] Carroll RJ et al. Portability of an algorithm to identify rheumatoid arthritis in electronic health records. J Am Med Inform Assoc: JAMIA 2012;19:e162–9.

[63] Peissig PL et al. Importance of multi-modal approaches to effectively identify cataract cases from electronic health records. J Am Med Inform Assoc 2012;19:225–34.

[64] Kho AN et al. Electronic Medical Records for Genetic Research: results of the eMERGE consortium. Sci Transl Med 2011;3:79re1.

[65] Hripcsak G, Rothschild AS. Agreement, the f-measure, and reliability in information retrieval. J Am Med Inform Assoc 2005;12:296–8.

[66] Hindorff LA et al. Potential etiologic and functional implications of genome-wide association loci for human diseases and traits. Proc Natl Acad Sci USA 2009;106:9362–7.

[67] Eriksson N et al. Novel associations for hypothyroidism include known autoimmune risk loci. PLoS ONE 2012;7:e34442.

[68] Roden DM, Xu H, Denny JC, Wilke RA. Electronic medical records as a tool in clinical pharmacology: opportunities and challenges. Clin Pharmacol Ther 2012;91:1083–6.

[69] Delaney JT et al. Predicting clopidogrel response using DNA samples linked to an electronic health record. Clin Pharmacol Ther 2012;91:257–63.

[70] Ramirez AH et al. Predicting warfarin dosage in European-Americans and African-Americans using DNA samples linked to an electronic health record. Pharmacogenomics 2012;13:407–18.

[71] Birdwell KA et al. The use of a DNA biobank linked to electronic medical records to characterize pharmacogenomic predictors of tacrolimus dose requirement in kidney transplant recipients. Pharmacogenet Genomics 2012;22:32–42.

[72] Xu H et al. MedEx: a medication information extraction system for clinical narratives. J Am Med Inform Assoc 2010;17:19–24.

[73] Pendergrass SA et al. The use of phenome-wide association studies (PheWAS) for exploration of novel genotype-phenotype relationships and pleiotropy discovery. Genet Epidemiol 2011;35:410–22.

[74] Denny JC et al. Scanning the EMR phenome for gene-disease associations using natural language processing. In: Proceedings AMIA annual fall symposium; 2010.

[75] Ammenwerth E, Schnell-Inderst P, Machan C, Siebert U. The effect of electronic prescribing on medication errors and adverse drug events: a systematic review. J Am Med Inform Assoc 2008;15:585–600.

[76] Mega JL et al. Reduced-function CYP2C19 genotype and risk of adverse clinical outcomes among patients treated with clopidogrel predominantly for PCI: a meta-analysis. JAMA 2010;304:1821–30.

[77] Link E et al. SLCO1B1 variants and statin-induced myopathy–a genomewide study. N Eng J Med 2008;359:789–99.

[78] Forbes SA et al. The Catalogue of Somatic Mutations in Cancer (COSMIC), Curr Protoc Hum Genet, Unit 10.11, 2008 [chapter 10].

[79] Masys DR et al. Technical desiderata for the integration of genomic data into Electronic Health Records. J Biomed Inform 2012;45:419–22.

[80] Scheuner MT et al. Are electronic health records ready for genomic medicine? Genet Med 2009;11:510–7.

[81] Hicks JK et al. A clinician-driven automated system for integration of pharmaco-genetic interpretations into an electronic medical record. Clini Pharmacol Ther 2012;92:563–6.

[82] Pulley JM et al. Operational implementation of prospective genotyping for personal-ized medicine: the design of the Vanderbilt PREDICT project. Clin Pharmacol Ther 2012. <http://dx.doi.org/10.1038/clpt.2011.371>

[83] Deshmukh VG, Hoffman MA, Arnoldi C, Bray BE, Mitchell JA. Efficiency of CYP2C9 genetic test representation for automated pharmacogenetic decision sup-port. Methods Inf Med 2009;48:282–90.

[84] Aronson SJ et al. The GeneInsight suite: a platform to support laboratory and pro-vider use of DNA-based genetic testing. Hum Mutat 2011;32:532–6.

[85] Clinical Genomics. <http://www.hl7.org/special/Committees/clingenomics/>.

[86] Relling MV et al. Clinical Pharmacogenetics Implementation Consortium guidelines for thiopurine methyltransferase genotype and thiopurine dosing. Clin Pharmacol Ther 2011;89:387–91.

[87] McLeod HL, Lin JS, Scott EP, Pui CH, Evans WE. Thiopurine methyltransfer-ase activity in American white subjects and black subjects. Clin Pharmacol Ther 1994;55:15–20.

[88] Rundell JR, Harmandayan M, Staab JP. Pharmacogenomic testing and outcome among depressed patients in a tertiary care outpatient psychiatric consultation prac-tice. Transl Psychiatry 2011;1:e6.

[89] Kullo IJ, Ding K, Jouni H, Smith CY, Chute CG. A genome-wide association study of red blood cell traits using the electronic medical record. PLoS ONE 2010;5.

[90] Denny JC et al. Identification of genomic predictors of atrioventricular conduc-tion: using electronic medical records as a tool for genome science. Circulation 2010;122:2016–21.

FURTHER READING

[1] Shortliffe EH, Cimino JJ, editors. Biomedical informatics: computer applications in health care and biomedicine. 3rd ed. Springer; 2006. p. 1064.

Chapters of particular relevance: Chapter 2 ("Biomedical data: their acquisition, storage, and use"), Chapter 8 ("Natural language and text processing in biomedicine"), Chapter 12 ("Electronic health record systems")

[2] Hristidis V, editors. Information discovery on electronic health records. 1st ed. Chapman and Hall/CRC; 2009. p. 331.

Chapters of particular relevance: Chapter 2 ("Electronic health records"), Chapter 4 ("Data quality and integration issues in electronic health records"), 7 ("Data mining and knowledge discovery on EHRs").

[3] Wilke RA, Xu H, Denny JC, Roden DM, Krauss RM, et al. The emerging role of electronic medical records in pharmacogenomics. Clin Pharmacol Ther 2011;89:379–86.

[4] Roden DM, Xu H, Denny JC, Wilke RA. Electronic medical records as a tool in clinical pharmacology: opportunities and challenges. Clin Pharmacol Ther 2012. <http://www.ncbi.nlm.nih.gov/pubmed/22534870>. Accessed 30 June 2012.

[5] Kohane IS. Using electronic health records to drive discovery in disease genomics. Nat Rev Genet 2011;12:417–28.

[6] Denny JC. Chapter 13: mining electronic health records in the genomics era. PLoS Comput Biol 2012;8(12):e1002823.

Putting Theory into Practice

Indra Neil Sarkar

Center for Clinical and Translational Science, University of Vermont, Burlington, VT, USA

13.1 ENTERING THE ERA OF BIG DATA

This book has introduced a sampling of biomedical informatics methodologies that span the entire continuum of biomedicine. As suggested in Chapter 1, a unifying theme throughout the description of each methodology is the underlying concept of transforming biomedical data into biomedical wisdom (as can be conceptualized through the DIKW framework). The concept of transforming data into knowledge is, of course, not new. From the earliest days of recorded civilization, the ability to gather, catalog, interpret, and share knowledge based on available data has been an essential element of progress. The ability to develop tools to help with data transformation has similarly been seen as an essential step toward progress in the sciences. Indeed, the modern computer traces its lineage to Charles Babbage, who was driven (along with John Herschel) to develop the concept of a machine (the "difference engine") to facilitate the calculation of error-free tables from astronomy data for use as nautical almanacs [1,2]. The theoretical need for machine-based analytics to analyze greater amounts of data to solve additional problems later led Babbage to conceive of the notion of an "analytic machine" (and abandon the original idea of the difference engine) [2,3]. While Babbage never actually was able to develop a functional machine for performing the desired calculations, he laid the framework for modern computing and enshrined its role in the transformation of data into wisdom.

The many advances in computing since Babbage's early concept have affected the ability to transform data from a wider spectrum of sources than was probably every truly contemplated. There are very few activities in modern times that do not involve some computation to gather relevant data and make them useful for a range of purposes. In biomedicine, data are gathered to enable a better understanding of disease processes, diagnosis, prognosis, progress, and overall societal impact. At the molecular level, one can contemplate the sequencing of an entire individual's genome (for thousands of US dollars, with the promise of a sub-US$1000 complete genome within a decade of this writing [4,5]) or set of genomic markers (at the cost of a few hundred US dollars, or just less than US$100 from direct-to-consumer organizations like 23andMe [6]). At the clinical level, the increased adoption of electronic health record systems supports the ability of clinicians [7] (and patients, via personal health record systems that interface with electronic health record systems [8]) to electronically catalog the full complement of clinical data. Finally, at the population level, electronic systems are enabling the gathering of general population health indicator [9], healthcare outcome [10,11], as well as health utilization and cost data [12]. The avalanche of data being gathered across the spectrum of biomedicine has resulted in the need for an unprecedented amount of computational analysis to enable their transformation into wisdom. To this end, the theoretical application of biomedical informatics methodologies, such as those presented in this book, is directly challenged by the practicality of their application in real-world scenarios.

The general term that has recently been used to refer to data in computationally challenging contexts is "Big Data." Big Data is defined according to four criteria [13,14]: (1) *Volume*—the raw amount of bytes that data need to be considered relative to the computational time available; (2) *Velocity*—the rate at which data are generated and the possibility to be processed with the available computational power to produce meaningful interpretations that are actionable; (3) *Variety*—the inherent complexity of data types that need to be considered within the context of a defined hypothesis; and (4) *Veracity*—the ability to have trust in the data from which interpretations may be made in support of a given hypothesis. The emergence of Big Data as a formal concept reflects a data paradox: the ability to generate data at higher rates continues to increase with advances in computing and related technologies, while the ability to interpret these data is of increasing difficulty due to at least one of the four aforementioned Big Data criteria. The rate of data increase is often compared to Moore's Law, which states that available computing power doubles every 18 months [15]. For Big Data, it is often the case that the ability to generate data far outstrips the rate at which advances are made in computing power [14]. Simply put, the available computing power is an increasingly limiting step when considering any of the Big Data four criteria: the available computing power cannot accommodate the volume, velocity, variety, and veracity of the data that need to be processed.

In the context of biomedicine, designing approaches that can leverage the appropriate data at the appropriate time to enable appropriate care or appropriate understanding of care regimens has always been of paramount importance. However, when considering Big Data and its impact or utility for biomedicine, the issues encapsulated by the four aforementioned criteria further underscore the importance of the application and development of methodological approaches for managing and using data that can lead to actionable knowledge or wisdom [16]. The sheer volume of data, taken in combination with the velocity of their availability and the variety of sources they may originate, make it almost humanly impossible to have full confidence (veracity) in any interpretations that may affect patient care. Thus it is essential for the modern healthcare professional to understand and appreciate both the advantages and challenges of Big Data [16,17].

Equally important is the appreciation of traditional approaches to data interpretation that have been ingrained into healthcare (e.g., the ability to discern whether a patient is having a clinically urgent myocardial infarction or is experiencing a less clinically urgent panic attack). It is important to again emphasize the Scientific Method and the hypothetico-deductive approach that is often used in clinical diagnosis. Instead of being overwhelmed by the many possible data points, the clinician must first make a statement of hypothesis (e.g., "the patient is experiencing a myocardial infarction") along with a prediction (e.g., "the patient will have an abnormal electrocardiogram"), followed by a series of validating/refuting tests (e.g., "perform an electrocardiogram"), and then evaluation and possible reformulation of hypothesis based on the analysis of the tests (e.g., "the results indicate an abnormal electrocardiogram with an elevated ST, therefore there is strong evidence that the patient is experiencing a myocardial infarction"). Big Data challenges the practicality of the hypothetico-deductive approach, especially when attempting to make decisions that can be of life or death for a patient in an emergent clinical situation, where every second or minute contributes to the ultimate outcome (e.g., to process all the possible data points that are available in time to make the diagnosis of a myocardial infarction may take too long and lead to the ultimate same conclusion that could have been made days, hours, or even minutes earlier). This is not to suggest that the hypothetico-deductive approach is no longer relevant or not possible in a Big Data environment. Big Data may very well offer revolutionary biomedical insights; however, there is a need for approaches to leverage the data born from Big Data to be clinically usable and ultimately actionable in a timely manner.

The scientific grounding of biomedical informatics and its transdisciplinary approach uniquely position the field to leverage Big Data from a multitude of sources across the entire spectrum of biomedicine for the betterment of human health. Within the context of biomedicine, the four criteria for Big Data need to be approached pragmatically. For example, in the context of Big Data, biomedical informatics methods focus on: (1) Identifying those data from a voluminous data stream that are most biomedically or clinically relevant; (2) Processing rapidly available data so as to identify the highest amount of biomedically or clinically relevant data in a manner that is actionable; (3) Distinguishing data gathered from multiple sources in a manner to identify the most plausible patterns; and (4) Providing adequate interpretation and transparency about the data interpretation that allow for a human to make the most informed decision. In the application of existing and new methodologies, the focus of biomedical informatics methods on Big Data further underscores the importance of the field's grounding in the Scientific Method. That is, methodologies are not developed for the sake of developing some interpretation of the data (a classic problem with many solutions that are canonically referred to as "hammers looking for nails"). Methodologies developed in biomedical informatics must serve the purpose to improve the understanding, diagnosis, and treatment of health conditions.

The juxtaposition of the DIKW framework and the Scientific Method aligned with the formal, basic, and applied sciences introduced in Chapter 1 (and graphically depicted in Figure 1.2) is ever more relevant in biomedical contexts. Building on the DIKW framework, the successful application of biomedical informatics approaches to Big Data will lead to Big Information, Big Knowledge, and Big Wisdom. Transforming Big Data into Big Information, Big Knowledge, and Big Wisdom follows the same general principles of transforming data into information, knowledge, and wisdom as introduced in Chapter 1. The framework that incorporates the DIKW principles in a "Big" context ("BigDIKW") needs to consider the aforementioned challenges with volume, velocity, variety, and veracity. As one approaches Big Wisdom in a biomedical scenario, one must consider the ability to record the ascertained knowledge into a form that can be leveraged in a manner to accommodate subsequent availability of Big Data.

The realization of Big Wisdom promises to establish a foundation for unprecedented advances in biomedicine. However, the necessary advances in infrastructure to allow for the BigDIKW framework to be of clinical utility remain unknown. The scientific community is mostly focused now on identifying the needed advances in formal sciences to make use of Big Data. One of the outcomes of this focus has been the emergence of "Data Science" that combines and augments the formal sciences to address Big

Data challenges [13]. Within a biomedical context, the grounding in the Scientific Method is paramount: What possible hypotheses might be supported or refuted by the available data? As was alluded to in Chapter 1, a possible pitfall of the sole focus on data analysis will result in an exclusive reliance on the Baconian Method toward addressing a scientific question. However, given the challenges to be considered in a Big Data context, it is highly possible that aiming to arrive at solutions in only an empirical manner may result in one only addressing the challenges of volume, velocity, and variety before ever beginning to address the veracity of the data and ultimately the utility or actionability of any interpretations.

13.2 PROSPECTIVE APPLICABILITY OF BIOMEDICAL INFORMATICS METHODOLOGIES

Does the emergence of the BigDIKW framework in place of the traditional DIKW framework immediately make the methods described in this book obsolete? No. In fact, it underscores the fundamental tenet of biomedical informatics that methodologies applied in one domain may very well be applied to another domain. The biomedical informatics methodologies introduced in this book, therefore, are ever more applicable in a BigDIKW framework. The volume, velocity, variety, and veracity of data do not imply that changes are required in any of the topics discussed in the preceding chapters. However, the challenges that are to be faced by contemporary biomedical researchers now and in the future will further require grounding in the Scientific Method. In addition to hypothesis testing, which has been described as the core of the biomedical data to wisdom transformation process, the BigDIKW framework provides additional support for the *generation* of hypotheses. In this sense, the Baconian Method and the Scientific Method can be viewed no longer as competing approaches to science. The Baconian Method provides a systematic process (called *reductionism* [18]) for reducing Big Data into tractable units of Big Information, Big Knowledge, and Big Wisdom that can be used as the substrate for further investigation. The reduction of Big Data to Big Knowledge forms the basis of "Actionable Knowledge," which are units of knowledge that one might be able to arrive at testable hypotheses that are used as the starting point for the Scientific Method and the corresponding DIKW framework.

Implicitly, we have relied on human intuition and curiosity for Big Data to Big Knowledge reduction (and embossed as Big Wisdom for anchoring future experiences with similar Big Data)—if a patient walks into the emergency department complaining about chest pain, clinicians immediately reduce the space of all possible diagnostic hypotheses to those that are just associated with the chest and subsequently test the short list of possible

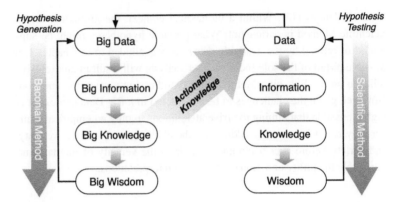

■ FIGURE 13.1 Overall Framework of BigDIKW and DIKW. The interrelationship of the BigDIKW (Big Data, Big Information, Big Knowledge, Big Wisdom) and DIKW (Data, Information, Knowledge, Wisdom) frameworks enables both the process of hypothesis generation (using the Baconian Method) and hypothesis testing (using the Scientific Method). Actionable knowledge, an artifact of reducing Big Data to Big Wisdom in the BigDIKW framework, forms the basis for new hypotheses that may be tested within the DIKW framework.

hypotheses instead of the universe of all possible hypotheses (e.g., clinicians would not test hypotheses related to a broken leg in this scenario). The technological advances that are associated with Big Data have necessitated the concerted effort of the scientific community to develop approaches for utilizing Big Data. In addition to Data Science, which aims to provide new formal science methods, the complement of existing biomedical informatics methods are highly relevant in reductionism of Big Data to Big Wisdom. As shown in Figure 13.1, the BigDIKW and DIKW frameworks can be viewed as an overall framework to develop synergy between the Baconian Method of reductionism (for *hypothesis generation*) and the Scientific Method (for *hypothesis testing*) described in Chapter 1.

13.3 A FINAL CHALLENGE TO THE READER

The methodologies described in each of the chapters of this book therefore offer techniques that are essential for both hypothesis generation and hypothesis testing. The contexts and scenarios described by the authors of the respective chapters focus mostly on the DIKW framework (i.e., to support or refute a hypothesis that may have been generated from available data), but they can just as easily be applied in a BigDIKW framework (i.e., to generate plausible hypotheses from Big Data that might be later be supported or refuted). The history of biomedical informatics is strongly aligned with the clinical need to support patient care (especially in the context of health informatics); however, the partnership with basic research is an essential aspect of the field that enables the appropriate leveraging of available data to support an understanding of the underpinning phenomena associated with health states. For each clinical decision that can be supported by biomedical informatics techniques that have been described in this book, it would be equally important to consider the applicability of the same techniques for filtering through the realm of possibly hypotheses. A useful exercise might thus be to reexamine each chapter in this book and consider how the described methodologies can be used for both hypothesis generation and hypothesis testing.

A final consideration that must be emphasized is the clinical utility of a given biomedical informatics methodology. For each of the methodologies described in this book, consider how practical the application of a given approach would be in a given clinical scenario. One of the most significant challenges in biomedical informatics is the design and development of approaches that are not only able to provide knowledge or wisdom, but also in an appropriate manner. For example, if developing a system to diagnose a myocardial infarction, it would be of limited utility to use a sophisticated but 100% accurate methodology that took two weeks to generate a result. On the other hand, if doing a post hoc analysis of available clinical data to identify potentially interesting patterns associated with patients who have been diagnosed with myocardial infarctions, then two weeks might not be considered unacceptable. The challenge put forth to the biomedical community by the BigDIKW framework is the ability to leverage available data in an appropriate manner while not compromising patient care; more data is not necessarily better in all contexts. Advances in biomedical informatics methodologies will be required to enhance the current suite of approaches and techniques (such as described in this book) with the latest in formal, basic, and applied science approaches. The reader is therefore challenged to identify at least one aspect of a given biomedical informatics methodology described in the previous chapters that might be enhanced with a formal, basic, or applied science method. By addressing this concluding challenge, biomedical informatics methodologies will continue to advance to better meet the challenges faces in the ever-expanding, complicated, and complex biomedicine ecosystem.

REFERENCES

[1] Campbell-Kelly M, Aspray W. 2nd. ed. In: Computer: a history of the information machine Boulder, Colorado: Westview Press; 2004. 325 pp.
[2] Snyder LJ. The philosophical breakfast club: four remarkable friends who transformed science and changed the world. 1st ed. New York: Broadway Books; 2011. 439 pp.

[3] Collier B, MacLachlan JH. Charles Babbage and the engines of perfection. New York: Oxford University Press; 1998. 123 pp.

[4] Mardis ER. Anticipating the 1,000 dollar genome. Genome biol 2006;7(7):112.

[5] Service RF. Gene sequencing. The race for the $1000 genome. Science 2006;311 (5767):1544–6.

[6] 23andMe; July 10, 2013. Available from: <https://http://www.23andme.com/>.

[7] Patel V, Jamoom E, Hsiao CJ, Furukawa MF, Buntin M. Variation in electronic health record adoption and readiness for meaningful use: 2008–2011. J Gen Intern Med 2013;28(7):957–64.

[8] Caligtan CA, Dykes PC. Electronic health records and personal health records. Semin Oncol Nurs 2011;27(3):218–28.

[9] Health Indicators Warehouse. July 10, 2013. Available from: <http://healthindicators.gov/>.

[10] Surveillance Epidemiology and End Results. July 10, 2013. Available from: <http://seer.cancer.gov/>.

[11] Patient Reported Outcomes Measurement Information System. July 10, 2013. Available from: <http://www.nihpromis.org/>.

[12] Healthcare Cost and Utilization Project. July 10, 2013. Available from: <http://www.hcup-us.ahrq.gov/>.

[13] Zikopoulos P. In: Understanding big data: analytics for enterprise class Hadoop and streaming data. New York: McGraw-Hill; 2012. 141 pp.

[14] Franks B. Taming the big data tidal wave: finding opportunities in huge data streams with advanced analytics. Hoboken, New Jersey: John Wiley and Sons; 2012. 304 pp.

[15] Moore GE. Cramming more components onto integrated circuits. Electron Mag 1965;38(8):4–7.

[16] Murdoch TB, Detsky AS. The inevitable application of big data to health care. JAMA: J Am Med Assoc 2013;309(13):1351–2.

[17] Larson EB. Building trust in the power of "big data" research to serve the public good. JAMA: J Am Med Assoc 2013;309(23):2443–4.

[18] Bacon F, Jardine L, Silverthorne M. In: The new organon. Cambridge UK, New York: Cambridge University Press; 2000. 252 pp.

Unix Primer

Elizabeth S. Chen

Center for Clinical and Translational Science, University of Vermont, Burlington, VT, USA
Department of Medicine, Division of General Internal Medicine, University of Vermont, Burlington, VT, USA
Department of Computer Science, University of Vermont, Burlington, VT, USA

Given the prevalence of Unix-based software used in biomedical informatics, there is significant value in gaining basic Unix knowledge and skills. The history of UNIX® dates back to 1969, when it was created by Dennis Ritchie and Ken Thompson at Bell Laboratories. The UNIX® operating system is characterized as being multi-tasking, multi-user, and text command based. Over the last few decades, numerous Unix variants or Unix-like systems have emerged (e.g., Linux, Solaris, AIX, and OS X). On Windows, Cygwin is a program that provides a Unix-like environment.

This primer serves as a brief introduction to working in the Unix environment and a set of commonly used commands for getting started. It is assumed that the reader has access to a Unix environment, either locally or by logging into a remote Unix server using an SSH (Secure Shell) client.

A.1 UNIX FILE SYSTEM

The Unix file system organizes files and directories into a hierarchical structure like an upside-down tree. The top of this hierarchy is called the *root directory*, which is represented as "/". Within the root directory, there are a number of standard directories such as /bin and /usr/bin that contain commands needed by system administrators and users, /etc that contains system-wide configuration files and system databases, and /home that contains the *home directory* for each user represented as "~" (in some systems, the location of home directories may be in a different location such as /users). For example, the home directories for the three users shown in Figure A.1 are /home/user1, /home/user2, and /home/user3.

As users traverse directories, the directory that they are currently in is referred to as the *working directory* (represented as ".") and the directory above this is the *parent directory* (represented as ".."). A *path* or *pathname* specifies where a user is in the file system. The *full path* or *absolute path* points to the same location regardless of the working directory (i.e., it is written in reference to the root directory). The *relative path* is the path relative to the working directory. For example, if the working directory is the home directory for user2, the full path for the scripts directory is /home/user2/scripts while the relative path is just scripts. If scripts

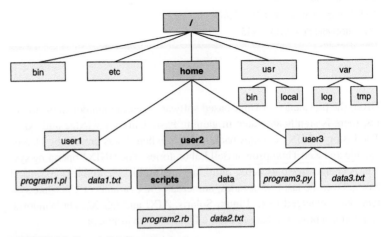

■ FIGURE A.1 Example Unix file system structure.

then becomes the working directory, the full path for the data directory from there is /home/user2/data while the relative path is ../data.

A.2 **UNIX SHELL**

The Unix shell provides a command-line interface for interacting with the operating system and is where commands are entered. Depending on your shell (e.g., Bourne shell [sh], C shell [csh], or Bourne-Again shell [bash]) and configuration, the ***shell prompt*** or ***command-line prompt*** may look different. Default prompts include: "$", "%", and "#" (this latter prompt typically appears when logged in as the *superuser* or *root user* who can do anything on the system, so should be restricted to trusted users, used only when necessary and with caution). The shell prompt can be configured to include additional information such as hostname, username, and pathname followed by "$" (e.g., hostname:/home/user2/scripts user2 $).

A.3 **UNIX COMMAND SYNTAX**

There are many Unix commands. Some commands will display output and then return to the shell prompt (e.g., the pwd command for print working directory) while others will just return to the shell prompt to indicate that it has executed the last command (e.g., the cd command for changing the directory).

```
$ pwd
/home/user2/scripts
$ cd
$ pwd
/home/user2
```

Unix commands are case-sensitive (e.g., pwd ≠ PWD), may include a list of ***options*** that modify their function, and may involve one or more ***arguments*** such as files or directories to perform the function on. The general format is: command -options arguments. For example, the wc command displays the number of lines, words, and bytes contained in a file that is specified as an argument. This command includes options for displaying number of bytes (-c), number of lines (-l), and number of words (-w); these options can be used individually (e.g., wc -l) or together (e.g., wc -c -w or wc -cw). In the example below, wc determines that the file data2.txt has 41 lines, 199 words, and 1275 bytes.

```
$ wc data2.txt
     41     199    1275 data2.txt
$ wc -l data2.txt
     41 data2.txt
```

```
$ wc -c -w data2.txt
     199    1275 data2.txt
$ wc -cw data2.txt
     199    1275 data2.txt
```

Unix manual pages (commonly referred to as ***man pages***) provide detailed documentation for commands and are a useful resource for learning about their functionality and usage. The basic format for using the man command is: man command.

```
$ man wc
    WC(1)              BSD General Commands Manual            WC(1)

    NAME
        wc -- word, line, character, and byte count

    SYNOPSIS
        wc [-clmw] [file ...]

    DESCRIPTION
        The wc utility displays the number of lines, words, and bytes contained in
        each input file, or standard input (if no file is specified) to the standard
        output.  A line is defined as a string of characters delimited by a <new-
        line> character. Characters beyond the final <newline> character will not
        be included in the line count.

        A word is defined as a string of characters delimited by white space char-
        acters.  White space characters are the set of characters for which the
        iswspace(3) function returns true. If more than one input file is specified,
        a line of cumulative counts for all the files is displayed on a separate line
        after the output for the last file.

    The following options are available:

        -c      The number of bytes in each input file is written to the standard output.
                This will cancel out any prior usage of the -m option.

        -l      The number of lines in each input file is written to the standard output.

        -m      The number of characters in each input file is written to the standard
                output. If the current locale does not support multi-byte characters,
                this is equivalent to the -c option.  This will cancel out any prior
                usage of the -c option.
        -w      The number of words in each input file is written to the standard output.

    :
```

Notice the ":" at the bottom of the page. This indicates that the manual page is longer than what can fit in the window. To scroll through the content, use the spacebar on the keyboard (or up and down arrows) and then press "q" (for quit) to return to the shell prompt at anytime. These keystrokes apply to other commands that may return more content than can fit in the window (e.g., the more command will show ":" or "--More--" to indicate additional content).

There are several useful keyboard shortcuts to keep in mind as you are working in the Unix environment. To *cancel or interrupt a command*, press the "control" key and then lowercase "c" key (referred to as Control-C or Ctrl-C or ^C). If you need to make some edits at the command-line, use Control-A (Ctrl-A or ^A) to go to the front of the line, Control-E (Ctrl-E or ^E) to go to the end, Control-F (Ctrl-F or ^F) to go one character forward, and Control-B (Ctrl-B or ^B) to go one character backward.

As you start to use more commands, it may be useful to scroll through the *command history* using the up ($\uparrow$) or down ($\downarrow$) arrows on the keyboard to find previously executed commands to either re-execute or modify. *Command completion* is also a useful shortcut that allows you to type the first few letters of a command or filename and then press the "tab" key to either complete it for you or display matching options.

A.4 BASIC COMMANDS

You may be wondering about what kind of Unix environment you have. Try out the following commands: hostname for printing the name of the current host system, uname for printing the operating system name, who to display who is logged in, and finger to display information about system users. To learn more about your username and the groups you belong to, use the id command. Try the date command to display the system date and time and cal to view a calendar. To find the path of a particular program or command, use the which command.

```
$ uname
Linux
$ date
Mon Mar  4 14:27:30 EST 2013
$ cal 1 2013
     January 2013
Su Mo Tu We Th Fr Sa
       1  2  3  4  5
 6  7  8  9 10 11 12
13 14 15 16 17 18 19
20 21 22 23 24 25 26
27 28 29 30 31
$ which date
/bin/date
$ which cal
/usr/bin/cal
```

Use clear to clear the screen and exit or logout to terminate all processes.

For more information about options and usage, refer to the man pages for each of these commands (as well as any others included in this primer).

A.5 TRAVERSING DIRECTORIES AND FILES

pwd and cd were introduced earlier for printing the working directory and changing directories. The absolute or relative path of a directory can be provided as an argument to the cd command. Just cd or cd ~ will change to the home directory, cd .. will change to the parent directory, and cd - will change to the previous directory.

```
$ pwd
/home/user2
$ cd scripts
$ pwd
/home/user2/scripts
$ cd ../data
$ pwd
/home/user2/data
$ cd -
/home/user2/scripts
$ cd ~
$ pwd
/home/user2/
```

The ls command can be used to list the contents of directories as well as get information for specified files. This command has several options including: -1 (number "1") for listing one entry per line, -a for listing all files including hidden files, -l (letter "l") for long format listing (includes file type, permissions, number of hard links, owner, group, size, date, and filename), -h for printing file sizes in human readable format, and -F that appends characters such as "/" to indicate directories and "*" to indicate executable files. Similar to other commands, these options can be used individually (e.g., ls -l) or in combination (e.g., ls -a -l or ls -al).

```
$ ls
data    scripts
$ ls -F
data/           scripts/
$ ls -F1
data/
scripts/
$ ls -l
total 0
```

```
drwxr-xr-x  3 user2  users  102 Mar  4 13:20 data
drwxr-xr-x  3 user2  users  102 Mar  4 14:36 scripts
$ ls -lh data
total 8
-rw-r--r--@ 1 user2  users   1.2K Mar  4 13:20 data2.txt
```

A.6 **WORKING WITH DIRECTORIES AND FILES**

To create or remove a directory, use the mkdir (e.g., mkdir new_dir) or rmdir (e.g., rmdir new_dir) commands. The touch command is for changing file access and modification times, but can also be used to create a new empty file (e.g., touch new_file.txt). To copy or move an existing file or directory, use the cp and mv commands respectively. The basic format of these commands is: command source target. In the case where the target name is the same as the source name, ".", can be used as a shortcut in the target. To remove a file, use the rm command. For comparing files line by line, the diff command can be used (e.g., diff file1.txt file2.txt); other file comparison commands include cmp and comm.

```
$ touch data4.txt
$ touch data5.txt
$ ls -F
data/          data4.txt      data5.txt      scripts/
$ mv data4.txt data/.
$ cp data5.txt data/data6.txt
$ ls
data           data5.txt      scripts
$ rm data5.txt
$ cd data
$ ls -l
total 8
-rw-r--r--@ 1 user2  users  1275 Mar  4 13:20 data2.txt
-rw-r--r--  1 user2  users     0 Mar  4 15:33 data4.txt
-rw-r--r--  1 user2  users     0 Mar  4 15:34 data6.txt
```

There are a couple of commands that can be used to display or view the contents of files such as more, less, head, and tail. While more only allows for scrolling forward through a file (using the spacebar and then "q" to quit), less allows for scrolling both backward and forward (using the up and down arrow keys). The head and tail commands will display the first or last specified number of lines (-n) or bytes (-c) of a file. To determine the type of a file, use the file command.

```
$ file data2.txt
data2.txt: ASCII English text
$ more data2.txt
```

```
PMID- 18428775
OWN - NLM
STAT- MEDLINE
DA  - 20080422
DCOM- 20080520
IS  - 1934-340X (Electronic)
IS  - 1934-3396 (Linking)
VI  - Appendix 1
DP  - 2007 Jan
TI  - Unix survival guide.
PG  - Appendix 1C
LID - 10.1002/0471250953.bia01cs16 [doi]
AB  - For a mixture of historical and practical reasons,
      much of the bioinformatics software discussed in
      this series runs on Linux, Mac OSX, Solaris, or
      one of the many other Unix variants. This appendix
      provides the novice with easy-to-understand infor-
      mation needed to survive in the Unix environment.
AD  - Cold Spring Harbor Laboratory, Cold Spring Harbor,
      New York, USA.
FAU - Stein, Lincoln D
AU  - Stein LD
LA  - eng
PT  - Journal Article
PT  - Review
PL  - United States
TA  - Curr Protoc Bioinformatics
JT  - Current protocols in bioinformatics / editoral
      board, Andreas D. Baxevanis ...[et al.]
JID - 101157830
SB  - IM
MH  - Computational Biology/*methods
MH  - *Programming Languages
MH  - *Software
MH  - Software Design
MH  - *User-Computer Interface
RF  - 13
EDAT- 2008/04/23 09:00
MHDA- 2008/05/21 09:00
CRDT- 2008/04/23 09:00
AID - 10.1002/0471250953.bia01cs16 [doi]
PST - ppublish
SO  - Curr Protoc Bioinformatics. 2007 Jan;Appendix
      1:Appendix 1C. doi: 10.1002/0471250953.bia01cs16.
$ head -c 15 data2.txt
PMID- 18428775
$ tail -n 3 data2.txt
PST - ppublish
SO  - Curr Protoc Bioinformatics. 2007 Jan;Appendix
      1:Appendix 1C. doi: 10.1002/0471250953.bia01cs16.
```

A.7 **INPUT AND OUTPUT**

Unix commands can be combined using the pipe symbol ("`|`"). The standard output of the command to the left of the pipe becomes the standard input for the command on the right (e.g., `command1 | command2`). The example below uses the `history` command that lists recently executed commands to demonstrate how to "pipe" commands together.

```
$ history | more
   19  pwd
   20  cd
   21  cd -
   22  cd data
   23  wc data2.txt
   24  wc -l data2.txt
   25  wc -c -w data2.txt
--More--
$ history | more | wc -l
      30
$ history | wc -l
      31
```

An alternative to displaying the output of commands or programs on the screen is to redirect it to a file using the ">" or ">>" symbols for writing and appending respectively. The `cat` command can be used to print, concatenate, and create files. `cat > file` allows one to provide input from the keyboard to store in the specified file (when done, do `Control-D` or `^D` to terminate input). If the `-b` option is used, line numbers will be displayed at the beginning of each line. The example below demonstrates how to redirect output and use the `cat` command. This example also demonstrates use of wildcard characters such as "`*`" for matching any number of characters in a filename or directory name (e.g., `ls *.txt` will list all files ending with `.txt`).

```
$ history > temp.txt
$ cal 2013 >> temp.txt
$ cat > temp2.txt
Demonstrate use of ">"
Demonstrate use of ">>"
Demonstrate cat command
^D
$ cat -b temp2.txt
     1 Demonstrate use of ">"
     2 Demonstrate use of ">>"
     3 Demonstrate cat command
$ cat temp.txt temp2.txt > temp3.txt
$ wc -l temp*.txt
      71 temp.txt
```

```
         3 temp2.txt
        74 temp3.txt
       148 total
$ rm temp*
```

A.8 BASIC DATA ANALYSIS

Unix has a number of useful utilities that can be used to quickly perform some basic data analysis. These commands include wc (introduced earlier), cut, sort, uniq, and grep that can be used in various combinations to characterize or filter a dataset.

To demonstrate the use of these commands, we will use a dataset of 3388 clinical studies from ClinicalTrials.gov (http://www.clinicaltrials.gov). This dataset is based on an Advanced Search for "obesity" under "Conditions" conducted on March 5, 2013 that was downloaded using the option to download shown fields as tab-separated values (other formats include plain text, comma-separated values, and XML). The resulting file is called study_fields.tsv and includes the following fields: (1) Rank, (2) Title, (3) Recruitment Status, (4) Study Results, (5) Conditions, (6) Interventions, and (7) URL. Below are results of using the head command to see the first three lines in this file.

```
$ head -n 3 study_fields.tsv
RankTitle     Recruitment Study Results  Conditions  Interventions    URL
1       Course of Obesity and Extreme Obesity in Adolescents   Recruiting        No
Results Available Obesity|Extreme Obesity
        http://ClinicalTrials.gov/show/NCT01662271
2       State of Obesity Care in Canada Evaluation Registry       Terminated   No
Results Available Obesity|Morbid Obesity
        http://ClinicalTrials.gov/show/NCT00328081
```

Using wc, let's check how many lines are in the file (there should be 3388).

```
$ wc -l study_fields.tsv
    3389 study_fields.tsv
```

Why is there an additional line? The first line in the file is a header line containing the field names. This should be excluded in subsequent analyses and can be done by either using the more command to skip this line with each command or saving the file without this line into a new file (e.g., called obesity_studies.txt).

```
$ more +2 study_fields.tsv | wc -l
3388
$ more +2 study_fields.tsv > obesity_studies.txt
$ wc -l obesity_studies.txt
3388 obesity_studies.txt
```

Now we are ready to do some analysis. Let's focus on the Recruitment Status field (Field 3). The cut command can be used to select portions of each line in a file based on the default delimiter (tab character) or a specified delimiter using -d delim (where delim may be a comma, pipe, or other character) and specified list of fields using -f list (where list is a comma-separated list of field numbers).

```
$ cut -f3 obesity_studies.txt | more
Recruiting
Terminated
Recruiting
Active, not recruiting
Not yet recruiting
--More--
```

Now let's sort the Recruitment Status field and then find the unique set of values using sort to sort lines in a file and uniq to report or filter out repeated lines, respectively.

```
$ cut -f3 obesity_studies.txt | sort | more
Active, not recruiting
Active, not recruiting
Active, not recruiting
--More--
$ cut -f3 obesity_studies.txt | sort | uniq
Active, not recruiting
Completed
Enrolling by invitation
Not yet recruiting
Recruiting
Suspended
Terminated
Withdrawn
```

The -c option for uniq can be used to count the number of times a line appears. For sort, -r can be used for reverse sorting and -n for numerical sorting. Used in combination, these commands and options can determine the distribution of values for Recruitment Status in descending order.

```
$ cut -f3 obesity_studies.txt | sort | uniq -c | sort -rn
   1606 Completed
    931 Recruiting
    477 Active, not recruiting
    156 Not yet recruiting
    107 Terminated
     75 Enrolling by invitation
     26 Withdrawn
     10 Suspended
```

Let's move on to the Conditions field (Field 5) that can include one or more conditions separated by the pipe ("|") symbol (e.g., "Hypertension|Obesity|

Diabetes"). Here, cut, sort, and uniq are used to find the top five conditions that are listed as the first condition. Notice the slight variation in using sort, head, and tail below for getting the same answer.

```
$ cut -f5 obesity_studies.txt | cut -d"|" -f1 | sort |
uniq -c | sort -rn | head -n 5
   1489 Obesity
    172 Overweight
    127 Morbid Obesity
    105 Cardiovascular Diseases
     61 Type 2 Diabetes
$ cut -f5 obesity_studies.txt | cut -d"|" -f1 | sort |
uniq -c | sort -n | tail -n 5
     61 Type 2 Diabetes
    105 Cardiovascular Diseases
    127 Morbid Obesity
    172 Overweight
   1489 Obesity
```

Finally, grep (global regular expression print) searches a file for a specified pattern where -i can be used to ignore case, -v to display lines not matching the pattern, and -c to count matching lines. Let's use grep to find lines including "asthma" (1 match), then use the -i and -c options to count case insensitive matches such as "asthma," "Asthma," and "ASTHMA" (34 matches), and then use -v to count lines that are not asthma-related (3354 matches).

```
$ grep "asthma" obesity_studies.txt
308    Weight-reduction  Intervention  in  Asthmatic  Children  With
Overweight/Obesity    Active, not recruiting      No Results Available
      Asthma|Overweight|Obesity    Behavioral: Multifactoral
Intervention for Children with asthma and overweight
      http://ClinicalTrials.gov/show/NCT00998413
$ grep -ic "asthma" obesity_studies.txt
34
$ grep -icv "asthma" obesity_studies.txt
3354
```

For more advanced pattern matching, the -E option can be used for extended regular expressions (also equivalent to the egrep command). cut and grep -E can be combined to find studies that include "diabetes" or "hypertension" in the list of conditions (Field 5).

```
$ cut -f1,5 obesity_studies.txt | grep -iE
"diabetes|hypertension" | more
38     Obesity|Diabetes Mellitus, Type 2
41     Obesity|Hypertension
51     Type 2 Diabetes|Obesity
58     Obesity Surgery and Diabetes
68     Hypertension|Abdominal Obesity
--More--
```

grep -E or egrep can also be used to search for ClinicalTrials.gov identifiers with a particular format that is specified in what is called a *regular expression* (regex). These 8-digit NCT numbers can be found as part of the URL in Field 7 (e.g., "http://ClinicalTrials.gov/show/**NCT00608062**"). Let's search for NCT numbers that start with "NCT0," followed by a digit between 1 and 9, followed by six additional digits between 0 and 9. The "^" and "$" characters specify matching at the beginning and end of a string respectively.

```
$ cut -f7 obesity_studies.txt | cut -d"/" -f5 | egrep
"^NCT0[1-9][0-9]{6}$" | wc -l
1705
$ cut -f7 obesity_studies.txt | cut -d"/" -f5 | egrep
"^NCT0[1-9][0-9]{6}$" | head -n 5
NCT01662271
NCT01363193
NCT01380418
NCT01794429
NCT01703273
```

A.9 ACCESS PERMISSIONS

Every file and directory is associated with a set of permissions that specify what can be done to it and by whom. Permission types are read (r), write/modify (w), execute (x), or no permissions (-) while user types are user/owner (u), group (g), other/world (o), and all (a). Each permission type is also associated with a numeric notation: 4 for read, 2 for write, and 1 for execute, where these numbers can be combined to specify permissions for each user type. For example, 3 for write (2) + execute (1), 5 for read (4) + execute (1), 6 for read (4) + write (2), or 7 for read (4) + write (2) + execute (1).

user (owner)				group				other (world)			
r	w	x	-	r	w	x	-	r	w	x	-
4	2	1	0	4	2	1	0	4	2	1	0

To see how the permissions are set for a particular file or directory, use ls -l. Based on the permissions associated with the following two files, the first one is readable and writeable only by the owner (user2) while the second one is readable and executable by the owner, the owner's group (users), and anyone else on the system as well as writeable by the owner.

```
$ ls -l
total 1568
-rw------- 1 user2 users 801234 Mar  5 14:15 obesity_studies.txt
-rwxr-xr-x 1 user2 users 801300 Mar  5 14:04 study_fields.tsv*
```

The benefit of a multi-user environment such as Unix is the ability to share files and programs with other users. This also stresses the importance of protecting files that should not be shared by appropriately setting the permissions. The chmod (change mode) command can be used to change access permissions in a variety of ways as demonstrated below (chmod mode file). To change the owner or group of a file, use the chown (chown owner file) or chgrp (chgrp group file) commands.

Permission Set	Numeric Notation	Symbolic Notation
-rw-------	600	
-rwx------	chmod 700	chmod u+x
-rwxr--r--	chmod 744	chmod a+r or chmod go+r
-rwxr-xr-x	chmod 755	chmod +x or chmod go+x
-rw-r--r--	chmod 644	chmod ugo-x

A.10 TEXT EDITORS

For editing files in the Unix environment, common text editors to become familiar with are pico (or nano that emulates pico), emacs, or vi. These can all be launched from the command-line and are associated with their own set of keyboard commands. Each of these text editors is associated with documentation and tutorials (see "References and Resources" section at the end of this primer).

A.11 SUMMARY OF COMMANDS

Below is a summary of the Unix commands and options covered in this primer. There are many more commands for users and system administrators. Readers are encouraged to refer to the Unix man pages as well as various Unix books and on-line resources for more details (see "References and Resources" section at the end of this primer).

Basic Commands	Working with Files and Directories
`exit` – terminate all processes	`mkdir [dir]` – make a directory
`logout` – terminate all processes	`rmdir [dir]` – remove a directory
`man [command]` – manual or help pages	`touch [file]` – create new or modify file
`hostname` – current host system	`cp [source] [target]` – copy file
`uname` – current operating system	`mv [source] [target]` – move file
`who` – list of users currently logged in	`rm [file]` – remove file
`finger` – information about system users	`diff [file1] [file2]` – compare files
`id [userid]` – id and groups for user	`comm [file1] [file2]` – compare files
`which [command]` – location of command	`cmp [file1] [file2]` – compare files
`date` – print or set system date and time	`more [file]` – view contents of file
`cal` – display calendar	`less [file]` – view contents of file
`clear` – clear the screen	`head -n [n] [file]` – display first n lines
Traversing Directories and Files	`tail -n [n] [file]` – display last n lines
`pwd` – print current/working directory	`file [file]` – determine file type
`cd [dir]` – change to specified directory	**Input and Output**
`cd` – change directory to home directory	`command1	command2` – pipe commands
`cd ~` – change to home directory	`command > file` – redirect output (write)
`cd -` – change to previous directory	`command >> file` – redirect output (append)
`cd ..` – change to parent directory	`command < file` – redirect input
`ls [file/dir]` – list files or directories	`cat > file` – write standard input to file
`ls -l [file]` – list with details	`cat file1 file2 > file3` – concatenate
`ls -lalhF [file]` – other options for `ls`	`cat -b file` – display line numbers

Basic Data Analysis
`wc -clw [file]` – word, line, character count
`cut -d delim -f list [file]` – cut portion of file based on specified delimiter and fields
`sort -rn [file]` – sort lines of file; options for reverse and numeric sorting
`uniq -c [file]` – report or filter out repeated lines in a file; option for showing counts
`grep -ivcE [pattern] [file]` – search for a pattern; options for ignoring case, etc.
`egrep [pattern] [file]` – search for specific pattern in file; same as `grep -E`

Access Permissions	Text Editors
`chmod [mode] [file]` – change mode	`pico` or `nano`
`chown [owner] [file]` – change owner	`emacs`
`chgrp [group] [file]` – change group	`vi`

REFERENCES AND RESOURCES

There are numerous books and on-line resources covering Unix. Below are a few references and tutorials that provide additional details and examples for the commands covered in this primer as well as additional Unix commands.

History

- Ritchie DM, Thompson K. The UNIX time-sharing system. Communications of the ACM. 1974 July;17(7):365–75.
- The creation of the UNIX* operating system [Internet]. 2002 [cited 2013 April 15]. Available from: http://www.bell-labs.com/history/unix/.

Commands

- Robbins A. Unix in a nutshell. Fourth Edition. O'Reilly Media, Inc.; 2005.
- Stein LD. Unix survival guide. Curr Protoc Bioinformatics. 2007 January; Appendix 1: Appendix 1C.
- Unix tutorial for beginners [Internet]. 2001 [cited 2013 April 15]. Available from: http://www.ee.surrey.ac.uk/Teaching/Unix/.
- Unix tutorial [Internet]. [cited 2013 Apr 15]. Available from: http://www.tutorialspoint.com/unix/.
- Wikibooks contributors. A quick introduction to Unix [Internet]. Wikibooks, The Free Textbook Project; 2010 [updated 2012 November 11; cited 2013 May 30]. Available from: http://en.wikibooks.org/w/index.php?title=A_Quick_Introduction_to_Unix&oldid=2438222.
- Wikibooks contributors. Guide to Unix [Internet]. Wikibooks, The Free Textbook Project; 2004 [updated 2013 April 3; cited 2013 May 30]. Available from: http://en.wikibooks.org/w/index.php?title=Guide_to_Unix&oldid=2508273.
- Wikipedia contributors. List of Unix utilities [Internet]. Wikipedia, The Free Encyclopedia; 2006 [updated 2013 April 25; cited 2013 May 30]. Available from: http://en.wikipedia.org/w/index.php?title=List_of_Unix_utilities&oldid=552156361.
- Wikibooks contributors. Ad hoc data analysis from the Unix command line [Internet]. Wikibooks, The Free Textbook Project; 2006 [updated 2013 January 5; cited 2013 May 30]. Available from: http://en.wikibooks.org/w/index.php?title=Ad_Hoc_Data_Analysis_From_The_Unix_Command_Line&oldid=2473825.

Text Editors

- Wikibooks contributors. Guide to Unix/explanations/introduction to editors [Internet]. Wikibooks, The Free Textbook Project; 2005 [updated 2012 February 15; cited 2013 May 30]. Available from: http://en.wikibooks.org/w/index.php?title=Guide_to_Unix/Explanations/Introduction_to_Editors&oldid=2265745.
- Wikibooks contributors. A quick introduction to Unix/editing text [Internet]. Wikibooks, The Free Textbook Project; 2010 [updated 2010 September 30; cited 2013 May 30]. Available from: http://en.wikibooks.org/w/index.php?title=A_Quick_Introduction_to_Unix/Editing_Text&oldid=1941243.
- pico [Internet]. 1989 [updated 2005 January 14; cited 2013 April 15]. Available from: http://www.washington.edu/pine/man/#pico.

- GNU nano [Internet]. [updated 2009 November 30; cited 2013 April 15]. Available from: http://www.nano-editor.org/.
- The vi editor tutorial [Internet]. [cited 2013 April 15]. Available from: http://www.tutorialspoint.com/unix/unix-vi-editor.htm.
- Wikibooks contributors. Learning the vi editor [Internet]. Wikibooks, The Free Textbook Project; 2004 [updated 2010 August 19; cited 2013 May 30]. Available from: http://en.wikibooks.org/w/index.php?title=Learning_the_vi_Editor&oldid=191501.
- A guided tour of emacs [Internet]. 2007 [updated 2012 August 18; cited 2013 April 15]. Available from: http://www.gnu.org/software/emacs/tour/.
- EmacsWiki [Internet]. [updated 2013 March 29; cited 2013 April 15]. Available from: http://emacswiki.org/.

Ruby Primer

Elizabeth S. Chen

Center for Clinical and Translational Science, University of Vermont, Burlington, VT, USA
Department of Medicine, Division of General Internal Medicine, University of Vermont, Burlington, VT, USA
Department of Computer Science, University of Vermont, Burlington, VT, USA

Scripting languages such as Perl, Python, and Ruby have grown in popularity for supporting a variety of processing, analysis, and application development tasks. These open-source and platform-independent languages are characterized as being relatively easy to use and learn in addition to being less restrictive when compared with other programming languages.

Yukihiro Matsumoto ("Matz") sought to develop a scripting language that was "more powerful than Perl and more object-oriented than Python" and as a result developed and released Ruby in 1995. This interpreted object-oriented language is written in C, has interfaces to a variety of other languages (e.g., Java through JRuby), and supports the Ruby on Rails framework for Web application development. In Ruby, everything is an **object** where objects are instances of **classes** that include **properties** and **methods**.

This primer serves as a brief introduction to Ruby that starts with the classic "Hello World" program (Sections B.1 and B.2) followed by descriptions of classes and methods associated with **Numbers and Math** (Section B.3), **Strings** (Section B.4), **Conditional Statements** and **Control Structures** (Section B.5), **Directories** and **Files** (Section B.6), **Regular Expressions** (Section B.7), and **Arrays and Hashes** (Section B.8). Within these sections, generic examples as well as specialized scripts (e.g., involving resources such as PubMed/MEDLINE, ClinicalTrials.gov, and mortality records) are provided.

Readers are encouraged to try the various methods described using Interactive Ruby or irb (Section B.9) and follow along with the scripts by writing them in a plain text editor and then running them (as described in Section B.1). It should be noted that the scripts in this primer offer one solution, but as the Perl motto goes "There Is More Than One Way To Do It" and readers should feel free to try different variations.

The last section of the primer provides a brief discussion of "gems" that are packaged Ruby libraries providing additional functionality (Section B.10). Finally, a list of references and resources for learning more about Ruby is provided that includes core resources such as the Ruby Programming Language site (http://www.ruby-lang.org), Ruby Documentation Project site (http://ruby-doc.org/), and Ruby community's gem hosting service (http://rubygems.org/).

For this primer, it is assumed that Ruby has already been installed on a system running Windows, Mac OS X, or other Unix variant such as Linux. The examples here assume a Unix environment (see Appendix A: Unix Primer).

B.1 HELLO WORLD

The classic first program is "Hello World". Here is an example of this program written in Ruby:

```
#! /usr/local/bin/ruby

# hello.rb
# First Ruby program for "Hello World"

puts "Hello World!"
print "How are you? "              # Print question
print "Good-bye!\n"
```

The first line starting with #! is referred to as the **shebang line**. This line tells the system where to find the Ruby interpreter. In a Unix environment, the which command can be used to determine the location of Ruby (commonly found in /usr/bin/ruby or /usr/local/bin/ruby). The -v or --version option can then be used to determine the version of Ruby (latest version is 2.0.0).

```
$ which ruby
/usr/local/bin/ruby

$ ruby -v
ruby 1.9.1p378 (2010-01-10 revision 26273)
[i386-darwin10.4.0]

$ ruby --version
ruby 1.9.1p378 (2010-01-10 revision 26273)
[i386-darwin10.4.0]
```

The next set of lines starting with # are **comment lines**, which are hidden from the interpreter and thus ignored. The # can also be used within a line where everything after this symbol will be ignored. Comments are valuable for documentation and the ability to "comment out" lines is useful for debugging and testing. If several lines need to be commented, a **block comment** can be used, which starts with =begin and ends with =end.

```
# This is a comment
# This is a comment too
# Another comment

=begin
This is a comment
This is a comment too
Another comment
=end
```

The last three lines in the program are **statements** that specify what the program should do (in this case, how and what to output). The `puts` method automatically adds the newline character ("\n") at the end when printing whereas the newline needs to be specified when using the `print` method. There are other methods for printing output such as `printf` that allows for specific formatting (see Sections B.3, B.5, and B.8 for examples).

Now that we have described each line in this program, let's try running it. Use a plain text editor to write the program and then save it as `hello.rb`. The `.rb` extension is the convention for Ruby programs (similar to how `.pl` and `.py` are used for Perl and Python programs respectively). To run the program, type `ruby hello.rb` at the Unix prompt. Alternatively, if the file is made executable (e.g., using the `chmod` command), just type `hello.rb` or `./hello.rb` and the shebang line will be used to find the Ruby interpreter.

```
$ ruby hello.rb
Hello World!
How are you? Good-bye!
$
```

```
$ ls -l hello.rb
-rw-r--r-- 1 user2  users   195 Mar 22 16:06 hello.rb
$ chmod u+x hello.rb
$ ls -l hello.rb
-rwxr--r-- 1 user2  users   195 Mar 22 16:06 hello.rb
```

```
$ hello.rb
Hello World!
How are you? Good-bye!
$
```

B.2 EXTENSIONS TO HELLO WORLD

The next set of examples depict extensions to the Hello World program that demonstrate use of shell commands, variables, constants, expression substitution, arguments, input, and methods.

First, let's add some lines to `hello.rb` for executing some Unix shell commands and then re-run the program. Unix commands can be executed

within a Ruby script by enclosing the command to be run within backticks
("`") and the results are returned as "strings" that can be displayed. Also,
notice the "+" in these lines that is used to append strings (we'll learn more
about strings in Section B.4).

```
# Run a Unix shell command with backticks (`command`)
puts "Where is Ruby? " + `which ruby`
puts "What version of Ruby? " + `ruby -v`
```

```
$ ruby hello.rb
Hello World!
How are you? Good-bye!
Where is Ruby? /usr/local/bin/ruby
What version of Ruby? ruby 1.9.1p378 (2010-01-10 revision 26273)
[i386-darwin10.4.0]
```

The following script for hello_var.rb is a variation of hello.rb that
includes use of variables, constants, and expression substitution. **Variables**
are used to assign a value to a name (e.g., $x = 5$ where is x is the variable name and 5 is the value). There are different types of variables such
as local, global, instance, and class. A **local variable** is one that has a local
scope or context (e.g., if a variable is defined within a method or loop, it is
only available within that method or loop); these variable names must begin
with a lowercase letter or underscore. The scope of a **global variable** is the
entire program; these names begin with "$" (e.g., $y = 10$). **Constants**
are variables that maintain the same value throughout a program; the names
of constants are capitalized or all uppercase (e.g., $Z = 25$). **Expression
substitution** can be used to include the value of a variable in a string. This is
represented by #{...} where "..." can be a variable name (e.g., #{x} would
produce 5) or an expression (e.g., #{x*Z} would produce 125).

```
#! /usr/local/bin/ruby

# hello_var.rb
# Personalized greeting using constants, variables,
# and expression substitution

Greeting = "Hello"                  # This is a constant
name1 = "World"                     # This is a variable (local)
name2 = "Matz"                      # This is another variable (local)
puts Greeting + " " + name1         # Concatenating values of variables
puts "#{Greeting} #{name2}"         # Using expression substitution
```

```
$ ruby hello_var.rb
Hello World
Hello Matz
```

The next two examples demonstrate use of command-line arguments and user input for the Hello World program. An **argument** is a variable that is passed to a program or method. Ruby has a predefined variable called ARGV for storing one or more command-line arguments in an array where ARGV[0] refers to the first argument, ARGV[1] the next, and so on (see Section B.8 for more information about arrays).

```
#! /usr/local/bin/ruby

# hello_arg.rb
# Personalized greeting using arguments

name = ARGV[0]                 # Get argument from the command line
puts "Hello #{name}!"
```

```
$ ruby hello_arg.rb user2
Hello user2!
```

A program can also receive **input** using the gets method that prompts the user to enter input from the keyboard.

```
#! /usr/local/bin/ruby

# hello_input.rb
# Personalized greeting using input

print "What is your name? "                    # Prompt user for name

# Get inputted name (gets) and remove newline from input (chomp)
name = gets.chomp

print "What is your favorite color? "          # Prompt user for color
color = gets.chomp                             # Get inputted color
puts "Hello #{name}! Your favorite color is  #{color}."
```

```
$ ruby hello_input.rb
What is your name? user2
What is your favorite color? blue
Hello user2! Your favorite color is blue.
```

Finally, **methods** can be used to gather code that performs a particular function or set of functions into one place for convenient and repeated use. When defining a method, it can have zero or more arguments and may explicitly return a value using the `return` statement. This last example demonstrates how methods can be created and used for the Hello World program.

```
#! /usr/local/bin/ruby

# hello_method.rb
# Personalized greeting using methods

def hello                          # This method has no arguments
  puts "Hello World! "
end

def hello_color (name, color)   # This method has two arguments
  puts "Hello #{name}! Your favorite color is #{color}."
end

name1 = "user1"
color1 = "green"

hello                           # Call the hello method
hello_color(name1, color1)      # Call the hello_color method with variables
hello_color("user2", "blue")    # Call the hello_color method with values
```

```
$ ruby hello_method.rb
Hello World!
Hello user1! Your favorite color is green.
Hello user2! Your favorite color is blue
```

B.3 NUMBERS AND MATH

Ruby includes several classes for numbers including **Integer** for whole numbers (e.g., -3, -2, -1, 0, 1, 2, and 3) and **Float** for real or floating-point numbers (e.g., -2.14, 0.0, and 3.7777).

Basic **math operations** can be applied to these numbers such as addition (+), subtraction (-), multiplication (*), division (/), exponent (**), and modulo (%). There are also equivalent methods for some of these operations such as `div` and `modulo`.

```ruby
#! /usr/local/bin/ruby

# math.rb
# Demonstrates different math operations

n1 = 7      # First number
n2 = 3      # Second number

# Output results of different math operations
puts "#{n1} + #{n2} = #{n1 + n2}"             # Addition
puts "#{n1} - #{n2} = #{n1 - n2}"             # Subtraction
puts "#{n1} * #{n2} = #{n1 * n2}"             # Multiplication
puts "#{n1} / #{n2} = #{n1 / n2}"             # Division
puts "#{n1} / #{n2} = #{n1.to_f / n2.to_f}"
printf "#{n1} / #{n2} = %.2f\n", n1.to_f / n2.to_f
puts "#{n1} ** #{n2} = #{n1 ** n2}"           # Power/Exponent
puts "#{n1} % #{n2} = #{n1 % n2}"             # Modulo
```

```
$ ruby math.rb
7 + 3 = 10
7 - 3 = 4
7 * 3 = 21
7 / 3 = 2
7 / 3 = 2.33333333333333
7 / 3 = 2.33
7 ** 3 = 343
7 % 3 = 1
```

Notice the three statements in `math.rb` for the division calculation. The first statement shows that when dividing integers, the result will be an integer. To ensure that the result is not truncated (i.e., missing the part after the decimal point), at least one of the numbers should be converted to a floating point using the `to_f` method; there are similar methods for converting to integers (`to_i`) and strings (`to_s`). For formatting the output, `printf` can be used to specify how many numbers after the decimal point to print (e.g., `%.2f` indicates two positions after the decimal).

Several **comparison operators** are available for testing if numbers are equal (== and eql?), not equal (!=), less than or equal to (< or <=), or greater than or equal to each other (> or >=) that return a Boolean value (true or false). There is also the spaceship operator (<=>) that returns −1 if the first value is less than the second, 0 if the values are equal, or 1 if the first value is greater than the second. Another operator, ===, can be used to determine if a value is within a range of numbers where a range can either be inclusive (represented as n..m that covers numbers from n to m including m) or exclusive (represented as n...m that covers n to m excluding m).

```ruby
#! /usr/local/bin/ruby

# compare.rb
# Demonstrate comparison operators

# Assign values to variables using parallel assignment
c1, c2, c3, c4 = 25, 50, 75, 50
print "c1 = #{c1}, c2 = #{c2}, c3 = #{c3}, c4 = #{c4}\n"

# Output results of different comparison operations

# Testing equality
print "  c1 = c3 is ", c1 == c3, "\n"
print "  c2 = c4 is ", c2.eql?(c4), "\n"

print "  c1 != c3 is ", c1 != c3, "\n"
print "  c2 != c4 is ", !c2.eql?(c4), "\n"

print "  c1 <=> c2 is ", c1 <=> c2, "\n"
print "  c4 <=> c2 is ", c4 <=> c2, "\n"
print "  c3 <=> c2 is ", c3 <=> c2, "\n"
# Changing values using abbreviated assignment operators

c1 *= 3          # Shorthand for c1 = c1 * 3
c4 += 1          # Shorthand for c4 = c4 + 1

print "c1 = #{c1}, c2 = #{c2}, c3 = #{c3}, c4 = #{c4}\n"

# Testing less than and greater than
print "  c1 < c2 is ", c1 < c2, "\n"
print "  c4 <= c2 is ", c4 <= c2, "\n"
```

```
print "  c1 > c2 is ", c1 > c2, "\n"
print "  c3 >= c2 is ", c3 >= c2, "\n"

# Testing inclusion in range
print "  (50..75) === c1 is ", (50..75) === c1, "\n"
print "  (50...75) === c1 is ", (50...75) === c1, "\n"
```

```
$ ruby compare.rb
c1 = 25, c2 = 50, c3 = 75, c4 = 50
  c1 = c3 is false
  c2 = c4 is true
  c1 != c3 is true
  c2 != c4 is false
  c1 <=> c2 is -1
  c4 <=> c2 is 0
  c3 <=> c2 is 1
c1 = 75, c2 = 50, c3 = 75, c4 = 51
  c1 < c2 is false
  c4 <= c2 is false
  c1 > c2 is true
  c3 >= c2 is true
  (50..75) === c1 is true
  (50...75) === c1 is false
```

In addition to demonstrating different comparison operators, compare.rb also highlights **parallel assignment** for assigning values to multiple variables in one statement and **abbreviated assignment operators** as a shorthand way for performing basic math operations on variables. For example, the statement x = x + 1 can be abbreviated as x += 1.

B.4 STRINGS

Working with **strings** (sequences of one or more characters) is a common programming task. This section covers methods for manipulating and transforming strings using methods in the String class while Section B.7 focuses on **regular expressions** for matching patterns in strings.

A new string can be created by using the new method or just directly assigning a value. Either a pair of double quotes or single quotes can be used; however, the former will interpret any escaped characters (e.g., \n for newline, \t for tab, \\ for backslash, or \" for double quote) while the latter will preserve them. For example, "\"hello\"\n" will display hello followed by a newline while '\"hello\"\n' will display \"hello\"\n.

```
title = String.new
title = String.new("Methods in Biomedical Informatics")
title = "Methods in Biomedical Informatics"
```

The empty? method can be used to determine if a string is empty (title.
empty? returns false) and length or size methods will return the
number of characters in a string (title.length or title.size
returns 33).

Strings can be "sliced" using the slice or [ ] method to obtain substrings.
To find the location of a particular character or substring, use the index
method. Remember, that in strings, the first character is at index position 0
(not 1). In the examples below and throughout the rest of this primer, the
notation "# =>" is used to indicate the output to expect.

```
title[4] or title.slice(4)        # => "o"
title[8, 2]                       # =>"in"
title[11...20]                    # => "Biomedica"
title[11..20]                     # => "Biomedical"
title.index("I")                  # => 22
```

Methods for transforming the case of a string include capitalize for capi-
talizing the first letter, downcase for lowercasing the entire string, upcase
for uppercasing the entire string, swapcase for swapping uppercase letters
with lowercase and vice versa, and reverse for reversing a string. These
methods can be used individually or combined (e.g., title.downcase.
capitalize will return "Methods in biomedical informat-
ics"). There are also "destructive" versions of these methods with the same
name followed by an "!", which will alter the string in place (capitalize!, downcase!, upcase!, swapcase!, and reverse!).

```
#! /usr/local/bin/ruby

# question.rb
# Demonstrate methods for string manipulation and transformation

question = "How Are You?"
answer = "I Am Fine."

# Length or size
puts "Question: #{question} (#{question.length})"
puts "Answer: #{answer} (#{answer.size})"
```

```
# Concatenate strings
puts question + " " + answer
puts question + " " + answer * 3
puts question[0, 3] + "---" + answer[5..8]
puts question << " " << answer

# Transform case
puts question.upcase + " -> " + question.swapcase + " -> " + question
puts question.downcase.capitalize + " -> " + question
puts question.downcase!.capitalize! + " -> " + question
puts question.upcase!.reverse! + " -> " + question
```

```
$ ruby question.rb
Question: How Are You? (12)
Answer: I Am Fine. (10)
How Are You? I Am Fine.
How Are You? I Am Fine.I Am Fine.I Am Fine.
How---Fine
How Are You? I Am Fine.
HOW ARE YOU? I AM FINE. -> hOW aRE yOU? i aM fINE. -> How Are You? I Am Fine.
How are you? i am fine. -> How Are You? I Am Fine.
How are you? i am fine. -> How are you? i am fine.
.ENIF MA I ?UOY ERA WOH -> .ENIF MA I ?UOY ERA WOH
```

The chop (or chop!) method will remove the last character of a string while the chomp (or chomp!) method can be used to remove the record separator (e.g., \n, \r, or \r\n). Whitespace can be added using the rjust, ljust, and center methods or removed from strings using lstrip, rstrip, and strip (or lstrip!, rstrip!, or strip!).

```
title.rjust(35)          # =>    "  Methods in Biomedical Informatics"
title.center(35, "-")    # =>    "-Methods in Biomedical Informatics-"
title.ljust(35, "*")     # =>    "Methods in Biomedical Informatics**"
```

To replace a substring, the gsub (or gsub!) method can be used. This method takes a string or pattern as the first argument to be substituted with the string specified in the second argument. For example, title. gsub("i", "I") replaces any lowercase "i" with the uppercase "I" and returns "Methods In BIomedIcal InformatIcs".

The split (or split!) method can be used to divide a string into substrings based on a specified delimiter (string or pattern), which are returned as an array of elements (see Section B.8 for more about arrays). For example, `title.split(" ")` or `title.split("\s")` will return "Methods", "in", "Biomedical", and "Informatics" based on using the space as a delimiter for splitting the string.

In the previous examples, a specific substring was specified for substitution and splitting; however, a regular expression or pattern (indicated by `/pattern/`) could also be specified such as in `title.gsub(/[aeiou]/, "*")`, which returns "M*th*ds *n B**m*d*c*l Inf*rm*t*cs" (see Section B.7 on Regular Expressions).

Similar to numbers, comparison operators can be applied to strings to determine if they are the same or not. For example, `==`, `<=>`, and `eql?` can all be used to test the equality of two strings.

```ruby
#! /usr/local/bin/ruby

# colors.rb
# Demonstrates use of comparison operators, split, and gsub

primary_colors = "Red^Yellow^Blue"
secondary_colors = "Green|Purple|Orange"

# Compare strings
print "#{primary_colors} = #{secondary_colors}? ", primary_colors ==
secondary_colors, "\n"

# Substitute strings
puts primary_colors + " -> " + primary_colors.gsub("^", "***") + " -> " +
primary_colors
puts secondary_colors + " -> " + secondary_colors.gsub!("|", "---") + " ->
" + secondary_colors

# Split strings
color1, color2, color3 = primary_colors.split("^")
puts "Primary Colors: #{color1}, #{color2}, #{color3}"

colors = secondary_colors.split("---")
puts "Secondary Colors: " + colors[0] + ", " + colors[1] + ", " + colors[2]

# Add whitespace to strings
```

```
puts "Primary Colors".center(40)
puts color1.ljust(40, ".")
puts color2.center(40, ".")
puts color3.rjust(40, ".")
```

```
$ ruby colors.rb
Red^Yellow^Blue = Green|Purple|Orange? false
Red^Yellow^Blue -> Red***Yellow***Blue -> Red^Yellow^Blue
Green|Purple|Orange -> Green---Purple---Orange -> Green---Purple---Orange
Primary Colors: Red, Yellow, Blue
Secondary Colors: Green, Purple, Orange
              Primary Colors
Red......................................
................Yellow...................
.........................................Blue
```

B.5 CONDITIONAL STATEMENTS AND CONTROL STRUCTURES

Like other programming languages, Ruby provides **control structures** for guiding the flow of execution in a program. These include **conditional statements** that test if a specified expression is true or false and **loops** for repeating a block of code a specified number of times or until some condition is met.

The basic if statement can be used to perform a particular action or set of actions if one or more conditions hold (i.e., evaluated as true). In the case of multiple conditions, the "&&" or "and" **logical operators** can be used to test if <u>all</u> of the conditions are true while the "||" or "or" logical operators are used to test if <u>any</u> of the conditions is true. To test if a condition is <u>not</u> true, the "!" or "not" operators can be applied. The unless statement is the opposite of an if statement where actions are performed when a condition does <u>not</u> hold (i.e., evaluated as false).

```
#! /usr/local/bin/ruby

# conditions.rb
# Demonstrates use of if statement

x, y, z = 100, 200, 300
puts "x = #{x}, y = #{y}, z = #{z}"

# Test if x equals 100
```

```ruby
if x == 100
  puts "#{x} equals 100"
end

# Same logic as above but in one line
puts "#{x} equals 100 again" if x == 100

# Test if y does not equal z
puts "#{y} does not equal #{z}" if !(y == z)

# Same logic as above but using unless statement
unless y == z
  puts "#{y} does not equal #{z} again"
end

# Testing multiple conditions using "and" or "&&"
puts "#{x} is less than #{y} and #{z}" if x < y && x < z

# Testing multiple conditions using "or" or "||"
if y < x || y < z
  puts "#{y} is less than #{x} or #{z}"
end
```

```
$ ruby conditions.rb
x = 100, y = 200, z = 300
100 equals 100
100 equals 100 again
200 does not equal 300
200 does not equal 300 again
100 is less than 200 and 300
200 is less than 100 or 300
```

An if statement can be expanded to form an if-else statement that uses the else keyword for specifying an alternative set of actions if the specified if condition does not hold or if-elsif-else statement that uses the elsif keyword for testing additional conditions after the initial if. A case statement provides a shorthand alternative to the if-elsif-else statement. Let's expand conditions.rb to include if-else, if-elsif-else, and case statements (and comment out the previous puts statements before running again).

```
# if-else statement
if x < 100
  puts "#{x} less than 100"
else
  puts "#{x} is equal to or greater than 100"
end

# Same logic as above but using the ternary or base three operator (?:)
print "#{x} is " + (x < 100 ? "less than 100 again\n" : "equal to or
greater than 100 again\n")

# if-elsif-else statement
if y < 100
  puts "#{y} is less than 100"
elsif y < 200
  puts "#{y} is less than 200"
elsif y < 300
  puts "#{y} is less than 300"
else
  puts "#{y} is greater than or equal to 300"
end

# case statement
case y
when 0..99    then puts "#{y} is less than 100 again"
when 100..199 then puts "#{y} is less than 200 again"
when 200..299 then puts "#{y} is less than 300 again"
  else puts "#{y} is greater than or equal to 300 again"
end
```

```
$ ruby conditions.rb
100 is equal to or greater than 100
100 is equal to or greater than 100 again
200 is less than 300
200 is less than 300 again
```

There are several types of loops in Ruby. A `while` loop can be used to execute code within it until a specified condition is true while the `until` loop executes the code until the specified condition is false. A `for` loop will iterate over code a specified number of times. The `times`, `upto`, and `downto` methods provide similar functionality to the `for` loop.

```ruby
#! /usr/local/bin/ruby

# loops.rb
# Demonstrates use of loops

i = 0

# while loop for incrementing i by 1 from 0 to 3
while i <= 3 do
  puts "while: #{i}"
  i += 1
end

# until loop for incrementing until i equals 5
until i == 5
  puts "until: #{i}"
  i += 1
end

# for loop
for j in 1..3 do
  puts "for: #{j}"
end

# nested for loop
for j in 1...3
  for k in 1...3
    puts "nested for: #{j} * #{k} = #{j*k}"
  end
end

# times
3.times do |t|
  puts "times: #{t} * 5 = #{t*5}"
end

# upto
10.upto(12) {|m| puts "upto: #{m}"}

# downto
20.downto(18) {|n| puts "downtoto: #{n}"}
```

```
$ ruby loops.rb
while: 0
while: 1
while: 2
while: 3
until: 4
for: 1
for: 2
for: 3
nested for: 1 * 1 = 1
nested for: 1 * 2 = 2
nested for: 2 * 1 = 2
nested for: 2 * 2 = 4
times: 0 * 5 = 0
times: 1 * 5 = 5
times: 2 * 5 = 10
upto: 10
upto: 11
upto: 12
downtoto: 20
downtoto: 19
downtoto: 18
```

Finally, the simple `loop` method continuously executes code until terminated using the `break` keyword to exit the loop (this can also be used for `while`, `until`, and `for` loops). Other keywords include `next` to skip the current iteration and `redo` that restarts the iteration.

B.5.1 **Calculating Body Mass Index (BMI)**

The last example program in this section demonstrates use of the `loop` method and `if-elsif-else` statement for an interactive body mass index (BMI) calculator for adults. This program prompts the user for a weight in pounds and height in inches,[1] calculates the BMI, and determines weight status based on the calculated BMI ("underweight" if below 18.5, "normal" is between 18.5 and 24.9, "overweight" if between 25 and 29.9, and "obese" if 30 and above).

```
#! /usr/local/bin/ruby

# bmi_calc.rb
# Interactive Body Mass Index (BMI) Calculator
```

---

[1] http://www.cdc.gov/healthyweight/assessing/bmi/adult_bmi.

```ruby
loop do
  print "Weight [lb]? "
  weight = gets.chomp  # Get weight in pounds as entered by the user

  print "Height [in]? "
  height = gets.chomp  # Get height in inches as entered by the user

  # Calculate BMI based on provided weight and height
  bmi = (weight.to_f / height.to_f ** 2) * 703

  # Determine weight status based on calculated BMI
  if bmi < 18.5
    status = "Underweight"
  elsif bmi < 25.0
    status = "Normal Weight"
  elsif bmi < 30.0
    status = "Overweight"
  else
    status = "Obese"
  end

  # Print BMI value and Status
  printf "BMI = %.2f and Status = #{status}\n", bmi

  # Prompt user to either continue or quit
  print "\nPress any key to continue or 'q' to quit: "
  command = gets

  # Exit the program
  if command =~ /q|Q/
    puts "For more information about BMI, go to:"
    puts "http://www.cdc.gov/healthyweight/assessing/bmi/"
    break
  end
end
```

```
$ ruby bmi_calc.rb
Weight [lb]? 200
Height [in]? 70
BMI = 28.69 and Status = Overweight

Press any key to continue or 'q' to quit: c
```

```
Weight [lb]? 130
Height [in]? 62
BMI = 23.77 and Status = Normal Weight

Press any key to continue or 'q' to quit: q
For more information about BMI, go to:
http://www.cdc.gov/healthyweight/assessing/bmi/
```

B.6 DIRECTORIES AND FILES

So far, the examples provided in this primer have involved using input specified within the program (e.g., as values assigned to variables) or provided by a user (e.g., as part of an interactive program). In addition, the output has primarily been displayed on the screen (e.g., using `puts` or `print` statements). Another source of input and output is files that can be read from and written to. In Ruby, the `Dir` and `File` classes include methods for working with directories and files respectively.

The `Dir` class includes methods for creating (`mkdir`), removing (`mkdir`), and changing (`chdir`) directories as well as getting the path of the directory (`pwd`). To get a list of files within a directory, the `entries` or `foreach` methods can be used, which will return all files, hidden files, and other directories (including "`.`" for the current directory and "`..`" for the parent directory). To only show files matching a particular pattern, the `glob` method can be used. All of these methods can either take the absolute path or relative path of a directory as an argument. In the following example, assume that there exists a directory called `data_files` that contains three files: `fruits.txt`, `vegetables.txt`, and `grains.txt`.

```ruby
#! /usr/local/bin/ruby

# read_dir.rb
# Demonstrates listing entries in a directory

# List files using entries method
puts "Listing 1:"
Dir.entries("data_files").each { |file| puts "  #{file}"}

# List files using foreach method
puts "Listing 2:"
Dir.foreach("data_files").each do |file|
  next if file == "." || file == ".."
```

```
   puts "  #{file}"
end
# List files using glob method
puts "Listing 3:"
Dir.glob("data_files/*.txt").each do |file|
   puts "  #{file.gsub("data_files/", "")}"
end
```

```
$ ruby read_dir.rb
Listing 1:
   .
   ..
   fruits.txt
   vegetables.txt
   grains.txt
Listing 2:
   fruits.txt
   vegetables.txt
   grains.txt
Listing 3:
   fruits.txt
   vegetables.txt
   grains.txt
```

For individual files, the File class has methods for creating (new), open-ing (open), and closing (close) files. The new and open methods take two arguments: the first is the filename and the second is the file mode (e.g., "w" for writing to a file anew [thus overwriting an existing file if it already exists] or "a" for appending to a file). The following example shows how to read lines from fruits.txt, add some additional text to each line, and then output the results to another file called fruits_modified.txt.

```
#! /usr/local/bin/ruby

# modify_file.rb
# Demonstrates how to read from, modify, and write to a file

input_file = "fruits.txt"
output_file = "fruits_modified.txt"

output = File.new(output_file, "w")
input = File.open(input_file)
```

```
input.each do |line|
  line.chomp!

# Add line number and "!" to the end of each line
  output.puts "#{input.lineno}: #{line}!"
end

input.close
output.close
```

```
$ ls
fruits.txt    grains.txt    modify_file.rb         vegetables.txt
$ more fruits.txt
apple
orange
banana
pear
grape
$ ruby modify_file.rb
$ ls
fruits_modified.txt  fruits.txt  grains.txt  modify_file.rb  vegetables.txt
$ more fruits_modified.txt
1: apple!
2: orange!
3: banana!
4: pear!
5: grape!
```

B.7 REGULAR EXPRESSIONS

Regular expressions (regex) are powerful tools for pattern matching and text processing. A regex is represented as /pattern/ where pattern consists of a special set of characters to search for in a string. To perform case-insensitive matches, the "i" option can be used (e.g., /pattern/i).

The Regexp class includes the match method for returning matches for a specified pattern in a string as a MatchData object that encapsulates all results (or nil if no match). The =~ operator can also be used that will return the character position for where the match starts while the !~ operator returns true if there is no match (and false otherwise). The String class also has the match method and =~ operator in addition to the scan

method that finds all matches for a pattern in a string and returns an array
(see Section B.8 for more details about arrays).

```
title = "Methods in Biomedical Informatics"

/in/.match(title)          # =>   #<MatchData "in">
/in/.match(title)[0]       # =>   "in"
/in/ =~ title              # =>   8

title.match(/in/)          # =>   #<MatchData "in">
title.match(/in/)[0]       # =>   "in"
title =~ /in/              # =>   8
title =~ /IN/              # =>   nil
title =~ /IN/i             # =>   8
title !~ /in/              # =>   false
title.scan(/in/i)          # =>   ["in", "In"]
```

A **character class** specifies a list of characters to match ([. . .] where . . .
represents the list) or not match ([^. . .]). For example, [aeiou] will
match any lowercase vowel, [0-9] any digit, [a-z] any lowercase letter,
[A-Z] any uppercase letter, and [a-zA-Z0-9] any digit, lowercase letter, or uppercase letter. On the other hand, [^aeiou] will match anything
except a lowercase vowel, [^0-9] anything except a digit, and [^] for
anything except a space.

```
title.match(/[aeiou]/)        # => #<MatchData "e">
title.match(/[aeiou]/)[0]     # => "e"
title.match(/[^0-9]/)[0]      # => "M"

title =~ /[a-zA-Z0-9]/        # => 0
title =~ /[^a-zA-Z\s]/        # => nil
title !~ /[1-5]/              # => true

title.scan(/[BMI]/)           # => ["M", "B", "I"]
title.scan(/[aeiou]/)         # => ["e", "o", "i",
                              #     "i", "o", "e", "i",
                              #     "a", "o", "a", "i"]
```

The following metacharacters behave like character classes: "." matches
any character except a newline, "\w" any word character (equivalent to
[a-zA-Z0-9_]), "\W" any non-word character (equivalent to [^a-zA-
Z0-9_]), "\d" a digit character (equivalent to [0-9]), "\D" any non-digit

character (equivalent to [^0-9]), "\s" any whitespace character (equivalent to [\t\r\n\f]), and "\S" any non-whitespace character (equivalent to [^\t\r\n\f]).

```
date = "1998-MAR-27"

date.match(/\w/)        # =>  #<MatchData "1">
date.match(/\W/)        # =>  #<MatchData "-">
date =~ /\s/            # =>  nil
date =~ /\S/            # =>  0
date.scan(/\d/)         # =>  ["1", "9", "9", "8", "2", "7"]
date.scan(/\D/)         # =>  ["-", "M", "A", "R", "-"]
date.scan(/./)          # =>  ["1", "9", "9", "8", "-", "M", "A",
                               R", "-", "2", "7"]
```

The pipe ("|") character can be used to specify **alternative** expressions to match. For example, the pattern /bio|med/ will try to match either "bio" or "med" in a string.

```
"medical".match(/bio|med/)       # =>  #<MatchData "med">
"biological" =~ /bio|med/        # =>  0
"biomedical".scan(/bio|med/)     # =>  ["bio", "med"]
```

Anchors are special characters that can be used to match a pattern at a specified position. For example, "^" specifies to match at the beginning of a line and "$" the end of a line while "\A" and "\Z" specify matching at the beginning and end of a string respectively. The following examples demonstrate the use of these anchors for a string that includes 5 lines delimited by the newline character ("\n").

```
list = "biological\nmedical\nbiomedical\npublic health\nhealth"

list.match(/^med/)               # =>  #<MatchData "med">
list.match(/\Amed/)              # =>  nil
list=~ /cal$/                    # =>  7
list=~ /cal\Z/                   # =>  nil
list.scan(/^bio|health$/)        # =>  ["bio", "bio", "health", "health"]
list.scan(/\Abio|health\Z/)      # =>  ["bio", "health"]
```

Repetition or **quantifier** characters can be used to specify the number of times to match a particular character or set of characters. Quantifiers include "*" for zero or more times, "+" for one or more times, "?" for zero or one time (optional), "{n}" for exactly n times, "{n,}" for n or more times,

"{,m}" for m or less times, and "{n,m}" for at least n and at most m times. By default, repetition performs greedy matching meaning it will try to match as many occurrences as possible. Non-greedy or lazy matching will try to find the fewest characters needed to match and can be specified by adding "?" to the end of the aforementioned quantifiers. The following examples demonstrate the use of different quantifier characters for finding patterns of digits in phone numbers and dates.

```
"555-788-2323".match(/5+/)        # =>  #<MatchData "555">
"555-788-2323".match(/5+?/)       # =>  #<MatchData "5">
"555-788-2323".scan(/[0-9]{3,}/)  # =>  ["555", "788", "2323"]
```

```
"1998-MAR-27".match(/[0-9]{2,4}-[A-Z]{3}-[0-9]{2}/)
# => #<MatchData "1998-MAR-27">

"98-MAR-27".match(/[0-9]{2,4}-[A-Z]{3}-[0-9]{2}/)
# => #<MatchData "98-MAR-27">

"98-MAR-27".match(/\d{2,4}-\w{3}-\d{2}/)
# => #<MatchData "98-MAR-27">
```

Parentheses can be used to **group** part of an expression and/or **capture** the text or substring matching a particular pattern. Text matching the first, second, and any additional capture groups are stored in global variables such as $1 and $2 where the number represents the order of parentheses.

```
"1998-MAR-27".match(/(\d{2,4})-(\w{3})-(\d{2})/)
# => #<MatchData "1998-MAR-27" 1:"1998" 2:"MAR" 3:"27">

puts "Year = " + $1        # =>  Year = 1998
puts "Month = " + $2       # =>  Month = MAR
puts "Day = " + $3         # =>  Day = 27

"1998-MAR-27".scan(/((\d{2,4})-(\w{3})-(\d{2}))/)
# => [["1998-MAR-27", "1998", "MAR", "27"]]

puts "Date = #{$1}, Year = #{$2}, Month = #{$3}, Day = #{$4}"
# => Date = 1998-MAR-27, Year = 1998, Month = MAR, Day = 27
```

Within a regular expression, there are several characters that have a specific meaning and must be "escaped" using the backslash ("\") to use them literally. These metacharacters include those that have been described throughout this section such as "(", ")", "[", "]", "{", "}", ".", "?", "+", and "*". For example, to match actual parentheses, the pattern would include "\ (" or "\ )"

```
"Multiplication: [5*2]" =~ /\[([0-9]\*[0-9])\]/      # =>    16
puts $1                                             # =>    5*2

"Addition: (7+3)" =~ /\(([0-9]\+[0-9])\)/           # =>    10
puts $1                                             # =>    7+3
```

The gsub (or gsub!) and split (or split!) methods were introduced in Section B.4 for performing string substitution and splitting. These methods can either take a specific substring or a pattern as arguments.

```
date = "1998-MAR-27"

date.gsub(/[0-9]/, "*")       # => "****-MAR-**"
date.split(/-[A-Z]{3}-/)      # => ["1998", "27"]
```

B.7.1 **Parsing PubMed/MEDLINE Records**

To demonstrate the use of regular expressions, let's parse and transform a file called pubmed_result.txt that includes a set of MEDLINE records from PubMed. The contents of this file are based on performing a search for "National Library of Medicine (U.S.)"[mh] and "PubMed"[mh] and "Teaching"[mh] in PubMed (http://www.ncbi.nlm.nih.gov/pubmed), choosing "File" as the Destination under "Send to", and selecting "MEDLINE" as the Format (other formats include Summary, Abstract, and XML). Below is an example of one record where descriptions of each element or field can be found at: http://www.nlm.nih.gov/bsd/mms/medlineelements.html. For example, "PMID" refers to the PubMed Unique Identifier, "DA" for date created, "TI" for title, "FAU" for full author name, "MH" for MeSH headings, and "MHDA" for the date MeSH headings were added. For the MeSH headings, subheadings are listed after the "/" and a "*" at the beginning of a heading or subheading indicates a major topic.

```
PMID- 20570844
OWN - NLM
STAT- MEDLINE
DA  - 20101122
DCOM- 20110406
LR  - 20111101
IS  - 1477-4054 (Electronic)
```

```
IS  - 1467-5463 (Linking)
VI  - 11
IP  - 6
DP  - 2010 Nov
TI  - Education resources of the National Center for Biotechnology
      Information.
PG  - 563-9
LID - 10.1093/bib/bbq022 [doi]
AB  - The National Center for Biotechnology Information (NCBI) hosts 39
      literature and molecular biology databases containing almost half
      a billion records. As the complexity of these data and associated
      resources and tools continues to expand, so does the need for edu-
      cational resources to help investigators, clinicians, information
      specialists and the general public make use of the wealth of public
      data available at the NCBI. This review describes the educational
      resources available at NCBI via the NCBI Education page (www.ncbi.
      nlm.nih.gov/Education/). These resources include materials designed
      for new users, such as About NCBI and the NCBI Guide, as well as
      documentation, Frequently Asked Questions (FAQs) and writings on the
      NCBI Bookshelf such as the NCBI Help Manual and the NCBI Handbook.
      NCBI also provides teaching materials such as tutorials, problem sets
      and educational tools such as the Amino Acid Explorer, PSSM Viewer
      and Ebot. NCBI also offers training programs including the Discovery
      Workshops, webinars and tutorials at conferences. To help users keep
      up-to-date, NCBI produces the online NCBI News and offers RSS feeds
      and mailing lists, along with a presence on Facebook, Twitter and
      YouTube.
AD  - NCBI/NLM/NIH, 45 Center Drive, Bethesda, MD 20892, USA. cooper@ncbi.
      nlm.nih.gov
FAU - Cooper, Peter S
AU  - Cooper PS
FAU - Lipshultz, Dawn
AU  - Lipshultz D
FAU - Matten, Wayne T
AU  - Matten WT
FAU - McGinnis, Scott D
AU  - McGinnis SD
FAU - Pechous, Steven
AU  - Pechous S
FAU - Romiti, Monica L
AU  - Romiti ML
FAU - Tao, Tao
```

```
AU  - Tao T
FAU - Valjavec-Gratian, Majda
AU  - Valjavec-Gratian M
FAU - Sayers, Eric W
AU  - Sayers EW
LA  - eng
PT  - Journal Article
PT  - Research Support, N.I.H., Intramural
PT  - Review
DEP - 20100622
PL  - England
TA  - Brief Bioinform
JT  - Briefings in bioinformatics
JID - 100912837
SB  - IM
MH  - Computational Biology/*education/methods
MH  - Databases, Factual
MH  - Internet
MH  - National Institutes of Health (U.S.)
MH  - *National Library of Medicine (U.S.)
MH  - PubMed
MH  - Teaching/*methods
MH  - United States
PMC - PMC2984538
OID - NLM: PMC2984538
EDAT- 2010/06/24 06:00
MHDA- 2011/04/07 06:00
CRDT- 2010/06/24 06:00
PHST- 2010/06/22 [aheadofprint]
AID - bbq022 [pii]
AID - 10.1093/bib/bbq022 [doi]
PST - ppublish
SO  - Brief Bioinform. 2010 Nov;11(6):563-9.
        doi: 10.1093/bib/bbq022. Epub 2010 Jun 22.
```

The script below performs the following tasks: (1) extracts the PubMed unique identifier from the PMID line; (2) extracts year from the DA line (format: YYYYMMDD); (3) extracts the title that may span one or more lines; (4) identifies authors from the FAU lines with a last name that ends with or first name that begins with "M" to "Z" and concatenates the author names with a ";"; (5) extracts and concatenates MeSH headings that begin with "A" to "L" from the MH lines; and, (6) extracts the year, month, and day from the MHDA line (format: YYYY/MM/DD HH:MM) and transforms the format to YYYY-MM-DD. The last step is to display the extracted and transformed information in a single pipe-delimited line for each record.

```ruby
#! /usr/local/bin/ruby

# parse_medline.rb
# Demonstrates use of regular expressions for parsing
# and transforming fields in MEDLINE records

first_record_flag = 0
field = ""
pmid = created_year = title = authors = mesh_headings = mesh_date = ""

File.open("pubmed_result.txt").each do |line|
      line.chomp!

      # Print information for each article after reaching
      # record separator (blank line)
      if line == ""
            # Print after first record has been processed
            if first_record_flag == 1
                  # Print information for each article
                  print "#{pmid}|#{created_year}|#{title}|#{authors}|"
                  print "#{mesh_headings}|#{mesh_date}\n\n"

                  # Clear values for variables
                  pmid = created_year = title = authors = ""
                  mesh_headings = mesh_date = ""
            end
            # Set flag for first record
            first_record_flag = 1
      end

      # Get field name ("PMID", "TI", "MH", etc.)
      if line =~ /^([A-Z]+)/
            field = $1
      end

      # Get PubMed unique identifier (PMID field)
```

```ruby
    # Example: PMID- 20570844
    if line =~ /PMID- ([0-9]*)/
          pmid = $1
    end

    # Get year from created date (DA field)
    # Example: DA  - 20101122
    if line =~ /^DA   - ([0-9]{4})[0-9]{2}[0-9]{2}/
          created_year = $1
    end

    # Get title (TI field)
    # Example:
    # TI  - Education resources of the National Center for Biotechnology …
    if line =~ /TI  - (.*)/
          title = $1
    end

    # Get title - if wraps onto multiple lines (TI field)
    # Example:
    # TI  - Searching MEDLINE free on the Internet using the National …
    #        PubMed.
    if line =~ /^\s{6}(.*)/ and field.eql?("TI")
          title = title + " " + $1
    end

    # Get list of authors (FAU field)
    # Only include those with last names ending with M to Z
    # or first names beginning with M to Z
    # Example formats:
    #   FAU - Sayers, Eric W
    #   FAU - Pechous, Steven
    #   FAU - DeGeorges, K M
    if line =~ /^FAU - ([^,]+),\s([^\s]+)\s?(.+)?/
          last_name = $1
          first_name = $2

          if first_name =~ /^[M-Z]/i or last_name =~ /[M-Z]$/i
                # Concatenate author names meeting criteria
                if authors == ""
```

```
                        authors = first_name + " " + last_name
                else
                        authors = authors + ", " + first_name + " " + last_name
                end
            end
        end


        # Get list of MeSH headings (MH field)
        # Only get headings that start with A to L
        # Example formats:
        #    MH  - Computational Biology/*education/methods
        #    MH  - *National Library of Medicine (U.S.)
        #    MH  - Databases, Factual
        if line =~ /MH   - \*?([A-L][^\/]*)/
            if mesh_headings == ""
                mesh_headings = $1
            else
                mesh_headings = mesh_headings + "^" + $1
            end
        end


        # Get MeSH date (MHDA field)
        # Example: MHDA- 2011/04/07 06:00
        if line =~ /MHDA- ([0-9]{4})\/([0-9]{2})\/([0-9]{2})\s[0-9]{2}\:[0-9]{2}/
            mesh_date = $1 + "-" + $2 + "-" + $3
        end
    end
end

# Print information for last record
print "#{pmid}|#{created_year}|#{title}|#{authors}|"
print "#{mesh_headings}|#{mesh_date}\n\n"
```

```
$ ruby parse_medline.rb
20570844|2010|Education resources of the National Center for Biotechnology
Information.|Peter Cooper, Dawn Lipshultz, Wayne Matten, Scott McGinnis,
Steven Pechous, Monica Romiti, Tao Tao, Majda Valjavec-Gratian, Eric
Sayers|Computational Biology^Databases, Factual^Internet|2011-04-07

12869862|2003|Recall to precision: retrieving clinical information with
MEDLINE.|Mollie Poynton|Computer User Training^Humans^Information Storage
and Retrieval|2003-10-04
```

```
11329561|2001|Using the National Library of Medicine's PubMed to improve
clinical practice.|D Dollar|Computer User Training^Humans^Interlibrary
Loans^Internet|2002-02-02

10455581|1999|Searching MEDLINE free on the Internet using the National
Library of Medicine's PubMed.|N Putnam|Computer User Training^Hotlines^Huma
ns^Internet|1999-08-24

9919086|1999|Help! I need a MEDLINE search!|K DeGeorges|Computer User Train
ing^Humans^Internet|1999-01-27

9803302|1999|The Healthnet project: extending online information resources
to end users in rural hospitals.|E Holtum, S Zollo|Computer User Training^
Databases, Bibliographic^Hospitals, Rural^Iowa|1998-11-06

9431431|1998|Health information networking via the Internet with the for-
mer Soviet Union.||Computer Communication Networks^Computer User Training^
Cross-Cultural Comparison^Data Collection^Databases, Bibliographic^Grateful
Med^Health Resources^Information Services^Information Storage and Retrieval^
International Cooperation|1998-02-12

8655874|1996|Accessing MEDLINE from the dental office.|W Lang|Automatic Data
Processing^CD-ROM^Computer Systems^Computer User Training^Dental Offices^De
ntists^Documentation^Humans|1996-04-01

8655874|1996|Accessing MEDLINE from the dental office.|W Lang|Automatic
Data Processing^CD-ROM^Computer Systems^Computer User Training^Dental Offic
es^Dentists^Documentation^Humans|1996-04-01
```

B.8 ARRAYS AND HASHES

Arrays and hashes are indexed collections of objects. An **array** is an ordered sequence of elements that are automatically indexed (consecutively numbered) by an integer starting with 0. A **hash** is an unordered collection of key-value pairs where the key serves as the index, can be any type of Ruby object (e.g., Integer, String, or Array), and must be unique. Figure B.1 depicts two arrays (season_array and semester_array) and two hashes (season_hash and semester_hash) that will be used to demonstrate methods for working with these types of data structures.

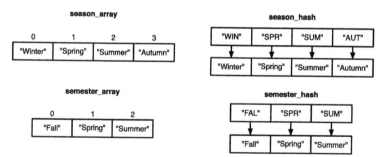

■ **FIGURE B.1** Example arrays and hashes.

B.8.1 **Creating Arrays and Hashes**

Arrays and hashes can be created using the `new` method. For arrays, this method can take two arguments that specify the size of the array and a default value. A default value can similarly be specified for hashes. Once created, use the `size` or `length` method to determine the number of elements or key-value pairs (e.g., `season_array.size` or `season_hash.length`).

```
season_array = Array.new
semester_array = Array.new(3, "semester")

season_hash = Hash.new
semester_hash = Hash.new("semester")
```

To remove all contents from an array or hash, use the `clear` method (e.g., `semester_array.clear` or `semester_hash.clear`). The `empty?` method can be used to determine if an array or hash is empty.

B.8.2 **Working with Arrays**

There are multiple ways to populate an array with the `[ ]` method:

```
season_array = Array.[]("Winter", "Spring", "Summer", "Autumn")
season_array = Array["Winter", "Spring", "Summer", "Autumn"]
season_array = ["Winter", "Spring", "Summer", "Autumn"]
season_array = %w[Winter Spring Summer Autumn]

semester_array = ["Fall", "Spring", "Summer"]
```

The [] or at method can be used to access elements within an array by specifying the index number. The first and last methods can be used to return the first and last elements respectively. Ranges can also be specified using [] or slice.

```
season_array[0]              # =>   "Winter"
season_array.at(2)           # =>   "Summer"
season_array[-1]             # =>   "Autumn"
season_array[-3]             # =>   "Spring"
season_array.first           # =>   "Winter"
season_array.last            # =>   "Autumn"
season_array[0, 2]           # =>   ["Winter", "Spring"]
season_array[1..3]           # =>   ["Spring", "Summer", "Autumn"]
season_array.slice(1...3)    # =>   ["Spring", "Summer"]
```

Alternatively, to determine if a particular value is in an array, the include? method tests if the array includes an element with a specified value. For determining where a particular value is in an array, index returns the first element that matches and rindex returns the last element that matches.

```
season_array.include? "Autumn"    # => true
season_array.include? "Fall"      # => false
season_array.index "Spring"       # => 1
season_array.rindex "Summer"      # => 2
```

There are several methods for adding, modifying, or deleting elements in an array. push and pop treat an array like a stack (Last In, First Out [LIFO]) by adding an element to the end and removing an element from the front, respectively. In the examples below and throughout this section, graphical representations of the resulting array (or hash) are shown.

```
season_array                        0         1         2         3
                                 +--------+--------+--------+--------+
                                 |"Winter"|"Spring"|"Summer"|"Autumn"|
                                 +--------+--------+--------+--------+

season_array.pop                    0         1         2
                                 +--------+--------+--------+
                                 |"Winter"|"Spring"|"Summer"|
                                 +--------+--------+--------+

season_array.push "Fall"            0         1         2         3
                                 +--------+--------+--------+--------+
                                 |"Winter"|"Spring"|"Summer"| "Fall" |
                                 +--------+--------+--------+--------+
```

`shift` and `unshift` treat an array like a queue (First In, First Out [FIFO])
by adding and removing an element to the beginning, respectively.

```
semester_array                              0         1        2
                                    +--------+--------+--------+
                                    |  "Fall" |"Spring"|"Summer"|
                                    +--------+--------+--------+
semester_array.shift                        0         1
                                    +--------+--------+
                                    |"Spring"|"Summer"|
                                    +--------+--------+
semester_array.unshift "Autumn"             0         1        2
                                    +--------+--------+--------+
                                    |"Autumn"|"Spring"|"Summer"|
                                    +--------+--------+--------+
```

The `delete` and `delete_at` methods will remove the element with a
specified value or at a specified location, respectively. The `insert` method
can be used to add one or more values before a specified index location. The
`[]` method can also be used to change values at a specific location or range.

```
semester_array.insert(1, "WINTER")          0         1        2        3
                                    +--------+--------+--------+--------+
                                    |"Autumn"|"WINTER"|"Spring"|"Summer"|
                                    +--------+--------+--------+--------+
semester_array[2] = "SPRING"                0         1        2        3
                                    +--------+--------+--------+--------+
                                    |"Autumn"|"WINTER"|"SPRING"|"Summer"|
                                    +--------+--------+--------+--------+
semester_array.delete "WINTER"              0         1        2
                                    +--------+--------+--------+
                                    |"Autumn"|"SPRING"|"Summer"|
                                    +--------+--------+--------+
```

Similar to other classes, comparison operators (`==`, `<=>`, or `eql?`) can be
used to compare arrays. There are also set operators for determining the
intersection (`&`), difference (`-`), and union (`|`) of arrays.

```
season_array == semester_array       # =>  false
season_array <=> semester_array      # =>  1
season_array & semester_array        # =>  ["Summer"]
season_array - semester_array        # =>  ["Winter", "Spring", "Fall"]
```

```
semester_array - season_array          # =>   ["Autumn", "SPRING"]
season_array | semester_array          # =>   ["Winter", "Spring", "Summer",
                                               "Fall", "Autumn", "SPRING"]
```

Similar to strings, arrays can be concatenated using the "+" operator. To identify unique elements in an array, use the uniq (or uniq!) method. For sorting, the sort (or sort!) method can be used.

```
combined_array = season_array + semester_array
# => ["Winter", "Spring", "Summer", "Fall", "Autumn", "SPRING", "Summer"]

combined_array.sort
# => ["Autumn", "Fall", "SPRING", "Spring", "Summer", "Summer", "Winter"]

combined_array.uniq
# => ["Winter", "Spring", "Summer", "Fall", "Autumn", "SPRING"]

combined_array.sort.uniq
# => ["Autumn", "Fall", "SPRING", "Spring", "Summer", "Winter"]
```

To convert an array to a string (e.g., for printing), use .to_s, inspect, or join. With the join method, a separator can be specified for delimiting each element.

```
season_array.join                      # =>   "WinterSpringSummerFall"
season_array.join", "                  # =>   "Winter, Spring, Summer, Fall"
season_array.join"---"                 # =>   "Winter---Spring---Summer---Fall"
```

B.8.3 Working with Hashes

Similar to arrays, hashes can be populated using the [ ] method or with { }.

```
semester_hash = Hash["FAL", "Fall", "SPR", "Spring", "SUM", "Summer"]
semester_hash = Hash["FAL" => "Fall", "SPR" => "Spring", "SUM" => "Summer"]
semester_hash = {"FAL" => "Fall", "SPR" => "Spring", "SUM" => "Summer"}

season_hash = {"WIN" => "Winter", "SPR" => "Spring", "SUM" => "Summer",
"AUT" => "Autumn"}
```

There are several ways of accessing keys and values in a hash. has_key?, key?, member?, or include? can be used to check for the existence of a particular key while has_value? or value? can be used to check for a particular value. The `keys` method will return an array of all keys in a hash, `values_at` will return an array of values based on one or more keys, and `[ ]` will retrieve a single value based on a specified key. The `values` method will return an array with all values and `key` will return a key for a specified value.

```
semester_hash.has_key? "SPR"              # =>  true
semester_hash.has_value? "Winter"         # =>  false
semester_hash.keys                        # =>  ["FAL", "SPR", "SUM"]
semester_hash.values                      # =>  ["Fall", "Spring", "Summer"]
semester_hash["SPR"]                      # =>  "Spring"
semester_hash.values_at "FAL", "SUM"      # =>  ["Fall", "Summer"]
semester_hash.key "Spring"                # =>  "SPR"
```

The `[ ]` or `store` method can also be used to add or change key-value pairs in a hash. To delete key-value pairs, use the `delete` method.

```
semester_hash                   +--------+        +--------+
                                | "FAL"  | ==> | "Fall" |
                                +--------+        +--------+
                                | "SPR"  | ==> |"Spring"|
                                +--------+        +--------+
                                | "SUM"  | ==> |"Summer"|
                                +--------+        +--------+
semester_hash.delete("FAL")     +--------+        +--------+
                                | "SPR"  | ==> |"Spring"|
                                +--------+        +--------+
                                | "SUM"  | ==> |"Summer"|
                                +--------+        +--------+
semester_hash["AUT"] = "Autumn" +--------+        +--------+
                                | "SPR"  | ==> |"Spring"|
                                +--------+        +--------+
                                | "SUM"  | ==> |"Summer"|
                                +--------+        +--------+
                                | "AUT"  | ==> |"Autumn"|
                                +--------+        +--------+
semester_hash["SPR"] = "SPRING" +--------+        +--------+
                                | "SPR"  | ==> |"SPRING"|
                                +--------+        +--------+
                                | "SUM"  | ==> |"Summer"|
                                +--------+        +--------+
                                | "AUT"  | ==> |"Autumn"|
                                +--------+        +--------+
```

Hashes can be combined using the merge (or merge!) method, which will remove duplicate keys by overwriting key-value pairs.

```
season_hash.merge semester_hash
# => {"WIN"=>"Winter", "SPR"=>"SPRING", "SUM"=>"Summer", "AUT"=>"Autumn"}

semester_hash.merge season_hash
# => {"SPR"=>"Spring", "SUM"=>"Summer", "AUT"=>"Autumn", "WIN"=>"Winter"}
```

To sort a hash by keys, use the sort method.

```
semester_hash
# => {"SPR"=>"SPRING", "SUM"=>"Summer", "AUT"=>"Autumn"}


semester_hash.sort
# => [["AUT", "Autumn"], ["SPR", "SPRING"], ["SUM", "Summer"]]
```

each (or each_pair), each_key, and each_value can be used to iterate over a hash (e.g., for printing).

```
semester_hash.each {|key, value| puts "#{key} = #{value}"}
# => SPR = SPRING
# => SUM = Summer
# => AUT = Autumn

semester_hash.each_key {|key| puts "Key = #{key}"}
# => Key = SPR
# => Key = SUM
# => Key = AUT

semester_hash.each_value {|value| puts "Value = #{value}"}
# => Value = SPRING
# => Value = Summer
# => Value = Autumn
```

B.8.4 Working with Multi-Dimensional Arrays and Hashes

The discussion thus far has focused on single-dimensional structures. Multi-dimensional arrays (array of arrays or array of hashes) and hashes (hash of hashes or hash of arrays) can also be created and used. Figure B.2 depicts

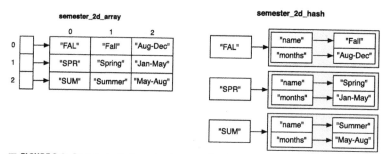

■ FIGURE B.2 Example multi-dimensional arrays and hashes.

a two-dimensional array (`semester_2d_array`) and a two-dimensional hash (`semester_2d_hash`) that will be used to demonstrate methods for working with these multi-dimensional structures, which can be viewed as a table or matrix with rows and columns.

Like single-dimensional arrays, a multi-dimensional array (two-dimensional, three-dimensional, etc.) can be created using the `new` method and elements can be accessed using [ ].

```
semester_2d_array = Array.new(Array.new)
semester_2d_array = [["FAL", "Fall", "Aug-Dec"], ["SPR", "Spring",
"Jan-May"], ["SUM", "Summer", "May-Aug"]]
```

```
semester_2d_array[0][1]           # =>  "Fall"
semester_2d_array[1][2]           # =>  "Jan-May"
semester_2d_array[2][0]           # =>  "SUM"
```

The `flatten` method will turn a multi-dimensional array into a single-dimensional array and `transpose` method will transpose the rows and columns in a two-dimensional array.

```
semester_2d_array.flatten
# => ["FAL", "Fall", "Aug-Dec", "SPR", "Spring", "Jan-May", "SUM", "Summer",
     "May-Aug"]

semester_2d_array.transpose
# => [["FAL", "SPR", "SUM"], ["Fall", "Spring", "Summer"], ["Aug-Dec",
     "Jan-May", "May-Aug"]]
```

Similarly, multi-dimensional hashes can be created using the new method and key-value pairs accessed using the various methods (e.g., [], keys, has_key?, and values).

```
semester_2d_hash = Hash.new{|hash, key| hash[key] = Hash.new}
semester_2d_hash = { "FAL" => { "name" => "Fall", "months" => "Aug-Dec" },
"SPR" => { "name" => "Spring", "months" => "Jan-May" }, "SUM" => { "name"
=> "Summer", "months" => "May-Aug" } }
```

```
semester_2d_hash.keys                       # =>  ["FAL", "SPR", "SUM"]
semester_2d_hash["FAL"].keys                # =>  ["name", "months"]
semester_2d_hash["FAL"].values              # =>  ["Fall", "Aug-Dec"]
semester_2d_hash["FAL"]["name"]             # =>  "Fall"
semester_2d_hash["SPR"]["months"]           # =>  "Jan-May"
semester_2d_hash["SUM"].has_key? "name"     # =>  true
semester_2d_hash["SUM"].has_value? "Summer" # =>  true
```

To print multi-dimensional arrays and hashes, nested each blocks (or each_pair, each_key, or each_value) can be used.

```
semester_2d_array.each do |row|
  row.each do |column|
    print "#{column}\t"
  end
  print "\n"
end
# => FAL      Fall     Aug-Dec
# => SPR      Spring   Jan-May
# => SUM      Summer   May-Aug
```

```
semester_2d_hash.each do |key, value|
  print "#{key}\t"
  value.each do |key2, value2|
    print "#{key2} = #{value2}\t"
  end
  print "\n"
end
# => FAL name = Fall      months = Aug-Dec
# => SPR name = Spring    months = Jan-May
# => SUM name = Summer    months = May-Aug
```

B.8.5 **Analyzing Conditions in Clinical Studies from ClinicalTrials.gov**

The following example demonstrates the use of single-dimensional arrays and hashes for analyzing a dataset of 3388 clinical studies related to obesity from ClinicalTrials.gov (http://www.clinicaltrials.gov) that was also used in Appendix A, Section A.8. The tab-delimited file study_fields.tsv includes the following fields: (1) Rank, (2) Title, (3) Recruitment Status, (4) Study Results, (5) Conditions, (6) Interventions, and (7) URL. Let's see how arrays and hashes can be used to obtain frequency counts for conditions listed in the Conditions field (Field 5) that may include one or more conditions separated by a "|" (e.g., "Hypertension|Obesity|Diabetes").

```ruby
#! /usr/local/bin/ruby

# count_conditions.rb
# Obtain frequency counts for conditions in the Conditions field (Field 5)
# of study_fields.tsv that contains information for 3,388 clinical studies
# related to obesity from ClinicalTrials.gov

# Create hash for counting frequency of each condition
# key = condition name, value = condition frequency (default value is 0)
count_hash = Hash.new(0)

# Open file with list of clinical studies
File.open("study_fields.tsv").each do |line|

    # Remove newline (\n) at end of line
    line.chomp!

    # Split line by "|" and store fields in an array
    fields_array = line.split("\t")

    # Get fifth element in array (Conditions field)
    conditions = fields_array[4]

    # Skip first line that includes field definitions
    next if conditions == "Conditions"

    # Split Conditions field by "|" and store conditions in an array
    # Example: Metabolic Syndrome|Abdominal Obesity|Heart Disease
    conditions_array = conditions.split("|")
```

```ruby
        # For each condition in the array, increment count
        conditions_array.each do |condition|
                # Increment count for specified condition
                count_hash[condition] += 1

                # Increment count for total number of conditions
                count_hash["TOTAL"] += 1
        end
end

# Print total number of unique conditions (i.e., key-value pairs)
print "Number of unique conditions: #{count_hash.size}\n\n"

# Print key-value pairs in hash in descending order based on frequency
count_hash.sort{|a,b| b[1] <=> a[1]}.each do |key, value|

        # Calculate proportion based on condition frequency and total frequency
        proportion = value.to_f / count_hash["TOTAL"].to_f

        # Print condition frequency, proportion, and name separated by tab (\t)
        printf "#{value}\t%.4f\t#{key}\n", proportion
end
```

```
$ ruby count_conditions.rb | more
Number of unique conditions: 1137

6726    1.0000   TOTAL
2283    0.3394   Obesity
306     0.0455   Overweight
164     0.0244   Hypertension
152     0.0226   Morbid Obesity
152     0.0226   Insulin Resistance
146     0.0217   Metabolic Syndrome
132     0.0196   Cardiovascular Diseases
121     0.0180   Diabetes
118     0.0175   Type 2 Diabetes
104     0.0155   Heart Diseases
67      0.0100   Type 2 Diabetes Mellitus
66      0.0098   Diabetes Mellitus
60      0.0089   Cardiovascular Disease
```

```
 60      0.0089  Weight Loss
 60      0.0089  Childhood Obesity
 59      0.0088  Diabetes Mellitus, Type 2
 48      0.0071  Healthy
 48      0.0071  Obese
 41      0.0061  Polycystic Ovary Syndrome
 35      0.0052  Metabolic Syndrome X
  :
```

B.8.6 **Analyzing Demographics in Mortality Records**

The following example demonstrates the use of single-dimensional arrays, single-dimensional hashes, and two-dimensional hashes for analyzing vital statistics, particularly mortality multiple cause-of-death public use records from 2010 (files and documentation accessible from http://www.cdc.gov/nchs/data_access/vitalstatsonline.htm). The file VS10MORT.DUSMCPUB includes 2,472,542 records (lines) with 488 characters per record where an individual field may be a single character or group of characters. For example, in the example record below, character 63 represents the code for education (e.g., "1" for "8th grade or less" and "9" for "Unknown"), character 84 represents the code for Marital Status (e.g., "S" for "Never married, single" and "M" for "Married"), and characters 146 to 149 include the ICD-10 code for the underlying cause of death (e.g., "E668" for "Other obesity" [E66.8] and "J459" for "Asthma, unspecified" [J45.9]).

```
                      1                               1101 M1048
  351507 M2M2                    2010U7BN
 E668E668169 111     37 0211I516 21E668

 02 E668 I516
 01   11                                    100 6
```

Let's focus on records with obesity as the underlying cause of death (ICD-10 codes starting with "E66"), determine the frequency of each ICD-10 code, and build a matrix containing frequencies by education and marital status for this population.

```ruby
#! /usr/local/bin/ruby

# create_matrix.rb
# For records with an obesity-related underlying cause of death
# (ICD-10 code starting with "E66"), determine distribution of each code
```

```ruby
# and build matrix of distribution by education and marital status
# for this population

# Create arrays and hashes for use as look-up tables
education_array = Array.new
marital_status_hash = Hash.new
icd10_codes_hash = Hash.new

# Create single- and two-dimensional hashes for keeping track of
# frequencies
count_hash = Hash.new(0)
matrix_hash = Hash.new{|hash, key| hash[key] = Hash.new(0)}

# Populate single-dimensional array for education descriptions
# Source: http://www.cdc.gov/nchs/nvss/mortality_public_use_data.htm
# Note: since there is no code "0", nil is used
education_array = [nil, "8th grade or less", "9 - 12th grade, no diploma",
"high school graduate or GED completed", "some college credit, but no
degree", "Associate degree", "Bachelor's degree", "Master's degree",
"Doctorate or professional degree", "Unknown"]

# Populate single-dimensional hash for marital status
# key = marital status code, value = marital status description
# Source: http://www.cdc.gov/nchs/nvss/mortality_public_use_data.htm
marital_status_hash = { "S" => "Never married, single", "M" => "Married",
"W" => "Widowed", "D" => "Divorced", "U" => "Marital Status unknown" }

# Populate single-dimensional hash for underlying cause of death
# Limited to ICD-10 codes starting with "E66" (obesity-related)
# Source: http://apps.who.int/classifications/icd10
icd10_codes_hash["E66"] = "Obesity"
icd10_codes_hash["E66.0"] = "Obesity due to excess calories"
icd10_codes_hash["E66.1"] = "Drug-induced obesity"
icd10_codes_hash["E66.2"] = "Extreme obesity with alveolar hypoventilation"
icd10_codes_hash["E66.8"] = "Other obesity"
icd10_codes_hash["E66.9"] = "Obesity, unspecified"

# File for 2010 mortality multiple cause-of-death public use records
mortality_file = "VS10MORT.DUSMCPUB"

# Open file and process each record (line)
```

```ruby
File.open(mortality_file).each do |line|

    line.chomp!                        # Remove newline (\n) at end of line

    education = line[62]               # Get education code (character 63)
    marital_status = line[83]          # Get marital status code (character 83)

    # Get ICD-10 code for underlying cause of death (characters 146 to 149)
    underlying_cause = line[145..148]

    # Determine if underlying cause of death is obesity-related
    # (focusing on ICD-10 codes starting with "E66")
    if underlying_cause =~ /^E66/
       # Reformat underlying cause of death code (e.g., E668 -> E66.8)
       underlying_cause.gsub!(/([A-Z0-9]{3})([0-9]+)/, '\1.\2')

       # Increment count for underlying cause of death code
       count_hash[underlying_cause] += 1

       # Increment count for education and marital status combination
       matrix_hash[education][marital_status] += 1
    end
end

# Print frequency of each underlying cause of death
puts "Distribution of Underlying Cause of Death".center(70, "*")
count_hash.sort{|a,b| b[1] <=> a[1]}.each do |cause_code, frequency|
      puts "#{frequency}\t#{cause_code}\t#{icd10_codes_hash[cause_code]}"
end

# Print matrix with frequencies for education and marital status
puts "Distribution of Education and Marital Status".center(70, "*")

# Print marital status codes (x-axis)
marital_status_hash.each_key do |status_code|
      print "#{status_code}\t"
end
print "\n"

# Print frequencies in each cell
```

```ruby
matrix_hash.each_key do |education_code|
      marital_status_hash.each_key do |status_code|
            if matrix_hash[education_code].has_key? status_code
                print "#{matrix_hash[education_code][status_code]}\t"
            else
                print "0\t"
            end
      end

      # Print education descriptions (y-axis)
      if education_code == " "
        puts "<empty value>"
      else
        puts "#{education_array[education_code.to_i]}\t"
      end
end

# Print key for marital status codes
puts "Key for Marital Status".center(70, "*")
marital_status_hash.each_key do |status_code|
      puts "#{status_code} = #{marital_status_hash[status_code]}"
end
```

```
$ ruby create_matrix.rb
***************Distribution of Underlying Cause of Death***************
3324    E66.8 Other obesity
2072    E66.9 Obesity, unspecified
128     E66.2 Extreme obesity with alveolar hypoventilation
24      E66.0 Obesity due to excess calories
*************Distribution of Education and Marital Status*************
S       M       W       D       U
414     622     223     298     7       <empty value>
518     625     205     367     7       high school graduate or GED completed
97      128     28      71      1       Bachelor's degree
65      75      67      37      2       8th grade or less
158     164     78      105     2       9 - 12th grade, no diploma
40      67      10      19      0       Master's degree
187     268     59      139     0       some college credit, but no degree
63      118     27      45      1       Associate degree
32      27      5       13      26      Unknown
```

```
10      16      6      6      0          Doctorate or professional degree
************************Key for Marital Status************************
S = Never married, single
M = Married
W = Widowed
D = Divorced
U = Marital Status unknown
```

B.9 **INTERACTIVE RUBY (irb)**

Interactive Ruby or irb provides an interactive command-line environment for Ruby that allows for real-time experimentation and is typically included with Ruby installations. In the Unix environment, the which command can be used to determine the location of irb and irb -v can be used to determine the version. At the Unix command prompt, type irb to enter the Interactive Ruby environment and exit or quit to exit.

```
$ which irb
/usr/local/bin/irb
$ irb -v
irb 0.9.5(05/04/13)
$ irb
irb(main):001:0> 1+2
=> 3
irb(main):002:0> exit
$
```

At the irb prompt, type in any Ruby statement or expression and see what results are returned. For example, try out the examples throughout this primer, particularly in Section B.4 (Strings), Section B.7 (Regular Expressions), and Section B.8 (Arrays and Hashes).

```
$ irb
irb(main):001:0> title = "Methods in Biomedical Informatics"
=> "Methods in Biomedical Informatics"
irb(main):002:0> /in/.match(title)
=> #<MatchData "in">
irb(main):003:0> title =~ /in/
=> 8
```

```
irb(main):004:0> title.scan(/in/i)
=> ["in", "In"]
irb(main):005:0> season_array = [ "Winter", "Spring", "Summer", "Autumn" ]
=> ["Winter", "Spring", "Summer", "Autumn"]
irb(main):006:0> season_array.size
=> 4
irb(main):007:0> season_array[0]
=> "Winter"
irb(main):008:0> season_array.pop
=> "Autumn"
irb(main):009:0> season_array
=> ["Winter", "Spring", "Summer"]
irb(main):010:0> season_array.push "Fall"
=> ["Winter", "Spring", "Fall"]
```

B.10 RUBY GEMS

A "gem" is a packaged Ruby application or library that may be used to address a particular requirement, solve a particular problem, or add specific functionality. The value of gems is that they can be shared and enhanced by the Ruby community, thus reducing duplicative efforts ("reinventing the wheel"). The RubyGems packaging system can be used to create, install, distribute, manage, and search gems using the gem command. For example, gem list will provide a list of locally installed gems while gem install gem_name (e.g., gem install bio) can be used to install a gem with the specified name.

```
$ which gem
/usr/local/bin/gem
$ gem list

*** LOCAL GEMS ***
bio (1.4.3)
htmlentities (4.3.1)
mysql (2.9.1, 2.8.1)
rest-client (1.6.7)
```

RubyGems.org, the community's gem hosting service, includes over 56,000 gems created since July 2009. These include the bio gem for the BioRuby library that provides access to resources such as PubMed/MEDLINE, `mysql` gem that provides an interface to MySQL databases, and `rest-client` gem that enables interaction with RESTful Web services (the use of these gems is demonstrated in Appendix C [Database Primer] and Appendix D [Web Services Primer]).

Gems can be used by "requiring" them at the beginning of a Ruby program. The following example demonstrates the use of the `htmlentities` gem for encoding and decoding HTML entities.

```
#! /usr/local/bin/ruby

# html.rb
# Demonstrate use of "htmlentities" gem
# for encoding and decoding HTML
require 'rubygems'
require 'htmlentities'

coder = HTMLEntities.new

text = "&quot;&lt;hello&gt;&quot;"
decoded_text = coder.decode(text)
puts "#{text} --> #{decoded_text}"

text = ">\"good-bye\"<"
encoded_text = coder.encode(text)
puts "#{text} --> #{encoded_text}"
```

```
$ ruby html.rb
&quot;&lt;hello&gt;&quot; --> "<hello>"
>"good-bye"< --> &gt;&quot;good-bye&quot;&lt;
```

REFERENCES AND RESOURCES

There are numerous books and on-line resources covering Ruby. Below are a few references and tutorials providing additional details and examples for the concepts covered in this primer as well as additional Ruby functionality.

Books and Articles

- Matsumoto Y. Ruby in a nutshell: a desktop quick reference. 1st Edition. O'Reilley Media, Inc.; 2001.
- Fitzgerald M. Learning Ruby. 1st Edition. O'Reilley Media, Inc.; 2007.

- Berman JJ. Ruby programming for medicine and biology. 1st Edition. Jones & Barlett Learning; 2007.
- Berman JJ. Methods in medical informatics: fundamentals of healthcare programming in Perl, Python, and Ruby. Taylor & Francis; 2010.
- Aerts J, Law A. An introduction to scripting in Ruby for biologists. BMC Bioinformatics. 2009 July 16;10:221.

Web Resources and Tutorials

- Ruby Programming Language [Internet]. [cited 2013 May 8]. Available from: http://www.ruby-lang.org.
- Documenting the Ruby Language [Internet]. [cited 2013 May 8]. Available from: http://ruby-doc.org/.
- Wikibooks contributors. Ruby Programming [Internet]. Wikibooks, The Free Textbook Project; 2003 [updated 2013 March 26; cited 2013 May 31]. Available from: http://en.wikibooks.org/w/index.php?title=Ruby_Programming&oldid=2506075.
- Ruby Essentials [Internet]. 2012 [cited 2013 May 8]. Available from: http://www.techotopia.com/index.php/Ruby_Essentials.
- Ruby Tutorial [Internet]. [cited 2013 May 8]. Available from: http://www.tutorialspoint.com/ruby/.
- Ruby Track (series of courses) [Internet]. [cited 2013 July 31]. Available from: http://www.codecademy.com/tracks/ruby.
- Rubular: a Ruby regular expression editor [Internet]. [cited 2013 May 8]. Available from: http://rubular.com/.
- RubyGems.org [Internet]. [cited 2013 May 8]. Available from: http://rubygems.org.
- RubyGems Manuals [Internet]. [cited 2013 May 8]. Available from: http://docs.rubygems.org/.
- JRuby [Internet]. [cited 2013 May 8]. Available from: http://jruby.org/.
- Ruby on Rails [Internet]. [cited 2013 May 8]. Available from: http://rubyonrails.org/.

Database Primer

Elizabeth S. Chen

Center for Clinical and Translational Science, University of Vermont, Burlington, VT, USA
Department of Medicine, Division of General Internal Medicine, University of Vermont, Burlington, VT, USA
Department of Computer Science, University of Vermont, Burlington, VT, USA

Databases provide a means for organizing and managing a collection of data. A Database Management System (DBMS) allows for the creation, update, querying, and administration of databases. There are several types of databases including relational, hierarchical, network, and object-oriented where relational DBMSs (RDBMSs) have been the predominant choice. In the relational model, introduced by Edgar F. Codd at IBM in 1970, data are stored in relations as tables that consist of columns and rows where keys can be used to link related tables. Within an RDBMS, the Structured Query Language (SQL), developed by Donald D. Chamberlin and Raymond F. Boyce at IBM in the early 1970s, is used for manipulating and retrieving data. Examples of RDMSs include IBM DB2, Microsoft SQL Server, Oracle,

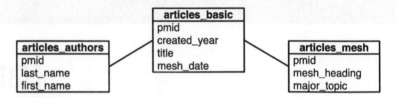

■ **FIGURE C.1** Database schema for example PubMed/MEDLINE database.

PostgreSQL, and MySQL where the latter two are open-source. For additional background on databases, see Chapter 2 (Data Integration) and particularly Section 2.3 (Database Basics) in this book.

This primer serves as a brief introduction to MySQL and basic SQL commands for creating, managing, and using a relational database. It is assumed that MySQL has already been downloaded and installed on a system running a Unix variant such as Mac OS X or Linux.[1] While MySQL can also be installed in a Windows environment, the examples here assume a Unix environment (see Appendix A: Unix Primer). Furthermore, the examples here show how to use MySQL from the command-line rather than through a Graphical User Interface (GUI) tool.

C.1 **EXAMPLE PubMed/MEDLINE DATABASE**

In this primer, we will create and use a simple database containing information from a set of PubMed/MEDLINE records (Figure C.1). This database will have three tables called: `articles_basic`—for basic information about each article that includes the PubMed unique identifier (PMID), year the record was created, title, and date that MeSH terms were added; `articles_authors`—includes the PMID, last name, and first name of each author for an article; `articles_mesh`—includes the PMID, MeSH headings, and indicator if the MeSH heading is a major topic.

The tables will be populated with information extracted and transformed from a file called `pubmed_result.txt` containing eight MEDLINE records for the following search: "National Library of Medicine (US)"[mh] and "PubMed"[mh] and "Teaching"[mh]. The following Ruby script is adapted from the one shown in Appendix B (see `parse_medline.rb` in Section B.7) and will output the results into three separate pipe-delimited files called `articles_basic.txt`, `articles_authors.txt`, and `articles_mesh.txt` to be loaded into the database (see Section C.5 on "Loading Data into Tables").

---

[1] http://www.mysql.com/.

```ruby
#! /usr/local/bin/ruby

# parse_medline_mysql.rb
# Parsing and transform fields in MEDLINE records
# for loading into MySQL database

first_record_flag = 0 # Flag for keeping track of first record
field = ""
pmid = created_year = title = mesh_date = ""

# Output files
articles_file = File.open("articles_basic.txt", "w")
authors_file = File.open("articles_authors.txt", "w")
mesh_headings_file = File.open("articles_mesh.txt", "w")

# Read each line of the MEDLINE file
File.open("pubmed_result.txt").each do |line|
    line.chomp!

    # Output information for each article
    if line == ""
        if first_record_flag == 1
            articles_file.puts "#{pmid}|#{created_year}|#{title}|#{mesh_date}"
        end
        first_record_flag = 1
    end

    # Get field name ("PMID", "TI", "MH", etc.)
    if line =~ /^([A-Z]+)/
        field = $1
    end

    # Get PubMed unique identifier (PMID field)
    # Example: PMID- 20570844
    if line =~ /PMID- ([0-9]*)/
        pmid = $1
    end

    # Get year from create date (DA field)
    # Example: DA  - 20101122
    if line =~ /^DA  - ([0-9]{4})[0-9]{2}[0-9]{2}/
        created_year = $1
    end

    # Get title (TI field)
    # Example:
    # TI  - Education resources of the National Center for Biotechnology …
    if line =~ /TI  - (.*)/
        title = $1
    end
```

```ruby
   # Get title - if wraps onto multiple lines (TI field)
   # Example:
   # TI  - Searching MEDLINE free on the Internet using the National …
   #        PubMed.
   if line =~ /^\s{6}(.*)/ and field.eql?("TI")
      title = title + " " + $1
   end

   # Get MeSH date (MHDA field)
   # Example: MHDA- 2011/04/07 06:00
   if line =~ /MHDA- ([0-9]{4})\/([0-9]{2})\/([0-9]{2})/
      mesh_date = $1 + "-" + $2 + "-" + $3
   end

   # Get authors (FAU) - first name and last name only
   # Examples:
   # FAU - Sayers, Eric W
   # FAU - Pechous, Steven
   # FAU - DeGeorges, K M
   if line =~ /^FAU - ([^,]+),\s([^\s]+)/
      authors_file.puts "#{pmid}|#{$1}|#{$2}"
   end

   # Get MeSH headings (MH field)
   # Examples:
   # MH  - Computational Biology/*education/methods
   # MH  - *National Library of Medicine (U.S.)
   # MH  - Databases, Factual
   if line =~ /MH  - (\*?)([^\/]*)/
      major_topic = $1
      mesh_heading = $2

      if major_topic == "*"
         mesh_headings_file.puts "#{pmid}|#{mesh_heading}|1"
      else
         mesh_headings_file.puts "#{pmid}|#{mesh_heading}|0"
      end
   end
 end

# Print information for last record
articles_file.puts "#{pmid}|#{created_year}|#{title}|#{mesh_date}"

# Close output files
articles_file.close
authors_file.close
mesh_headings_file.close
$ ruby parse_medline_mysql.rb
```

```
$ wc -l *.txt
       8 articles_basic.txt
      18 articles_authors.txt
      86 articles_mesh.txt
     432 pubmed_result.txt
     544 total
$ head -n 3 articles_basic.txt
20570844|2010|Education resources of the National Center for Biotechnology
Information.|2011-04-07
12869862|2003|Recall to precision: retrieving clinical information with
MEDLINE.|2003-10-04
11329561|2001|Using the National Library of Medicine's PubMed to improve clinical
practice.|2002-02-02
$ head -n 10 articles_authors.txt
20570844|Cooper|Peter
20570844|Lipshultz|Dawn
20570844|Matten|Wayne
20570844|McGinnis|Scott
20570844|Pechous|Steven
20570844|Romiti|Monica
20570844|Tao|Tao
20570844|Valjavec-Gratian|Majda
20570844|Sayers|Eric
12869862|Poynton|Mollie
$ head -n 10 articles_mesh.txt
20570844|Computational Biology|0
20570844|Databases, Factual|0
20570844|Internet|0
20570844|National Institutes of Health (U.S.)|0
20570844|National Library of Medicine (U.S.)|1
20570844|PubMed|0
20570844|Teaching|0
20570844|United States|0
12869862|Computer User Training|0
12869862|Humans|0
```

C.2 WORKING IN THE MySQL ENVIRONMENT

In a Unix environment, the `which` command can be used to determine the location of the MySQL client program and `mysql --version` can be used to determine the version (latest version is 5.7).

```
$ which mysql
/usr/local/mysql/bin/mysql

$ mysql --version
mysql  Ver 14.14 Distrib 5.1.48, for apple-darwin10.3.0
(i386) using readline 5.1
```

To connect to a MySQL server, the following parameters are needed: `-h` and *hostname* of the remote server (if the server is running locally, this does not need to be specified or `localhost` can be specified); `-u` and *username* of MySQL account; and `-p` that will prompt for the password for the specified username.

```
$ mysql -h hostname -u username -p
```

Once logged in, some introductory information will be provided followed by the `mysql>` prompt. To disconnect, type `exit`, `quit`, or `\q` (or `Control-D` in Unix).

```
$ mysql -h example.mysqlserver.edu -u user2 -p
Enter password:
Welcome to the MySQL monitor.  Commands end with ; or \g.
Your MySQL connection id is 6276964
Server version: 5.1.68-rel14.6-log Percona Server (GPL), 14.6, Revision 551

Copyright (c) 2000, 2013, Oracle and/or its affiliates. All rights reserved.

Oracle is a registered trademark of Oracle Corporation and/or its affiliates. Other
names may be trademarks of their respective owners.

Type 'help;' or '\h' for help. Type '\c' to clear the current input statement.

mysql> quit
$ mysql -u user2 -p
Enter password:
Welcome to the MySQL monitor.  Commands end with ; or \g.
Your MySQL connection id is 7
Server version: 5.1.48 MySQL Community Server (GPL)

Copyright (c) 2000, 2010, Oracle and/or its affiliates. All rights reserved.
This software comes with ABSOLUTELY NO WARRANTY. This is free software, and you are
welcome to modify and redistribute it under the GPL v2 license

Type 'help;' or '\h' for help. Type '\c' to clear the current input statement.

mysql> \q
```

In most cases, MySQL commands or queries should end with a semicolon ("`;`") and are case-insensitive (e.g., either `select` or `SELECT` will work). However, database and table names may be case-sensitive (e.g., `table 1` ≠ `TABLE1`). Query results will be returned in a tabular format where the first row contains the column names and the following rows include the actual results. The number of rows returned and execution time are also displayed. Multiple queries can be written in the same line separated by ";" and a single query can span multiple lines. In the latter case, the prompt will change from mysql> to -> and the query will not execute until the ";" is provided. To cancel a command, type \c. The following are a couple of basic queries for getting familiar with working in the MySQL environment.

```
mysql> SELECT CURRENT_DATE;
+--------------+
| CURRENT_DATE |
+--------------+
| 2013-05-14   |
+--------------+
1 row in set (0.00 sec)

mysql> SELECT VERSION(); SELECT NOW();
+-----------+
| VERSION() |
+-----------+
| 5.1.48    |
+-----------+
1 row in set (0.00 sec)

+---------------------+
| NOW()               |
+---------------------+
| 2013-05-14 12:12:24 |
+---------------------+
1 row in set (0.00 sec)

mysql> select 3+5,
    -> 3*5
    -> ;
+-----+-----+
| 3+5 | 3*5 |
+-----+-----+
|   8 |  15 |
+-----+-----+
1 row in set (0.00 sec)

mysql> select 5-3, 5/3\c
mysql>
```

C.3 CREATING, ACCESSING, AND DELETING A DATABASE

The SHOW DATABASES statement can be used to list what databases exist on the server. The USE statement can then be used for accessing a specified database. To display the list of tables within a database, type SHOW TABLES. If there are no tables in the database, it will return "Empty set."

```
mysql> SHOW DATABASES;
+--------------------+
| Database           |
+--------------------+
| information_schema |
| test               |
+--------------------+
2 rows in set (0.00 sec)

mysql> USE test;
Database changed

mysql> SHOW TABLES;
Empty set (0.00 sec)
```

To create or remove a database, use CREATE DATABASE or DROP DATABASE respectively. There are various commands for administering a database such as creating users, changing passwords, and granting permissions (for more details, see the "References and Resources" section at the end of this primer for links to MySQL documentation).

```
mysql> CREATE DATABASE primer;
Query OK, 1 row affected (0.00 sec)

mysql> CREATE DATABASE mysql_primer;
Query OK, 1 row affected (0.00 sec)

mysql> SHOW DATABASES;
+--------------------+
| Database           |
+--------------------+
| information_schema |
| mysql_primer       |
| primer             |
| test               |
+--------------------+
4 rows in set (0.00 sec)

mysql> DROP DATABASE primer;
Query OK, 0 rows affected (0.06 sec)

mysql> USE mysql_primer;
Database changed

mysql> SHOW TABLES;
Empty set (0.00 sec)
```

C.4 CREATING, MODIFYING, AND DELETING TABLES

Once a database has been created, the next step is to create tables. This process involves determining what tables are needed and how they should be structured. The CREATE TABLE statement requires that column names be defined and data types specified for each column. Table C.1 includes a listing of numeric, string, and date and time data types.

Table C.1   Numeric, string, and date and time data types.

Numeric Types *(M= total number of digits; D= number of digits following decimal point)*

Type	Description	Range
TINYINT(M)	Tiny integer	-128 to 127 (signed)
		0 to 255 (unsigned)
SMALLINT(M)	Small integer	-32768 to 32767 (signed)
		0 to 65535 (unsigned)
MEDIUMINT(M)	Medium integer	-8388608 to 8388607 (signed)
		0 to 16777215 (unsigned)
INT(M) or INTEGER(M)	Normal sized integer	-2147483648 to 2147483647 (signed)
		0 to 4294967295 (unsigned)
BIGINT(M)	Large integer	-9223372036854775808 to 9223372036854775807 (signed); 0 to 18446744073709551615 (unsigned)
FLOAT(M, D)	Small (single-precision) floating-point number	$-3.402823466E+38$ to $-1.175494351E-38, 0,$ and $1.175494351E-38$ to $3.402823466E+38$
DOUBLE(M, D)	Normal-size (double-precision) floating-point number	$-1.7976931348623157E+308$ to $-2.2250738585072014E-308, 0,$ and $2.2250738585072014E-308$ to $1.7976931348623157E+308$
DECIMAL(M, D)	Exact fixed-point number	M: max$=65$, default$=10$; D: max$=30$, default$=0$

String Types *(M= total number of characters)*

CHAR(M)	Fixed length string	0 to 255 characters
VARCHAR(M)	Variable length string	0 to 65,535 characters
BINARY(M)	Fixed length binary string	0 to 255 bytes
VARBINARY(M)	Variable length binary string	0 to 65,535 bytes
TINYTEXT	Text types	Up to 255 characters
TEXT		Up to 65,535 characters
MEDIUMTEXT		Up to 16,777,215 characters
LONGTEXT		Up to 4,294,967,295 characters
TINYBLOB	Binary large objects (blob) types	Up to 255 bytes
BLOB		Up to 65,535 bytes
MEDIUMBLOB		Up to 16,777,215 bytes
LONGBLOB		Up to 4,294,967,295 bytes
ENUM(X,Y,Z,…)	List of possible values	Up to 65,535 values

(Continued)

Table C.1 Numeric, string, and date and time data types (Continued).

String Types (M= total number of characters)

Type	Description	Range
SET(X,Y,Z,…)	List of possible values where more than one value can be specified	Up to 64 values

Date and Time Types

DATE	Date only (YYYY-MM-DD)	'1000-01-01' to '9999-12-31'
DATETIME	Date and time (YYY-MM-DD HH:MM:SS)	'1000-01-01 00:00:00' to '9999-12-31 23:59:59'
TIMESTAMP	Date and time (YYY-MM-DD HH:MM:SS)	'1970-01-01 00:00:01' UTC to '2038-01-09 03:14:07' UTC
TIME	Time only (HH:MM:SS)	'−838:59:59' to '838:59:59'
YEAR(4)	Four-digit year (YYYY)	'1901' to '2155'

Constraints for individual columns can be defined such as NOT NULL that specifies that there should be no NULL values, PRIMARY KEY that uniquely identifies each record, and FOREIGN KEY that points to a primary key in another table. These also serve as optimizations for improving query performance. Once created, the DESCRIBE statement can be used to see information about each column in a table.

In our example database, the articles_basic table is the main table with the pmid column serving as the primary key.

```
mysql> CREATE TABLE articles_basic (
    -> pmid INTEGER NOT NULL,
    -> created_year YEAR(4),
    -> title VARCHAR(200),
    -> mesh_date DATE,
    -> PRIMARY KEY (pmid)
    -> );
Query OK, 0 rows affected (0.02 sec)

mysql> DESCRIBE articles_basic;
+--------------+--------------+------+-----+---------+-------+
| Field        | Type         | Null | Key | Default | Extra |
+--------------+--------------+------+-----+---------+-------+
| pmid         | int(11)      | NO   | PRI | NULL    |       |
| created_year | year(4)      | YES  |     | NULL    |       |
| title        | varchar(200) | YES  |     | NULL    |       |
| mesh_date    | date         | YES  |     | NULL    |       |
+--------------+--------------+------+-----+---------+-------+
4 rows in set (0.00 sec)
```

The articles_authors table is linked to this table by pmid that is defined as a foreign key. Aside from the indexes for primary and foreign keys, additional indexes can be defined using INDEX, either when a table is created or afterwards. In this case, it is determined that it would be useful to have an additional multi-column index for the last_name and first_name fields. The SHOW INDEX statement can be used to return index information for a table.

```
mysql> CREATE TABLE articles_authors (
    -> pmid INTEGER NOT NULL,
    -> last_name VARCHAR(50),
    -> first_name VARCHAR(50),
    -> FOREIGN KEY (pmid) REFERENCES articles_basic(pmid)
    -> );
Query OK, 0 rows affected (0.03 sec)

mysql> CREATE INDEX name on articles_authors (last_name, first_name);
Query OK, 0 rows affected (0.02 sec)
Records: 0  Duplicates: 0  Warnings: 0

mysql> DESCRIBE articles_authors;
+------------+-------------+------+-----+---------+-------+
| Field      | Type        | Null | Key | Default | Extra |
+------------+-------------+------+-----+---------+-------+
| pmid       | int(11)     | NO   | MUL | NULL    |       |
| last_name  | varchar(50) | YES  | MUL | NULL    |       |
| first_name | varchar(50) | YES  |     | NULL    |       |
+------------+-------------+------+-----+---------+-------+
3 rows in set (0.00 sec)

mysql> SHOW INDEX FROM articles_authors;
+------------------+------------+----------+--------------+-------------+-----------+-------------+----------+--------+------+------------+---------+
| Table            | Non_unique | Key_name | Seq_in_index | Column_name | Collation | Cardinality | Sub_part | Packed | Null | Index_type | Comment |
+------------------+------------+----------+--------------+-------------+-----------+-------------+----------+--------+------+------------+---------+
| articles_authors |          1 | pmid     |            1 | pmid        | A         |           9 |     NULL | NULL   |      | BTREE      |         |
| articles_authors |          1 | name     |            1 | last_name   | A         |          18 |     NULL | NULL   | YES  | BTREE      |         |
| articles_authors |          1 | name     |            2 | first_name  | A         |          18 |     NULL | NULL   | YES  | BTREE      |         |
+------------------+------------+----------+--------------+-------------+-----------+-------------+----------+--------+------+------------+---------+
3 rows in set (0.00 sec)
```

The articles_mesh table is also linked to articles_basic by the pmid field that is defined as a foreign key. In the initial creation of this table, the mesh_heading column was defined as having a variable size of 25. It is determined that this is insufficient since some MeSH headings are longer than 25 characters and the ALTER TABLE statement is used to change the size of this column to 50.

```
mysql> CREATE TABLE articles_mesh (pmid INTEGER NOT NULL, mesh_heading VARCHAR(25),
major_topic TINYINT(1), FOREIGN KEY (pmid) REFERENCES articles(pmid));
Query OK, 0 rows affected (0.04 sec)

mysql> DESCRIBE articles_mesh;
+--------------+-------------+------+-----+---------+-------+
| Field        | Type        | Null | Key | Default | Extra |
+--------------+-------------+------+-----+---------+-------+
| pmid         | int(11)     | NO   | MUL | NULL    |       |
| mesh_heading | varchar(25) | YES  |     | NULL    |       |
| major_topic  | tinyint(1)  | YES  |     | NULL    |       |
+--------------+-------------+------+-----+---------+-------+
3 rows in set (0.00 sec)

mysql> ALTER TABLE articles_mesh MODIFY mesh_heading VARCHAR(50);
Query OK, 0 rows affected (0.01 sec)
Records: 0  Duplicates: 0  Warnings: 0

mysql> DESCRIBE articles_mesh;
+--------------+-------------+------+-----+---------+-------+
| Field        | Type        | Null | Key | Default | Extra |
+--------------+-------------+------+-----+---------+-------+
| pmid         | int(11)     | NO   | MUL | NULL    |       |
| mesh_heading | varchar(50) | YES  |     | NULL    |       |
| major_topic  | tinyint(1)  | YES  |     | NULL    |       |
+--------------+-------------+------+-----+---------+-------+
3 rows in set (0.00 sec)
```

To completely remove a table from a database, use the DROP TABLE statement.

```
mysql> CREATE TABLE tmp (id INTEGER,  name VARCHAR(10));
Query OK, 0 rows affected (0.02 sec)

mysql> SHOW TABLES;
+----------------------+
| Tables_in_mysql_primer |
+----------------------+
| articles_authors     |
| articles_basic       |
| articles_mesh        |
| tmp                  |
+----------------------+
```

```
4 rows in set (0.00 sec)

mysql> DROP TABLE tmp;
Query OK, 0 rows affected (0.01 sec)

mysql> SHOW TABLES;
+----------------------+
| Tables_in_mysql_primer |
+----------------------+
| articles_authors     |
| articles_basic       |
| articles_mesh        |
+----------------------+
3 rows in set (0.00 sec)
```

Often times, there is a need to just remove the contents of a table without completely deleting it. To do this, use the TRUNCATE TABLE statement or DELETE statement to completely empty out a table.

```
mysql> TRUNCATE TABLE table_name
Query OK, 0 rows affected (0.00 sec)

mysql> DELETE FROM table_name
Query OK, 0 rows affected (0.00 sec)
```

C.5 **LOADING DATA INTO TABLES**

Now that the tables have been created, the next step is to load data into them, which can be done by inserting records one at a time (INSERT) or inserting data from existing files (LOAD DATA). Records can be modified using the UPDATE statement.

Let's first insert a test record into the articles_basic table, make some updates to this record, and then remove it before loading more data. The SELECT statement can then be used to see the contents of this table (see Section C.6 for more details about SELECT).

```
mysql> INSERT INTO articles_basic VALUES (12345678, '2010', 'Title for test record',
'2010-04-12');
Query OK, 1 row affected (0.00 sec)

mysql> SELECT * FROM articles_basic;
+----------+--------------+-----------------------+------------+
| pmid     | created_year | title                 | mesh_date  |
+----------+--------------+-----------------------+------------+
| 12345678 |         2010 | Title for test record | 2010-04-12 |
+----------+--------------+-----------------------+------------+
1 row in set (0.00 sec)

mysql> UPDATE articles_basic
    -> SET created_year='2011', mesh_date='2011-04-12'
    -> WHERE pmid=12345678;
```

```
Query OK, 0 rows affected (0.00 sec)
Rows matched: 1  Changed: 1  Warnings: 0

mysql> SELECT * FROM articles_basic;
+----------+--------------+---------------------+------------+
| pmid     | created_year | title               | mesh_date  |
+----------+--------------+---------------------+------------+
| 12345678 |         2011 | Title for test record | 2011-04-12 |
+----------+--------------+---------------------+------------+
1 row in set (0.00 sec)

mysql> DELETE FROM articles_basic WHERE pmid=12345678;
Query OK, 1 row affected (0.00 sec)

mysql> SELECT * FROM articles;
Empty set (0.00 sec)
```

Let's now try loading data from the three files created earlier (see Section C.1). The fields in these files are separated by the pipe character ("|") and lines are terminated by the newline character ("\n"). The following statements assume that the full path to these files is: /home/user2/data.

```
mysql> LOAD DATA LOCAL INFILE '/home/user2/data/articles_basic.txt'
    -> INTO TABLE articles_basic
    -> FIELDS TERMINATED BY '|'
    -> LINES TERMINATED BY '\n';
Query OK, 8 rows affected (0.00 sec)
Records: 8  Deleted: 0  Skipped: 0  Warnings: 0

mysql> LOAD DATA LOCAL INFILE '/home/user2/data/articles_authors.txt' INTO TABLE
articles_authors FIELDS TERMINATED BY '|' LINES TERMINATED BY '\n';
Query OK, 18 rows affected (0.03 sec)
Records: 18  Deleted: 0  Skipped: 0  Warnings: 0

mysql> LOAD DATA LOCAL INFILE '/home/user2/data/articles_mesh.txt' INTO TABLE
articles_mesh FIELDS TERMINATED BY '|' LINES TERMINATED BY '\n';
Query OK, 86 rows affected (0.03 sec)
Records: 86  Deleted: 0  Skipped: 0  Warnings: 0
```

All three of the LOAD DATA statements executed successfully, loading the expected number of records in each table (the numbers match the number of lines from the Unix wc command in Section C.1). There were no skipped records (as indicated by "Skipped: 0") and no warnings (as indicated by "Warnings: 0"). To see warnings, use the SHOW WARNINGS command to see a list of warnings, which may be due to incompatible formats (e.g., more or less columns in the file than the table), incorrect column data type leading to truncated data (e.g., VARCHAR(25) specified for a column where data may be more than 25 characters long), or other reasons. These warning messages are helpful for determining if there need to be modifications to the data and/or table definitions.

C.6 RETRIEVING DATA FROM TABLES

With data loaded, the tables are now ready for querying. The SELECT statement is used to retrieve data from a database. The general format is as follows where the names of the columns to retrieve from a particular table are specified (or "*" to indicate all columns) and conditions for filtering particular rows can optionally be provided.

```
SELECT column1, column2
FROM table
WHERE conditions
```

Our first queries will involve retrieving all columns and rows from the articles_basic table, retrieving specified columns, and limiting the number of records returned using the LIMIT clause. To display only part of a string, SUBSTRING() can be used that takes the column name, starting position, and length as arguments. The UCASE() and LCASE() functions can be applied to convert values to all uppercase or lowercase respectively. Aliases can be created for tables and columns using AS.

```
mysql> SELECT * FROM articles_basic;
+----------+------------+------------------------------------------------------------------------------------------+------------+
| pmid     |created_year| title                                                                                    | mesh_date  |
+----------+------------+------------------------------------------------------------------------------------------+------------+
| 20570844 |       2010| Education resources of the National Center for Biotechnology Information.                 | 2011-04-07 |
| 12869862 |       2003| Recall to precision: retrieving clinical information with MEDLINE.                        | 2003-10-04 |
| 11329561 |       2001| Using the National Library of Medicine's PubMed to improve clinical practice.            | 2002-02-02 |
| 10455581 |       1999| Searching MEDLINE free on the Internet using the National Library of Medicine's PubMed.  | 1999-08-24 |
|  9919086 |       1999| Help! I need a MEDLINE search!                                                            | 1999-01-27 |
|  9803302 |       1999| The Healthnet project: extending online information resources to end users in rural hospitals. | 1998-11-06 |
|  9431431 |       1998| Health information networking via the Internet with the former Soviet Union.              | 1998-02-12 |
|  8655874 |       1996| Accessing MEDLINE from the dental office.                                                 | 1996-04-01 |
+----------+------------+------------------------------------------------------------------------------------------+------------+
8 rows in set (0.00 sec)

mysql> SELECT pmid, created_year, mesh_date FROM articles_basic LIMIT 3;
+----------+--------------+------------+
| pmid     | created_year | mesh_date  |
+----------+--------------+------------+
```

```
| 20570844 |              2010 | 2011-04-07 |
| 12869862 |              2003 | 2003-10-04 |
| 11329561 |              2001 | 2002-02-02 |
+----------+-------------------+------------+
3 rows in set (0.00 sec)3 rows in set (0.00 sec)

mysql> SELECT pmid, SUBSTRING(title, 1, 50) AS partial_title FROM
articles_basic LIMIT 3;
+----------+--------------------------------------------------+
| pmid     | partial_title                                    |
+----------+--------------------------------------------------+
| 20570844 | Education resources of the National Center for Bio |
| 12869862 | Recall to precision: retrieving clinical informati |
| 11329561 | Using the National Library of Medicine's PubMed to |
+----------+--------------------------------------------------+
3 rows in set (0.00 sec)

mysql> SELECT pmid, UCASE(SUBSTRING(title, 1, 50)) AS partial_title
FROM articles_basic LIMIT 3;
+----------+--------------------------------------------------+
| pmid     | partial_title                                    |
+----------+--------------------------------------------------+
| 20570844 | EDUCATION RESOURCES OF THE NATIONAL CENTER FOR BIO |
| 12869862 | RECALL TO PRECISION: RETRIEVING CLINICAL INFORMATI |
| 11329561 | USING THE NATIONAL LIBRARY OF MEDICINE'S PUBMED TO |
+----------+--------------------------------------------------+
3 rows in set (0.00 sec)

mysql> SELECT pmid, LCASE(SUBSTRING(title, 1, 50)) AS partial_title
FROM articles_basic LIMIT 3;
+----------+--------------------------------------------------+
| pmid     | partial_title                                    |
+----------+--------------------------------------------------+
| 20570844 | education resources of the national center for bio |
| 12869862 | recall to precision: retrieving clinical informati |
| 11329561 | using the national library of medicine's pubmed to |
+----------+--------------------------------------------------+
3 rows in set (0.00 sec)
```

To determine the number of records in a table, the COUNT() function can be used. The DISTINCT keyword can be used to identify unique records or unique column values in a table. The following queries are used to determine the total number of records in the articles_mesh table, number of unique values in the mesh_heading column, and display five of these unique values.

```
mysql> SELECT COUNT(*) FROM articles_mesh;
+----------+
| COUNT(*) |
```

```
+----------+
|       86 |
+----------+
1 row in set (0.00 sec)

mysql> SELECT COUNT(DISTINCT mesh_heading) FROM articles_mesh;
+----------------------------+
| COUNT(DISTINCT mesh_heading) |
+----------------------------+
|                         46 |
+----------------------------+
1 row in set (0.02 sec)

mysql> SELECT DISTINCT mesh_heading from articles_mesh LIMIT 5;
+----------------------------------+
| mesh_heading                     |
+----------------------------------+
| Computational Biology            |
| Databases, Factual               |
| Internet                         |
| National Institutes of Health (U.S.) |
| National Library of Medicine (U.S.) |
+----------------------------------+
5 rows in set (0.00 sec)
```

As introduced earlier, the WHERE clause can be added for specifying particular records to retrieve from a table based on one or more criteria. There are a number of comparison operators that can be used in a WHERE clause: equal (=), not equal (<> or !=), greater than (>), less than (<), greater than or equal to (>=), and less than or equal to (<=). There are also operators for determining if a value is within a specified range (BETWEEN), among a specified set of values (IN), or matches a particular pattern (LIKE, RLIKE, or REGEXP). The NOT keyword can be added to negate a particular operation (e.g., NOT BETWEEN, NOT IN, NOT LIKE, and NOT REGEXP).

First, let's identify articles (represented by PMID) that include "MEDLINE" as a MeSH heading, those with this heading as the major topic using the AND logical operator, and those where it is not the major topic (this can either be done by checking records where major_topic is 0 or major_topic is <u>not</u> 1).

```
mysql> SELECT * FROM articles_mesh WHERE mesh_heading = 'MEDLINE';
+----------+--------------+-------------+
| pmid     | mesh_heading | major_topic |
+----------+--------------+-------------+
| 12869862 | MEDLINE      |           0 |
```

```
| 11329561 | MEDLINE     |             0 |
| 10455581 | MEDLINE     |             1 |
|  9919086 | MEDLINE     |             1 |
|  9803302 | MEDLINE     |             0 |
|  9431431 | MEDLINE     |             0 |
|  8655874 | MEDLINE     |             1 |
+----------+-------------+------- ----+
7 rows in set (0.01 sec)

mysql> SELECT *
    -> FROM articles_mesh
    -> WHERE mesh_heading = 'MEDLINE' AND major_topic = 1;
+----------+--------------+-------------+
| pmid     | mesh_heading | major_topic |
+----------+--------------+-------------+
| 10455581 | MEDLINE      |           1 |
|  9919086 | MEDLINE      |           1 |
|  8655874 | MEDLINE      |           1 |
+----------+--------------+-------------+
3 rows in set (0.00 sec)

mysql> SELECT *
    -> FROM articles_mesh
    -> WHERE mesh_heading = 'MEDLINE' AND major_topic != 1;
+----------+--------------+-------------+
| pmid     | mesh_heading | major_topic |
+----------+--------------+-------------+
| 12869862 | MEDLINE      |           0 |
| 11329561 | MEDLINE      |           0 |
|  9803302 | MEDLINE      |           0 |
|  9431431 | MEDLINE      |           0 |
+----------+--------------+-------------+
4 rows in set (0.00 sec)
```

Next, let's identify articles where the year when the record was created (created_year) is: (1) greater than or equal to 2000, (2) is between 1997 and 2000, (3) is not between 1997 and 2000, (4) is in 1999, 2001, or 2003, and (5) is greater than 2005 or less than or equal to 1996 using the OR logical operator.

```
mysql> SELECT pmid, created_year, SUBSTRING(title, 1, 40) AS partial_title
    -> FROM articles_basic
    -> WHERE created_year >= 2000;
+----------+--------------+------------------------------------------+
| pmid     | created_year | partial_title                            |
+----------+--------------+------------------------------------------+
| 20570844 |         2010 | Education resources of the National Cent |
| 12869862 |         2003 | Recall to precision: retrieving clinical |
| 11329561 |         2001 | Using the National Library of Medicine's |
+----------+--------------+------------------------------------------+
3 rows in set (0.00 sec)
```

```
mysql> SELECT pmid, created_year, SUBSTRING(title, 1, 40) AS partial_title
    -> FROM articles_basic
    -> WHERE created_year BETWEEN 1997 AND 2000;
+----------+--------------+------------------------------------------+
| pmid     | created_year | partial_title                            |
+----------+--------------+------------------------------------------+
| 10455581 |         1999 | Searching MEDLINE free on the Internet u |
|  9919086 |         1999 | Help! I need a MEDLINE search!           |
|  9803302 |         1999 | The Healthnet project: extending online  |
|  9431431 |         1998 | Health information networking via the In |
+----------+--------------+------------------------------------------+
4 rows in set (0.00 sec)

mysql> SELECT pmid, created_year, SUBSTRING(title, 1, 40) AS partial_title
    -> FROM articles_basic
    -> WHERE created_year NOT BETWEEN 1997 AND 2000;
+----------+--------------+------------------------------------------+
| pmid     | created_year | partial_title                            |
+----------+--------------+------------------------------------------+
| 20570844 |         2010 | Education resources of the National Cent |
| 12869862 |         2003 | Recall to precision: retrieving clinical |
| 11329561 |         2001 | Using the National Library of Medicine's |
|  8655874 |         1996 | Accessing MEDLINE from the dental office |
+----------+--------------+------------------------------------------+
4 rows in set (0.00 sec)

mysql> SELECT pmid, created_year, SUBSTRING(title, 1, 40) AS partial_title
    -> FROM articles_basic
    -> WHERE created_year IN (1999, 2001, 2003);
+----------+--------------+------------------------------------------+
| pmid     | created_year | partial_title                            |
+----------+--------------+------------------------------------------+
| 12869862 |         2003 | Recall to precision: retrieving clinical |
| 11329561 |         2001 | Using the National Library of Medicine's |
| 10455581 |         1999 | Searching MEDLINE free on the Internet u |
|  9919086 |         1999 | Help! I need a MEDLINE search!           |
|  9803302 |         1999 | The Healthnet project: extending online  |
+----------+--------------+------------------------------------------+
5 rows in set (0.00 sec)

mysql> SELECT pmid, created_year, SUBSTRING(title, 1, 40) AS partial_title
    -> FROM articles_basic
    -> WHERE created_year > 2005 OR created_year <= 1996;
+----------+--------------+------------------------------------------+
| pmid     | created_year | partial_title                            |
+----------+--------------+------------------------------------------+
| 20570844 |         2010 | Education resources of the National Cent |
|  8655874 |         1996 | Accessing MEDLINE from the dental office |
+----------+--------------+------------------------------------------+
2 rows in set (0.00 sec)
```

If multiple OR and AND operators are used, it is good practice to use parentheses to indicate how to group the conditions.

```
mysql> SELECT pmid, created_year, mesh_date
    -> FROM articles_basic
    -> WHERE created_year = '1999'
    -> AND (mesh_date >= '1999-01-01' AND mesh_date <= '1999-12-31');
+----------+--------------+------------+
| pmid     | created_year | mesh_date  |
+----------+--------------+------------+
| 10455581 |         1999 | 1999-08-24 |
| 9919086  |         1999 | 1999-01-27 |
+----------+--------------+------------+
2 rows in set (0.00 sec)
```

What if we are interested in searching for a particular pattern within a column rather than a specific value? When using the LIKE operator, a pattern is specified that includes a specified set of characters and wildcard symbol ("%") before, after, or both before and after. In addition, the underscore character ("_") can be used to match any single character. Let's try to find article titles that start or end with "MEDLINE" or include "MEDLINE" within them.

```
mysql> SELECT title FROM articles_basic WHERE title LIKE 'MEDLINE%';
Empty set (0.00 sec)

mysql> SELECT title FROM articles_basic WHERE title LIKE '%MEDLINE.';
+--------------------------------------------------------------+
| title                                                        |
+--------------------------------------------------------------+
| Recall to precision: retrieving clinical information with MEDLINE. |
+--------------------------------------------------------------+
1 row in set (0.00 sec)

mysql> SELECT title FROM articles_basic WHERE title LIKE '%MEDLINE%';
+----------------------------------------------------------------------------+
| title                                                                      |
+----------------------------------------------------------------------------+
| Recall to precision: retrieving clinical information with MEDLINE.          |
| Searching MEDLINE free on the Internet using the National Library of Medicine's PubMed. |
| Help! I need a MEDLINE search!                                             |
| Accessing MEDLINE from the dental office.                                  |
+----------------------------------------------------------------------------+
4 rows in set (0.00 sec)

mysql> SELECT title FROM articles_basic WHERE title NOT LIKE '%MEDLINE%';
```

```
+------------------------------------------------------------------------+
| title                                                                  +
+------------------------------------------------------------------------+
| Education resources of the National Center for Biotechnology Information. |
| Using the National Library of Medicine's PubMed to improve clinical practice. |
| The Healthnet project: extending online information resources to end users |
| in rural hospitals.                                                    |
| Health information networking via the Internet with the former         |
| Soviet Union.                                                          |
+------------------------------------------------------------------------+
4 rows in set (0.00 sec)
```

For more complex pattern matching, RLIKE or REGEXP can be used for
identifying regular expressions (similar to the Unix grep command [see
Appendix A, Section A.8] and regular expressions in Ruby [see Appendix
B, Section B.7]). Now let's try to find articles that have authors with a first
name beginning with "M" and ending with "A," with a last or first name
beginning with a vowel, and a last name that is six characters long.

```
mysql> SELECT * FROM articles_authors WHERE first_name REGEXP '^M.*A$';
+----------+-----------------+-------------+
| pmid     | last_name       | first_name  |
+----------+-----------------+-------------+
| 20570844 | Romiti          | Monica      |
| 20570844 | Valjavec-Gratian | Majda      |
+----------+-----------------+-------------+
2 rows in set (0.00 sec)

mysql> SELECT *
    -> FROM articles_authors
    -> WHERE first_name REGEXP '^[aeiou]' OR last_name REGEXP '^[aeiou]';
+----------+-----------+-------------+
| pmid     | last_name | first_name  |
+----------+-----------+-------------+
| 20570844 | Sayers    | Eric        |
|  9803302 | Holtum    | E           |
|  8655874 | Ahluwalia | K           |
+----------+-----------+-------------+
3 rows in set (0.00 sec)

mysql> SELECT last_name
    -> FROM articles_authors
    -> WHERE last_name REGEXP '^.{6}$';
+-----------+
| last_name |
+-----------+
| Cooper    |
```

```
| Dollar    |
| Holtum    |
| Matten    |
| Putnam    |
| Romiti    |
| Sayers    |
+-----------+
7 rows in set (0.00 sec)
```

Often times, tables will contain NULL values that represent missing unknown data. To test for NULL values, use the IS NULL or NOT NULL operators. In this case, the three tables do not include any rows with NULL values and during table creation it was specified that the pmid column should not have any NULL values; however, the other fields could potentially have NULL values. Let's temporarily add a record that does include such values to demonstrate the use of IS NULL and how comparison operators do not work for NULL values.

```
mysql> SELECT * FROM articles_basic WHERE title IS NULL;
Empty set (0.00 sec)

mysql> INSERT INTO articles_basic VALUES (99999999, NULL, 'Title for testing for NULL values', NULL);
Query OK, 1 row affected (0.01 sec)

mysql> SELECT * FROM articles_basic where created_year IS NULL;
+-----------+--------------+-----------------------------------+------------+
| pmid      | created_year | title                             | mesh_date  |
+-----------+--------------+-----------------------------------+------------+
| 99999999  |         NULL | Title for testing for NULL values | NULL       |
+-----------+--------------+-----------------------------------+------------+
1 row in set (0.00 sec)

mysql> SELECT * FROM articles_basic where created_year = NULL or created_year = 'NULL';
Empty set, 1 warning (0.00 sec)

mysql> DELETE FROM articles_basic WHERE pmid = 99999999;
Query OK, 1 row affected (0.00 sec)
```

The ORDER BY clause can be added to sort results in one or more columns in a meaningful way. By default, values in the specified column will be ordered in ascending order. To sort in descending order, the DESC keyword can be added. Let's focus on the date fields in the articles_basic table and first sort by the created year and then by MeSH date (notice the difference in the order in rows where the created year is 1999).

```
mysql> SELECT pmid, created_year, mesh_date
    -> FROM articles_basic
    -> ORDER BY created_year;
+-----------+--------------+------------+
| pmid      | created_year | mesh_date  |
+-----------+--------------+------------+
|  8655874  |         1996 | 1996-04-01 |
|  9431431  |         1998 | 1998-02-12 |
| 10455581  |         1999 | 1999-08-24 |
|  9919086  |         1999 | 1999-01-27 |
|  9803302  |         1999 | 1998-11-06 |
| 11329561  |         2001 | 2002-02-02 |
| 12869862  |         2003 | 2003-10-04 |
| 20570844  |         2010 | 2011-04-07 |
+-----------+--------------+------------+
8 rows in set (0.00 sec)

mysql> SELECT pmid, created_year, mesh_date
    -> FROM articles_basic
    -> ORDER BY created_year, mesh_date;
+-----------+--------------+------------+
| pmid      | created_year | mesh_date  |
+-----------+--------------+------------+
|  8655874  |         1996 | 1996-04-01 |
|  9431431  |         1998 | 1998-02-12 |
|  9803302  |         1999 | 1998-11-06 |
|  9919086  |         1999 | 1999-01-27 |
| 10455581  |         1999 | 1999-08-24 |
| 11329561  |         2001 | 2002-02-02 |
| 12869862  |         2003 | 2003-10-04 |
| 20570844  |         2010 | 2011-04-07 |
+-----------+--------------+------------+
8 rows in set (0.00 sec)
```

To group values within a particular column, the GROUP BY clause can be used. This can be useful for obtaining distribution counts and characterizing the data. Within the articles_mesh table, there are 46 total unique headings and 11 major topic headings. Let's first group and sort the major headings and then all the headings. Let's also get the distribution of articles by year based on the created year.

```
mysql> SELECT mesh_heading, count(*) AS num
    -> FROM articles_mesh
    -> WHERE major_topic = 1
    -> GROUP BY mesh_heading
    -> ORDER BY num DESC;
+------------------------------------------+-----+
| mesh_heading                             | num |
+------------------------------------------+-----+
```

```
| MEDLINE                                 | 3 |
| Internet                                | 2 |
| Computer User Training                  | 2 |
| National Library of Medicine (U.S.)     | 1 |
| Telemedicine                            | 1 |
| Hospitals, Rural                        | 1 |
| Dental Offices                          | 1 |
| Computer Communication Networks         | 1 |
| Online Systems                          | 1 |
| Software                                | 1 |
| International Cooperation               | 1 |
+-----------------------------------------+---+
11 rows in set (0.00 sec)

mysql> SELECT mesh_heading, major_topic, count(*) AS num
    -> FROM articles_mesh
    -> GROUP BY mesh_heading, major_topic
    -> ORDER BY mesh_heading, major_topic, num DESC
    -> LIMIT 10;
+---------------------------------+-------------+-----+
| mesh_heading                    | major_topic | num |
+---------------------------------+-------------+-----+
| Automatic Data Processing       |           0 |   1 |
| CD-ROM                          |           0 |   1 |
| Computational Biology           |           0 |   1 |
| Computer Communication Networks |           1 |   1 |
| Computer Systems                |           0 |   1 |
| Computer User Training          |           0 |   5 |
| Computer User Training          |           1 |   2 |
| Cross-Cultural Comparison       |           0 |   1 |
| Data Collection                 |           0 |   1 |
| Databases, Bibliographic        |           0 |   2 |
+---------------------------------+-------------+-----+
10 rows in set (0.00 sec)

mysql> SELECT created_year, count(*) FROM articles_basic
GROUP BY created_year;
+--------------+----------+
| created_year | count(*) |
+--------------+----------+
|         1996 |        1 |
|         1998 |        1 |
|         1999 |        3 |
|         2001 |        1 |
|         2003 |        1 |
|         2010 |        1 |
+--------------+----------+
6 rows in set (0.00 sec)
```

MySQL includes several functions for performing math, text, and date calculations. For example, MAX() can be used to find the largest value in a specified column, MIN() to find the smallest value, AVG() to find the average value, and SUM() for the total sum.

```
mysql> SELECT MAX(created_year) AS max_year FROM articles_basic;
+----------+
| max_year |
+----------+
|     2010 |
+----------+
1 row in set (0.00 sec)

mysql> SELECT MIN(created_year) AS min_year FROM articles_basic;
+----------+
| min_year |
+----------+
|     1996 |
+----------+
1 row in set (0.01 sec)

mysql> SELECT AVG(created_year) AS avg_year FROM articles_basic;
+-----------+
| avg_year  |
+-----------+
| 2000.6250 |
+-----------+
1 row in set (0.00 sec)
```

As shown earlier, the SUBSTRING() or MID() function can be used to extract characters from a string field and LENGTH() can be used to determine the length of values in a text field.

```
mysql> SELECT pmid, LENGTH(title) AS title_length FROM articles_basic;
+----------+--------------+
| pmid     | title_length |
+----------+--------------+
| 20570844 |           73 |
| 12869862 |           66 |
| 11329561 |           77 |
| 10455581 |           87 |
|  9919086 |           30 |
|  9803302 |           94 |
|  9431431 |           76 |
|  8655874 |           41 |
+----------+--------------+
8 rows in set (0.00 sec)
```

For dates, the YEAR(), MONTH(), and DAYOFMONTH() functions can be used to extract different parts of dates. The TIMESTAMPDIFF() function can then be used to find the difference between two dates.

```
mysql> SELECT pmid, mesh_date, YEAR(mesh_date) AS mesh_year,
    -> MONTH(mesh_date) AS mesh_month, DAYOFMONTH(mesh_date) AS mesh_day
    -> FROM articles_basic;
+----------+------------+-----------+------------+-----------+
| pmid     | mesh_date  | mesh_year | mesh_month | mesh_date |
+----------+------------+-----------+------------+-----------+
| 20570844 | 2011-04-07 |      2011 |          4 |         7 |
| 12869862 | 2003-10-04 |      2003 |         10 |         4 |
| 11329561 | 2002-02-02 |      2002 |          2 |         2 |
| 10455581 | 1999-08-24 |      1999 |          8 |        24 |
|  9919086 | 1999-01-27 |      1999 |          1 |        27 |
|  9803302 | 1998-11-06 |      1998 |         11 |         6 |
|  9431431 | 1998-02-12 |      1998 |          2 |        12 |
|  8655874 | 1996-04-01 |      1996 |          4 |         1 |
+----------+------------+-----------+------------+-----------+
8 rows in set (0.00 sec)

mysql> SELECT pmid, mesh_date, CURDATE(),
    -> TIMESTAMPDIFF(YEAR, mesh_date, CURDATE()) AS date_diff
    -> FROM articles_basic
    -> ORDER BY date_diff DESC;
+----------+------------+------------+-----------+
| pmid     | mesh_date  | CURDATE()  | date_diff |
+----------+------------+------------+-----------+
|  8655874 | 1996-04-01 | 2013-05-17 |        17 |
|  9431431 | 1998-02-12 | 2013-05-17 |        15 |
|  9919086 | 1999-01-27 | 2013-05-17 |        14 |
|  9803302 | 1998-11-06 | 2013-05-17 |        14 |
| 10455581 | 1999-08-24 | 2013-05-17 |        13 |
| 11329561 | 2002-02-02 | 2013-05-17 |        11 |
| 12869862 | 2003-10-04 | 2013-05-17 |         9 |
| 20570844 | 2011-04-07 | 2013-05-17 |         2 |
+----------+------------+------------+-----------+
8 rows in set (0.00 sec)
```

C.7 JOINING MULTIPLE TABLES

The previous set of queries involved just one table. To combine data from two or more tables, the JOIN keyword can be used. To demonstrate the different types of "joins," let's create another table called mesh_lookup that includes a mapping of unique identifiers to names for a small set of MeSH headings (that can be generated by searching the MeSH Browser[2] or parsing the MeSH files in ASCII or XML format[3]).

---

[2] http://www.nlm.nih.gov/mesh/MBrowser.html.

[3] http://www.nlm.nih.gov/mesh/filelist.html.

```
mysql> CREATE TABLE mesh_lookup (id VARCHAR(10), name VARCHAR(50));
Query OK, 0 rows affected (0.01 sec)

mysql> LOAD DATA LOCAL INFILE '/home/user2/data/mesh_lookup.txt' INTO TABLE mesh_
lookup FIELDS TERMINATED BY '|' LINES TERMINATED BY '\n';
Query OK, 9 rows affected (0.00 sec)
Records: 9  Deleted: 0  Skipped: 0  Warnings: 0

mysql> SELECT * FROM mesh_lookup;
+---------+----------------------------------+
| id      | name                             |
+---------+----------------------------------+
| D019295 | Computational Biology            |
| D016208 | Databases, Factual               |
| D009316 | National Institutes of Health (U.S.) |
| D009317 | National Library of Medicine (U.S.) |
| D039781 | PubMed                           |
| D013663 | Teaching                         |
| D008523 | MEDLARS                          |
| D016239 | MEDLINE                          |
| D012984 | Software                         |
+---------+----------------------------------+
9 rows in set (0.00 sec)
```

Let's also create a "view" of the articles_mesh table that is a virtual table and only includes the MeSH headings associated with a particular article (PMID 20570844).

```
mysql> CREATE VIEW 20570844_mesh AS
    -> SELECT * FROM articles_mesh WHERE pmid=20570844;
Query OK, 0 rows affected (0.01 sec)

mysql> SELECT * FROM 20570844_mesh;
+----------+----------------------------------+-------------+
| pmid     | mesh_heading                     | major_topic |
+----------+----------------------------------+-------------+
| 20570844 | Computational Biology            |           0 |
| 20570844 | Databases, Factual               |           0 |
| 20570844 | Internet                         |           0 |
| 20570844 | National Institutes of Health (U.S.) |       0 |
| 20570844 | National Library of Medicine (U.S.) |       1 |
| 20570844 | PubMed                           |           0 |
| 20570844 | Teaching                         |           0 |
| 20570844 | United States                    |           0 |
+----------+----------------------------------+-------------+
8 rows in set (0.01 sec)
```

Using JOIN or INNER JOIN will return records if there is at least one match in both tables (in this case, 20570844_mesh and mesh_lookup).

Notice that there are no rows for the MeSH headings "Internet" and "United States" that are associated with the article.

```
mysql> SELECT a.pmid, a.mesh_heading, m.id AS mesh_id
    -> FROM 20570844_mesh AS a
    -> INNER JOIN mesh_lookup AS m
    -> ON a.mesh_heading = m.name;
+----------+------------------------------------+---------+
| pmid     | mesh_heading                       | mesh_id |
+----------+------------------------------------+---------+
| 20570844 | Computational Biology              | D019295 |
| 20570844 | Databases, Factual                 | D016208 |
| 20570844 | National Institutes of Health (U.S.) | D009316 |
| 20570844 | National Library of Medicine (U.S.) | D009317 |
| 20570844 | PubMed                             | D039781 |
| 20570844 | Teaching                           | D013663 |
+----------+------------------------------------+---------+
6 rows in set (0.00 sec)
```

With LEFT JOIN, records from the left table (20570844_mesh) will be returned even if there are no matches in the right table (mesh_lookup). Here, all the MeSH headings for the article are listed, but there are NULL values for the two headings that are not included in mesh_lookup ("Internet" and "United States").

```
mysql> SELECT a.pmid, a.mesh_heading, m.id AS mesh_id FROM 20570844_mesh AS a LEFT
JOIN mesh_lookup AS m ON a.mesh_heading = m.name;
+----------+------------------------------------+---------+
| pmid     | mesh_heading                       | mesh_id |
+----------+------------------------------------+---------+
| 20570844 | Computational Biology              | D019295 |
| 20570844 | Databases, Factual                 | D016208 |
| 20570844 | Internet                           | NULL    |
| 20570844 | National Institutes of Health (U.S.) | D009316 |
| 20570844 | National Library of Medicine (U.S.) | D009317 |
| 20570844 | PubMed                             | D039781 |
| 20570844 | Teaching                           | D013663 |
| 20570844 | United States                      | NULL    |
+----------+------------------------------------+---------+
8 rows in set (0.00 sec)
```

A RIGHT JOIN will return records from the right table (mesh_lookup) even if there are no matches in the left table (20570844_mesh). In this case, all the MeSH headings in the mapping table are listed, but there are NULL values for the three headings that are not associated with the article ("MEDLARS" [D008523], "MEDLINE" [D016239], and "Software" [D012984]).

```
mysql> SELECT a.pmid, a.mesh_heading, m.id AS mesh_id FROM 20570844_mesh as a RIGHT
JOIN mesh_lookup AS m ON a.mesh_heading = m.name;
+----------+--------------------------------------+----------+
| pmid     | mesh_heading                         | mesh_id  |
+----------+--------------------------------------+----------+
| 20570844 | Computational Biology                | D019295  |
| 20570844 | Databases, Factual                   | D016208  |
| 20570844 | National Institutes of Health (U.S.) | D009316  |
| 20570844 | National Library of Medicine (U.S.)  | D009317  |
| 20570844 | PubMed                               | D039781  |
| 20570844 | Teaching                             | D013663  |
|     NULL | NULL                                 | D008523  |
|     NULL | NULL                                 | D016239  |
|     NULL | NULL                                 | D012984  |
+----------+--------------------------------------+----------+
9 rows in set (0.00 sec)
```

While MySQL does not support FULL JOIN, which will return records
when there is a match in either one of the tables, the functionality can be
emulated by using UNION with LEFT JOIN and RIGHT JOIN.

```
mysql> SELECT a.pmid, a.mesh_heading, m.id AS mesh_id
    -> FROM 20570844_mesh AS a
    -> LEFT JOIN mesh_lookup AS m
    -> ON a.mesh_heading = m.name
    -> UNION
    -> SELECT a.pmid, a.mesh_heading, m.id AS mesh_id
    -> FROM 20570844_mesh AS a
    -> RIGHT JOIN mesh_lookup AS m
    -> ON a.mesh_heading = m.name;
+----------+--------------------------------------+----------+
| pmid     | mesh_heading                         | mesh_id  |
+----------+--------------------------------------+----------+
| 20570844 | Computational Biology                | D019295  |
| 20570844 | Databases, Factual                   | D016208  |
| 20570844 | Internet                             | NULL     |
| 20570844 | National Institutes of Health (U.S.) | D009316  |
| 20570844 | National Library of Medicine (U.S.)  | D009317  |
| 20570844 | PubMed                               | D039781  |
| 20570844 | Teaching                             | D013663  |
| 20570844 | United States                        | NULL     |
|     NULL | NULL                                 | D008523  |
|     NULL | NULL                                 | D016239  |
|     NULL | NULL                                 | D012984  |
+----------+--------------------------------------+----------+
11 rows in set (0.00 sec)
```

C.8 **AUTOMATING MySQL QUERIES**

The examples provided in this primer thus far have involved typing in MySQL queries at the command line (mysql> prompt). For repeated or complex queries, one option is to save the queries in a text file that can then be executed within or outside the MySQL environment. For example, suppose the following queries are saved in a file called queries.sql.

```
USE mysql_primer;
SELECT COUNT(*) FROM articles_basic;
SELECT * FROM articles_basic WHERE pmid=9919086;
SELECT * FROM articles_authors WHERE pmid=9919086;
SELECT * FROM articles_mesh WHERE pmid=9919086;
```

Within MySQL, the SOURCE command can be used to execute the queries in this file.

```
mysql> SOURCE queries.sql
Reading table information for completion of table and column names
You can turn off this feature to get a quicker startup with -A

Database changed
+----------+
| COUNT(*) |
+----------+
|        8 |
+----------+
1 row in set (0.00 sec)

+----------+--------------+--------------------------------+------------+
| pmid     | created_year | title                          | mesh_date  |
+----------+--------------+--------------------------------+------------+
| 9919086  |         1999 | Help! I need a MEDLINE search! | 1999-01-27 |
+----------+--------------+--------------------------------+------------+
1 row in set (0.00 sec)

+----------+-----------+------------+
| pmid     | last_name | first_name |
+----------+-----------+------------+
| 9919086  | DeGeorges | K          |
+----------+-----------+------------+
1 row in set (0.00 sec)

+----------+-------------------------------+-------------+
| pmid     | mesh_heading                  | major_topic |
+----------+-------------------------------+-------------+
| 9919086  | Computer User Training        |           1 |
| 9919086  | Humans                        |           0 |
| 9919086  | Internet                      |           1 |
| 9919086  | MEDLINE                       |           1 |
| 9919086  | National Library of Medicine (U.S.) |     0 |
```

```
| 9919086 | Nurses                                         |           0 |
| 9919086 | United States                                  |           0 |
+---------+------------------------------------------------+-------------+
7 rows in set (0.00 sec)
```

The queries can also be executed outside of the MySQL environment (e.g., at the Unix command line) and results saved to an output file.

```
$ mysql -u user2 -p < queries.sql > output.txt
Enter password:
$ more output.txt
COUNT(*)
8
pmid      created_year    title    mesh_date
9919086 1999    Help! I need a MEDLINE search!  1999-01-27
pmid      last_name          first_name
9919086 DeGeorges          K
pmid      mesh_heading       major_topic
9919086 Computer User Training  1
9919086 Humàns  0
9919086 Internet        1
9919086 MEDLINE 1
9919086 National Library of Medicine (U.S.)     0
9919086 Nurses  0
9919086 United States   0
```

Applications involving database queries can be written in a variety of languages including Ruby. The following Ruby script is an interactive program that uses the mysql gem[4] (see Appendix B, Section B.10) that prompts the user for a PMID and then returns the associated title, authors, and MeSH headings. For the purposes of this example, the MySQL password is included in the script; however, this is generally not good practice. Options include saving credentials in a separate file or requiring that the password be entered at runtime.

```
#! /usr/local/bin/ruby

# query_pmid.rb
#
# Demonstrates how to query a MySQL database from a Ruby script
# using the "mysql" gem.

require "rubygems"
require "mysql"

# Parameters for database
```

---

[4]mysql gem: http://rubygems.org/gems/mysql.

```ruby
host = "localhost"          # Replace with your MySQL server name
user = "user2"              # Replace with your MySQL username
password = "xxxxxxxx"       # Replace with your MySQL password
db = "mysql_primer"         # Replace with your MySQL database name

# Get user-specified PMID
print "PMID? "
pmid = gets.chomp

# Print header
puts "Information for PMID #{pmid}".center(70, "*")

# Connect to database
dbh = Mysql.connect(host, user, password, db)

# Get basic article information
article_results = dbh.query("SELECT * FROM articles_basic WHERE pmid = #{pmid}")

# Print out basic article information
article_results.each do |row|
        puts "PMID:\t\t\t#{row[0]}"
        puts "Created Year:\t\t#{row[1]}"
        puts "Title:\t\t\t#{row[2]}"
        puts "MeSH Date:\t\t#{row[3]}"
end
article_results.free

# Get MeSH headings (major topics only)
mesh_query = "SELECT mesh_heading FROM articles_mesh
                WHERE pmid = #{pmid} AND major_topic = 1"
mesh_results = dbh.query(mesh_query)

# Print out MeSH headings
mesh_results.each do |row|
        puts "MeSH Heading (*):\t#{row[0]}"
end

# Close database connection
dbh.close
```

```
$ ruby query_pmid.rb
PMID? 9919086
*********************Information for PMID 9919086*********************
PMID:                  9919086
Created Year:          1999
Title:                 Help! I need a MEDLINE search!
MeSH Date:             1999-01-27
MeSH Heading (*):      Computer User Training
MeSH Heading (*):      Internet
MeSH Heading (*):      MEDLINE
```

```
$ ruby query_pmid.rb
PMID? 8655874
**********************Information for PMID 8655874*********************
PMID:                   8655874
Created Year:           1996
Title:                  Accessing MEDLINE from the dental office.
MeSH Date:              1996-04-01
MeSH Heading (*):       Dental Offices
MeSH Heading (*):       MEDLINE
```

REFERENCES AND RESOURCES

There are numerous books and on-line resources covering SQL and MySQL. Below are a few references and tutorials providing additional details and examples for the commands covered in this primer as well as additional SQL commands.

Articles

- Codd EF. A relational model of data for large shared data banks. Communications of the ACM 1970;13(6):377–387.
- Chamberlin DD, Boyce RF. SEQUEL: A structured English query language. Proceedings of the 1974 ACM SIFFIDET (now SIGMOD) Workshop on Data Description, Access and Control. 1974:249–264.
- Jamison DC. Structured Query Language (SQL) fundamentals. Curr Protoc Bioinformatics. 2003 February;Chapter 9:Unit9.2.
- Stein L. Creating databases for biological information: an introduction. Curr Protoc Bioinformatics. 2002 August;Chapter 9:Unit 9.1.

Web Resources and Tutorials

- MySQL [Internet]. [cited 2013 May 13]. Available from: http://www.mysql.com/.
- MySQL Documentation: MySQL Reference Manuals [Internet]. [cited 2013 May 13]. Available from: http://dev.mysql.com/doc/.
  See Section 3 (Tutorial) in the MySQL Reference Manual for any version.
- SQL Tutorial [Internet]. [cited 2013 May 13]. Available from: http://www.w3schools.com/sql/.
- SQL Database Language Tutorial [Internet]. [cited 2013 May 13]. Available from: http://www.tutorialspoint.com/sql/.
- MySQL News, Books, Conferences, Courses, and Community [Internet]. [cited 2013 May 13]. Available from: http://oreilly.com/mysql/.

Web Services

Elizabeth S. Chen

Center for Clinical and Translational Science, University of Vermont, Burlington, VT, USA
Department of Medicine, Division of General Internal Medicine, University of Vermont, Burlington, VT, USA
Department of Computer Science, University of Vermont, Burlington, VT, USA

A Web service, as defined by the World Wide Web Consortium (W3C), is a "a software system designed to support interoperable machine-to-machine interaction over a network."[1] These services can convert applications into Web applications, allow for sharing of reusable application components, and allow for exchange of data between different applications and platforms.[2]

There are two major approaches to Web services: SOAP (originally standing for Simple Object Access Protocol) and REST (Representational State Transfer). SOAP was originally designed in 1998 by Dave Winer, Don Box, Bob Atkinson, and Mohsen Al-Ghosein for Microsoft and is characterized as a standards-based protocol for accessing a Web service that uses XML

---

[1] Web Services Glossary: http://www.w3.org/TR/2004/NOTE-ws-gloss-20040211/

[2] Web Services Tutorial: http://www.w3schools.com/webservices.

(eXtensible Markup Language) and HTTP (Hypertext Transfer Protocol).[3] SOAP-based Web services are often associated with WSDL (Web Services Description Language), an XML-based language for describing Web services and how to access them.[4] The REST approach, introduced by Roy Fielding in 2000, offers a simpler alternative and provides an architectural style rather than a set of standard protocols.[5] A "RESTful" Web service is implemented using HTTP (accommodating the request methods GET, POST, PUT, and DELETE) and the principles of REST.

This primer serves as a brief introduction to Web services by demonstrating use of two services that can be accessed using the REST approach: (1) **NCBI E-utilities** for interfacing with databases such as PubMed and (2) **NCBO Annotator** for annotating text with biomedical ontology concepts. While these services are platform-independent and language-independent, the examples here assume a Unix environment (see Appendix A: Unix Primer) and use of the Ruby programming language (see Appendix B: Ruby Primer).

D.1 NCBI E-UTILITIES

The Entrez Programming Utilities (E-utilities) are a set of server-side programs providing interfaces into the Entrez query and database system at the National Center for Biotechnology Information (NCBI) that includes databases such as PubMed, PubMed Central, and GenBank. Table D.1 includes a listing of the eight utilities that each involve a standard set of input parameters for determining how to search for and retrieve the requested data from a specified database. These utilities can be used individually or combined to create a data pipeline.

Let's focus on ESearch and EFetch and building an ESearch → EFetch pipeline for first identifying a list of Unique Identifiers (UIDs) from a specified database for a particular query and then retrieving the full record for each UID. For example, ESearch will return a set of PubMed Unique Identifiers (PMID) for a given PubMed query and EFetch will return the full records for each PMID in the specified format (e.g., MEDLINE or XML).

The basic format of an ESearch query is:

```
esearch.fcgi?db=<database>&term=<query>
```

---

[3] SOAP Tutorial: http://www.w3schools.com/soap.
[4] WSDL Tutorial: http://www.w3schools.com/wsdl.
[5] REST: http://www.ics.uci.edu/~fielding/pubs/dissertation/rest_arch_style.htm.

Table D.1   List of NCBI E-utilities.[a]

Utility	Brief Description	Base URL
EInfo	Database Statistics	http://eutils.ncbi.nlm.nih.gov/entrez/eutils/einfo.fcgi
ESearch	**Text Searches**	http://**eutils.ncbi.nlm.nih.gov/entrez/eutils/esearch.fcgi**
EPost	UID Uploads	http://eutils.ncbi.nlm.nih.gov/entrez/eutils/epost.fcgi
ESummary	Document Summary Downloads	http://eutils.ncbi.nlm.nih.gov/entrez/eutils/esummary.fcgi
EFetch	**Data Record Downloads**	http://**eutils.ncbi.nlm.nih.gov/entrez/eutils/efetch.fcgi**
ELink	Entrez Links	http://eutils.ncbi.nlm.nih.gov/entrez/eutils/elink.fcgi
EGQuery	Global Query	http://eutils.ncbi.nlm.nih.gov/entrez/eutils/egquery.fcgi
ESpell	Spelling Suggestions	http://eutils.ncbi.nlm.nih.gov/entrez/eutils/espell.fcgi

[a]*A General Introduction to the E-utilities: http://www.ncbi.nlm.nih.gov/books/NBK25497/.*

where database is the name of the Entrez database (e.g., "pubmed" for PubMed and "pmc" for PubMed Central) and term is the text query to perform on that database. Optional parameters include retmax that specifies the maximum number of UIDs to return (default is 20). For a listing of database names and UIDs, see Table 1 in Chapter 2 ("A General Introduction to the E-utilities") of the NCBI Help Manual "Entrez Programming Utilities Help."[6]

The basic format for an Efetch query is:

```
efetch.fcgi?db=<database>&id=<uid_list>&rettype=<retrieval
_type>&retmode=<retrieval_mode>
```

where database is the name of the Entrez database and id is the list of UIDs (e.g., as obtained from ESearch). Optional parameters include rettype that specifies the retrieval type for each returned record (e.g., "Abstract" or "MEDLINE" for PubMed) and retmode that specifies the retrieval mode or format for the returned records (e.g., plain text or XML for PubMed). For a listing of valid rettype and retmode values for each database, see Table 1 in Chapter 4 ("The E-utilities In-Depth: Parameters,

---

[6]http://www.ncbi.nlm.nih.gov/books/NBK25497/table/chapter2.chapter2_table1/.

Syntax and More") of the NCBI Help Manual "Entrez Programming Utilities Help."[7]

Now let's try out these queries for the following PubMed search: "National Library of Medicine (US)"[mh] and "PubMed"[mh] and "Teaching"[mh]. Open up a Web browser and type in (or copy) the following ESearch URL:

```
http://eutils.ncbi.nlm.nih.gov/entrez/eutils/
esearch.fcgi?db=pubmed&term=%22National%20Library%20
of%20Medicine%20%28U.S.%29%22[mh]%20and%20
%22PubMed%22[mh]%20and%20%22Teaching%22[mh]
```

This will return the following XML results in the browser where the number between the <count> and </count> tags is the number of results followed by the list of PMIDs between the <Id> and </Id> tags and various statistics about the search.

```
<eSearchResult>
    <Count>8</Count>
    <RetMax>8</RetMax>
    <RetStart>0</RetStart>
    <IdList>
        <Id>20570844</Id>
        <Id>12869862</Id>
        <Id>11329561</Id>
        <Id>10455581</Id>
        <Id>9919086</Id>
        <Id>9803302</Id>
        <Id>9431431</Id>
        <Id>8655874</Id>
    </IdList>
    <TranslationSet/>
    <TranslationStack>
        <TermSet>
            <Term>"National Library of Medicine
(U.S.)"[mh]</Term>
            <Field>mh</Field>
            <Count>1682</Count>
            <Explode>Y</Explode>
        </TermSet>
        <TermSet>
            <Term>"PubMed"[mh]</Term>
            <Field>mh</Field>
            <Count>5131</Count>
            <Explode>Y</Explode>
        </TermSet>
        <OP>AND</OP>
```

[7]http://www.ncbi.nlm.nih.gov/books/NBK25499/table/chapter4.chapter4_table1/.

```
    <TermSet>
        <Term>"Teaching"[mh]</Term>
        <Field>mh</Field>
        <Count>63723</Count>
        <Explode>Y</Explode>
    </TermSet>
    <OP>AND</OP>
    </TranslationStack>
  <QueryTranslation>
     "National Library of Medicine (U.S.)"[mh] AND
"PubMed"[mh] AND "Teaching"[mh]
  </QueryTranslation>
  <WarningList>
     <PhraseIgnored>and</PhraseIgnored>
  </WarningList>
</eSearchResult>
```

To get the full records for each of these PMIDs in MEDLINE format, type in (or copy) the following EFetch URL in a Web browser (see Appendix B, Section B.7 for an example MEDLINE record):

```
http://eutils.ncbi.nlm.nih.gov/entrez/eutils/efetch.fcgi?
db=pubmed&id=0570844,12869862,11329561,10455581,9919086,9
803302,9431431,8655874&rettype=medline&retmode=text
```

The Entrez History Server allows for temporary storage of results from an E-utility request for subsequent use by other E-utilities. To use the History Server, the usehistory parameter should be added to the ESearch URL. The results will include a Web Environment string (WebEnv) and query key (query_key) that are specific to that search and should then be included as input parameters in the EFetch URL. Now let's perform the same ESearch → EFetch pipeline as before except using the History Server this time.

```
http://eutils.ncbi.nlm.nih.gov/entrez/eutils/esearch.
fcgi?db=pubmed&term=%22National%20Library%20of%20
Medicine%20%28U.S.%29%22[mh]%20and%20%22PubMed%22[mh]%20
and%20%22Teaching%22[mh]&usehistory=y
```

This will return the same XML results as before, but will include additional lines near the beginning for the Web Environment string and query key (note that these will be different for each E-utility request).

```
<eSearchResult>
  <Count>8</Count>
  <RetMax>8</RetMax>
  <RetStart>0</RetStart>
  <QueryKey>1</QueryKey>
  <WebEnv>
```

```
NCID_1_4918728_130.14.18.97_5555_1369154518_1133174232
</WebEnv>
<IdList>
    <Id>20570844</Id>
    <Id>12869862</Id>
    <Id>11329561</Id>
    <Id>10455581</Id>
    <Id>9919086</Id>
    <Id>9803302</Id>
    <Id>9431431</Id>
    <Id>8655874</Id>
</IdList>
...
```

The EFetch request would then look as follows (be sure to replace the values for `WebEnv` and `query_key` with the ones you obtained from the previous ESearch request). The results should be the same as those returned by the first EFetch example that did not involve the History Server.

```
http://eutils.ncbi.nlm.nih.gov/entrez/eutils/efetch.
fcgi?db=pubmed&query_key=1&WebEnv=NCID_1_4918728_130.1
4.18.97_5555_1369154518_1133174232&rettype=medline&ret
mode=text
```

Now that we have gained some familiarity with ESearch and EFetch through a Web browser (which is often a good way to experiment with the different parameters for formulating and testing URLs; there is also an HTML client called E-Bench that can be used[8]), how can they be incorporated into an automated application such as a Ruby script? While the E-utilities can be accessed using both SOAP[9] and REST, the following two scripts will demonstrate the REST method.

The first Ruby script called `esearch_efetch.rb` involves use of the `rest-client` gem,[10] a simple HTTP and REST client for Ruby. This script performs the ESearch query, parses the XML results to extract the list of PMIDs, performs the EFetch query using the PMID list, and then parses the record in MEDLINE format for each PMID to get the PMID and title (adapted from the `parse_medline.rb` script in Appendix B, Section B. 7).

---

[8] E-Bench: http://www.ncbi.nlm.nih.gov/Class/wheeler/eutils/eu.html.
[9] Overview of the E-utility Web Service (SOAP): http://www.ncbi.nlm.nih.gov/books/NBK43082/.
[10] Rest-client gem: http://rubygems.org/gems/rest-client.

```ruby
#! /usr/local/bin/ruby

# esearch_efetch.rb
#
# Demonstrates use of rest-client gem for interacting with
# NCBI E-utilities - particularly ESearch and EFetch
require 'rubygems'
require 'rest_client'

#######################################################################
# Perform ESearch request for specified PubMed query
#######################################################################

query = "\"National Library of Medicine (U.S.)\"[mh] and
         \"PubMed\"[mh] and \"Teaching\"[mh]"

# Perform ESearch for specified database and query term
esearch_result =
RestClient.post 'http://eutils.ncbi.nlm.nih.gov/entrez/eutils/esearch.fcgi?',
                :db => 'pubmed',
                :term => query

#######################################################################
# Parse XML results to get list of PMIDs from ESearch results
#######################################################################

# Array for PMID list
pmid_array = Array.new

# Read each line from ESearch results
esearch_result.split("\n").each do |line|
  line.chomp!

  # Get PMID from XML output: e.g., <Id>22996180</Id>
  if line =~ /<Id>([^\<]+)<\/Id>/
    pmid = $1

    # Add PMID to pmid_array
    pmid_array.push(pmid)
  end
end

# Print PMID list
pmid_list = pmid_array.join(",")
puts "PMID List: #{pmid_list}\n\n" # Concatenate PMIDs separated by ','

#######################################################################
# Perform EFetch request to get full MEDLINE record for each PMID
#######################################################################
# Perform EFetch for specified database, PMID list, and output format
efetch_result =
```

```ruby
RestClient.post 'http://eutils.ncbi.nlm.nih.gov/entrez/eutils/efetch.fcgi?',
                :db => 'pubmed',
                :id => pmid_list,
                :rettype => 'medline',
                :retmode => 'text'

###################################################################
# Parse EFetch results for PMID, created year, and title from
# each MEDLINE record
###################################################################

# Initialize variables
first_record_flag = 0       # Flag for keeping track of first record
field = pmid = created_year = title = ""

# Read each line from EFetch results
efetch_result.split("\n").each do |line|
  # Remove newline
  line.chomp!

  # Print information for each article
  if line == ""
    if first_record_flag == 1
      puts "#{pmid}|#{created_year}|#{title}"
      pmid = created_year = title = ""
    end
    first_record_flag = 1
  end

  # Get field name ("PMID", "TI", "MH", etc.)
  if line =~ /^([A-Z]+)/
    field = $1
  end

  # Get PubMed unique identifier (PMID field)
  # Example: PMID- 20570844
  if line =~ /PMID- ([0-9]*)/
    pmid = $1
  end

  # Get year from create date (DA field)
  # Example: DA  - 20101122
  if line =~ /^DA  - ([0-9]{4})[0-9]{2}[0-9]{2}/
    created_year = $1
  end

  # Get title (TI field)
  if line =~ /TI  - (.*)/
    title = $1
  end
```

```
  # Get title - if wraps onto multiple lines (TI field)
  if line =~ /^\s{6}(.*)/ and field.eql?("TI")
    title = title + " " + $1
  end
end

# Print last record
puts "#{pmid}|#{created_year}|#{title}"
```

```
$ ruby esearch_efetch.rb
PMID List:
20570844,12869862,11329561,10455581,9919086,9803302,9431431,8655874

20570844|2010|Education resources of the National Center for Biotechnology
Information.
12869862|2003|Recall to precision: retrieving clinical information with
MEDLINE.
11329561|2001|Using the National Library of Medicine's PubMed to improve clinical
practice.
10455581|1999|Searching MEDLINE free on the Internet using the National Library
of Medicine's PubMed.
9919086|1999|Help! I need a MEDLINE search!
9803302|1999|The Healthnet project: extending online information resources to end
users in rural hospitals.
9431431|1998|Health information networking via the Internet with the former Soviet
Union.
8655874|1996|Accessing MEDLINE from the dental office.
```

The second Ruby script called `query_pubmed.rb` involves use of the `bio` gem[11] for the BioRuby project that provides tools and libraries for bioinformatics and molecular biology (other programming languages have similar libraries—e.g., BioPerl, BioPython, and BioJava). BioRuby has a variety of components (e.g., for sequence analysis, pathway analysis, protein modeling, and phylogenetic analysis) and provides easy access to databases and public Web Services including the NCBI E-utilities.[12] The functionality and results provided by `query_pubmed.rb` are the same as `esearch_efetch.rb` except that it uses the `bio` gem instead of the `rest-client` gem. Also, in this version, the parsing functionality is provided by a method called `parse_medline` that is in a separate script called `parse_medline_method.rb` (not shown below, but essentially the same code as above).

---

[11] Bio gem: http://rubygems.org/gems/bio.
[12] BioRuby: http://www.bioruby.org/.

```
#! /usr/local/bin/ruby

# query_pubmed.rb
# Demonstrates use of BioRuby for interacting with
# NCBI E-utilities - particularly ESearch and EFetch
#
# http://bioruby.org/rdoc/Bio/NCBI/REST/ESearch/Methods.html
# http://bioruby.org/rdoc/Bio/NCBI/REST/EFetch/Methods.html


# Include needed gems/files
require 'rubygems'
require 'bio'
require 'parse_medline_method.rb'

# Set default email address for E-utilities
Bio::NCBI.default_email = "user@institution.edu"

# Instantiate the ncbi_search and ncbi_fetch variables
ncbi_search = Bio::NCBI::REST::ESearch.new
ncbi_fetch  = Bio::NCBI::REST::EFetch.new

# ESearch request to retrieve list of PMIDs from PubMed for a query
query = "\"National Library of Medicine (U.S.)\"[mh] and
         \"PubMed\"[mh] and \"Teaching\"[mh]"
pmid_list = ncbi_search.search("pubmed", query, 0)  # 0 = return all results

# Print out number of PMIDs returned and PMID list
puts "Number of Results: #{pmid_list.length}"
puts "PMID List: #{pmid_list.join(",")}\n\n"

# EFetch request to get MEDLINE records for each PMID
efetch_output = ncbi_fetch.pubmed(pmid_list, "medline")

# Parse MEDLINE output: pmid|created_date|title
parse_medline(efetch_output)
```

D.2 NCBO ANNOTATOR

The National Center for Biomedical Ontology (NCBO) BioPortal provides Web-based access and use of an open repository of biomedical ontologies (almost 350 as of May 22, 2013).[13] Among the features of BioPortal is the ability to browse, search, and visualize ontologies as well as annotate free-text with ontology terms using the NCBO Annotator tool and determine the most relevant ontologies using the NCBO Ontology Recommender tool. These features are also associated with a set of RESTful Web services. The focus of this section is to learn more about Annotator and the Annotator Web service.

---

[13] BioPortal: http://bioportal.bioontology.org/.

Within BioPortal, the Annotator tool can be found at: http://bioportal.bioontology.org/annotator. Go to this page in your Web browser and use the following article title (PMID 22928177) as the input text: *A sense of calling and primary care physicians' satisfaction in treating smoking, alcoholism, and obesity.* After clicking "Get Annotations," a list of almost 100 annotations are returned representing terms from numerous ontologies. The results can be filtered by adding restrictions such as limiting to terms from specific ontologies or with particular semantic types. For example, if "SNOMED Clinical Terms" is selected as the ontology and "Disease or Syndrome" (T047), "Mental or Behavioral Dysfunction" (T048), and "Individual Behavior" (T055) are selected as the UMLS (Unified Medical Language System) Semantic Types, the number of annotations returned is now eight for "smoking," "alcoholism," and "obesity."

The base URL for the Annotator Web service is:

```
http://rest.bioontology.org/obs/annotator
```

A number of parameters can be specified for customizing the workflow and filtering results. For the full listing of parameters and their descriptions and values (including default values), see the Annotator User Guide.[14] One of the required parameters is `apikey` that is user-specific and used to track Web service usage. To obtain this key, create a BioPortal account and then go to the "API Key" section under "Account." Try specifying the following parameters and values in the test HTML page[15] that can be used to formulate and test an Annotator request (be sure to replace the `apikey` value with your API key):

```
textToAnnotate=A sense of calling and primary care
physicians' satisfaction in treating smoking, alco-
holism, and obesity.&format=tabDelimited&ontologiesT
oKeepInResult=1353&withDefaultStopWords=true&levelM
ax=0&semanticTypes=T047,T055,T048&mappingTypes=&who
leWordOnly=true&isVirtualOntologyId=true&apikey=xxxxx
xxx-xxxx-xxxx-xxxx-xxxxxxxxxxxx
```

A brief description of these parameters: `textToAnnotate` is the text to be annotated, `format` is the format of the returned results (i.e., `xml` [default], `text`, or `tabDelimited`), `ontologiesToKeepInResult` is the list

---

[14] Annotator User Guide: http://www.bioontology.org/wiki/index.php/Annotator_User_Guide.

[15] Annotator Test Page: http://rest.bioontology.org/test_oba.html.

of virtual identifiers of the ontologies to keep in the results (e.g., 1353 for SNOMED CT), isVirtualOntologyId specifies if the virtual ontology identifier is used instead of a version-specific ontology identifier (e.g., 46896 for SNOMED CT), withDefaultStopWords is either true or false indicating whether or not to use default stop words, levelMax is an integer specifying the maximum level of parent concepts to expand to in the is_a hierarchy for the concept, semanticTypes is the list of codes for the semantic types to keep in the results, mappingTypes specifies the mapping expansion type where an empty value is the default for all mapping types, and wholeWordOnly is a true or false value for matching whole words only or not.

Now that we have gained some familiarity with Annotator and its parameters, let's try writing and running a Ruby script that first obtains annotations for a specified piece of text and then parses specific information from each tab-delimited annotation (format=tabDelimited). This format includes fields for: score, identifiers (includes ontology identifier and concept identifier separated by a "/"), preferred name, link, synonyms, semantic types, context name, and other context properties. The following is an example of one annotation:

```
10      46896/414916001 Obesity

        http://purl.bioontology.org/ontology/
SNOMEDCT/414916001    Obesity (disorder) /// Adiposity
/// Adiposis  [T047, Disease or Syndrome] /// [T032,
Organism Attribute] MGREP [name: Obesity, concept:
{[localConceptId: 46896/414916001, conceptId: 36258806,
localOntologyId: 46896, isTopLevel: 0, fullId: http://
purl.bioontology.org/ontology/SNOMEDCT/414916001, pre-
ferredName: Obesity, definitions: [], synonyms: [Obesity
(disorder),    Adiposity,    Adiposis],    semanticTypes:
[[id: 33, semanticType: T047, description: Disease or
Syndrome], [id: 96, semanticType: T032, description:
Organism Attribute]]]}, isPreferred: true]
```

The following run_annotator.rb script demonstrates use of the rest-client gem (there is also an Annotator-specific gem called oba-client that can be used).

```
#! /usr/local/bin/ruby

# run_annotator.rb
# Demonstrates use of NCBO Annotator Web service

require 'rubygems'
```

```
require 'rest_client'

# Text to annotate
text = "A sense of calling and primary care physicians' satisfaction in
treating smoking, alcoholism, and obesity"

###############################################
# Run NCBO Annotator Web service
###############################################
annotations = RestClient.post 'http://rest.bioontology.org/obs/annotator?',
                    :textToAnnotate => text,
                    :format => 'tabDelimited',
                    :ontologiesToKeepInResult => '1353',
                    :withDefaultStopWords => 'true',
                    :levelMax => '0',
                    :semanticTypes => 'T047,T055,T048',
                    :mappingTypes => '',
                    :wholeWordOnly => 'true',
                    :isVirtualOntologyId => 'true',
                    :apikey => 'xxxxxxxx-xxxx-xxxx-xxxx-xxxxxxxxxxxx'

###############################################
# Parse annotations in tab-delimited format
###############################################

# Hash with mapping of version-specific ontology identifiers to names
ontology_hash = Hash.new
ontology_hash["46896"] = "SNOMED Clinical Terms"

annotations.split("\n").each do |annotation|
  annotation.chomp!

  # Get each field in annotation separated by tab (\t)
  score, identifiers, preferredName, link, synonyms, semanticType, contextName,
otherContext = annotation.split("\t")

  # Get ontology ID and concept ID
  ontologyID, conceptID = identifiers.split("/")

  # Outputs score, ontology ID and name, conceptID, preferred name, and
  # semantic type(s) for each annotation
  print "#{score}|#{ontologyID}|#{ontology_hash[ontologyID]}|"
  print "#{conceptID}|#{preferredName}|#{semanticType}\n"
end
```

```
$ ruby run_annotator.rb
10|46896|SNOMED Clinical Terms|154776002|Obesity|[T047, Disease or Syndrome]
10|46896|SNOMED Clinical Terms|414916001|Obesity|[T032, Organism Attribute]
/// [T047, Disease or Syndrome]
10|46896|SNOMED Clinical Terms|190963004|Obesity|[T047, Disease or Syndrome]
```

```
10|46896|SNOMED Clinical Terms|7200002|Alcoholism|[T048, Mental or Behavioral
Dysfunction]
8|46896|SNOMED Clinical Terms|228484007|Tobacco smoking behavior|[T055,
Individual Behavior]
8|46896|SNOMED Clinical Terms|5476005|Adiposity|[T032, Organism Attribute]
/// [T047, Disease or Syndrome]
8|46896|SNOMED Clinical Terms|365981007|Tobacco smoking behavior -
finding|[T055, Individual Behavior]
8|46896|SNOMED Clinical Terms|191801006|(Alcohol dependence syndrome
[including alcoholism]) or (alcohol problem drinking)|[T048, Mental or
Behavioral Dysfunction]
```

REFERENCES AND RESOURCES

There are numerous books and on-line resources covering Web services. Below are a few references and tutorials that provide additional details and examples for the topics covered in this primer.

Book and Articles

- Henderson C. Building scalable web sites. O'Reilly Media, Inc. 2006.
- Fielding RT, Naylor RN. Principled design of the modern Web architecture. ACM Transactions on Internet Technology. 2002 May;2(2):115–150.
- Steinberg RM, Zwies R, Yates C, Stave C, Pouliot Y, Heilemann HA. SmartSearch: automated recommendations using librarian expertise and the National Center for Biotechnology Information's Entrez programming utilities. J Med Libr Assoc. 2010 April;98(2):171–5.
- Whetzel PL, Noy NF, Shah NH, Alexander PR, Nyulas C, Tudorache T, Musen MA. BioPortal: enhanced functionality via new Web services from the National Center for Biomedical Ontology to access and use ontologies in software applications. Nucleic Acids Res. 2011 July;39(Web Server issue):W541–5.
- Jonquet C, Shah NH, Musen MA. The open biomedical annotator. Summit on Translat Bioinforma. 2009 March 1;2009:56–60.Jonquet C, Musen MA, Shah NH. Building a biomedical ontology recommender web service. J Biomed Semantics. 2010 June 22;1 Suppl 1:S1.

Web Resources and Tutorials

- Entrez Programming Utilities Help [Internet]. Bethesda (MD): National Center for Biotechnology Information (US); 2010- [cited 2013 May 28]. Available from: http://www.ncbi.nlm.nih.gov/books/NBK25501/.
- Annotator Web Service [Internet]. 2009 [updated 2012 Aug 16; cited 2013 May 28]. Available from: http://www.bioontology.org/wiki/index.php/Annotator_Web_service.
- Web Services Tutorial [Internet]. [cited 2013 May 28]. Available from: http://www.w3schools.com/webservices/.
- Web Services Tutorial [Internet]. [cited 2013 May 28]. Available from: http://www.tutorialspoint.com/webservices/.

- SOAP Tutorial [Internet]. [cited 2013 May 28]. Available from: http://www.w3schools.com/soap/.
- SOAP Tutorial [Internet]. [cited 2013 May 28]. Available from: http://www.tutorialspoint.com/soap/.
- WSDL Tutorial [Internet]. [cited 2013 May 28]. Available from: http://www.w3schools.com/wsdl/.
- WSDL Tutorial [Internet]. [cited 2013 May 28]. Available from: http://www.tutorialspoint.com/wsdl/.
- Learn REST: A tutorial [Internet]. [cited 2013 May 28]. Available from: http://rest.elkstein.org/.

Author Index

Index

Printed and bound by CPI Group (UK) Ltd, Croydon, CR0 4YY

03/10/2024

01040329-0004